# PROLOG

## PATIENT MANAGEMENT IN THE OFFICE

### FIFTH EDITION

## CRITIQUE BOOK

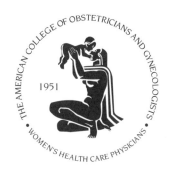

THE AMERICAN COLLEGE OF OBSTETRICIANS AND GYNECOLOGISTS

1951

WOMEN'S HEALTH CARE PHYSICIANS

ISBN 978-1-932328-28-8

2345/3210

The American College of Obstetricians and Gynecologists
409 12th Street, SW
PO Box 96920
Washington, DC 20090-6920

# Contributors

**PROLOG Editorial and Advisory Committee**

**CHAIR**

Ronald T. Burkman Jr, MD
    Chair, Department of Obstetrics and
      Gynecology
    Baystate Medical Center
    Springfield, Massachusetts
    Deputy Chair and Professor
    Department of Obstetrics and
      Gynecology
    Tufts University School of Medicine
    Boston, Massachusetts

**MEMBERS**

Bernard Gonik, MD
    Professor and Fann Srere Chair of
      Perinatal Medicine
    Division of Maternal–Fetal Medicine
    Department of Obstetrics and Gynecology
    Wayne State University School of
      Medicine
    Detroit, Michigan
Louis Weinstein, MD
    Paula and Elloise B. Bowers Professor
      and Chair
    Department of Obstetrics and Gynecology
    Thomas Jefferson University
    Philadelphia, Pennsylvania
Sterling B. Williams, MD
    Vice President, Education
    The American College of Obstetricians
      and Gynecologists
    Washington, DC

**PROLOG Task Force for *Patient Management in the Office*, Fifth Edition**

**COCHAIRS**

Sabine A. Kelischek, MD
    Clinical Associate Professor
    Department of Obstetrics and
      Gynecology
    University of North Carolina at Chapel
      Hill School of Medicine
    Women's Medical Associates, PA
    Asheville, North Carolina
Thomas C. C. Peng, MD
    Professor
    Division of Maternal and Fetal
      Medicine
    Department of Gynecology and
      Obstetrics
    Virginia Commonwealth University
      Medical Center
    Richmond, Virginia

**MEMBERS**

Janice L. Bacon, MD
    Professor and Chair
    Department of Obstetrics and Gynecology
    University of South Carolina
    Columbia, South Carolina
Daniel M. Breitkopf, MD
    Associate Professor
    Department of Obstetrics and Gynecology
    University of Texas Medical Branch,
      Galveston
    Galveston, Texas
Andrew M. Kaunitz, MD
    Professor and Assistant Chairman
    Department of Obstetrics and Gynecology
    University of Florida Health Science
      Center—Jacksonville
    Jacksonville, Florida
Susan M. Mou, MD
    Kansas City Ob-Gyn Physicians, PC
    Kansas City, Missouri
    Clinical Associate Professor of Obstetrics
      and Gynecology
    Department of Obstetrics and Gynecology
    University of Kansas School of Medicine
    Kansas City, Kansas

*Continued on next page*

**PROLOG Task Force for *Patient Management in the Office*, Fifth Edition (*continued*)**

Neil J. Murphy, MD
  Chief Clinical Consultant, Indian
    Health Service
  Southcentral Foundation
  Women's Medical Service
  Alaska Native Medical Center
  Anchorage, Alaska
John G. Pierce Jr, MD
  Associate Professor
  Departments of Obstetrics and
    Gynecology and Internal Medicine
  Virginia Commonwealth University
    Medical Center
  Richmond, Virginia
Patricia J. Sulak, MD
  Professor, Texas A&M College of
    Medicine
  Director, Sex Education Program
  Director, Division of Ambulatory Care
  Department of Obstetrics and
    Gynecology
  Scott and White Clinic—Memorial
    Hospital
  Temple, Texas

Carmen J. Sultana, MD
  Associate Professor
  Residency Program Director
  Department of Obstetrics and
    Gynecology
  Thomas Jefferson University
  Philadelphia, Pennsylvania
Amy L. Van Blaricom, MD
  Assistant Professor and Associate
    Residency Program Director
  Division of Education
  Department of Obstetrics and Gynecology
  University of Washington
  Seattle, Washington
Jeffrey W. Wall, MD
  Director of Ambulatory Care
  Department of Obstetrics and Gynecology
  Truman Medical Centers—Kansas City
  Kansas City, Missouri

**ACOG STAFF**
Sallye B. Brown, RN, MN
  Director, Educational Development and
    Testing
  Division of Education
Christopher T. George, MA
  Editor, PROLOG

This PROLOG unit was developed under the direction of the PROLOG Advisory Committee and the Task Force for *Patient Management in the Office*, Fifth Edition. PROLOG is planned and produced in accordance with the Standards for Enduring Materials of the Accreditation Council for Continuing Medical Education. Any discussion of unapproved use of products is clearly cited in the appropriate critique.

Current guidelines state that continuing medical education (CME) providers must ensure that CME activities are free from the control of any commercial interest. The task force and advisory committee members declare that neither they nor any business associate nor any member of their immediate families has material interest, financial interest, or other relationships with any company manufacturing commercial products relative to the topics included in this publication or with any provider of commercial services discussed in the unit except for **Daniel M. Breitkopf, MD**, who is a clinical investigator of Orion, Inc.; **Ronald T. Burkman Jr, MD**, who has conducted research through the National Institute for Child Health and Human Development, has consulted with Pfizer Inc. and Ortho-McNeil Pharmaceutical, and has received research support from Ortho-McNeil Pharmaceutical, Berlex Inc., and Organon, Inc.; **Andrew M. Kaunitz, MD**, who has conducted clinical trials through the University of Florida Research Foundation with funding from Barr Laboratories, Inc., Berlex Inc., Galen, Johnson & Johnson, Pfizer Inc., and the National Institutes of Health, has consulted with or been a speaker for Barr Laboratories, Inc., Berlex Inc., Johnson & Johnson, Pfizer, Inc., Proctor & Gamble Pharmaceuticals, and owns stock in Noven; **Patricia J. Sulak, MD**, who is a member of advisory boards for Berlex Inc., Barr Laboratories, Inc., Wyeth Pharmaceuticals, has received research grants from Berlex Inc., Barr Laboratories, Inc., and is a speaker and has received honoraria from Barr Laboratories, Inc., Berlex Inc., Ortho-McNeil Pharmaceutical, and Wyeth Pharmaceuticals. All potential conflicts have been resolved through multiple task force and advisory committee review of all content.

# Preface

## Purpose

PROLOG (Personal Review of Learning in Obstetrics and Gynecology) is a voluntary, strictly confidential, self-evaluation program. PROLOG was developed specifically as a personal study resource for the practicing obstetrician–gynecologist. It is presented as a self-assessment mechanism that, with its accompanying performance information, should assist the physician in designing a personal, self-directed life-long learning program. It may be used as a valuable study tool, reference guide, and a means of attaining up-to-date information in the specialty. The content is selected carefully and presented in multiple-choice questions that are clinically oriented. The questions are designed to stimulate and challenge physicians in areas of medical care that they confront in their practices or when they work as consultant obstetrician–gynecologists.

PROLOG also provides the American College of Obstetricians and Gynecologists (ACOG) with one mechanism to identify the educational needs of the Fellows. Individual scores are reported only to the participant; however, cumulative performance data and evaluation comments obtained for each PROLOG unit help determine the direction for future educational programs offered by the College.

## Process

The PROLOG series offers the most current information available in five areas of the specialty: obstetrics, gynecology and surgery, reproductive endocrinology and infertility, gynecologic oncology and critical care, and patient management in the office. A new PROLOG unit is produced annually, addressing one of those subject areas. *Patient Management in the Office*, Fifth Edition, is the fifth unit in the fifth 5-year PROLOG series.

Each unit of PROLOG represents the efforts of a special task force of subject experts under the supervision of an advisory committee. PROLOG sets forth current information as viewed by recognized authorities in the field of women's health. This educational resource does not define a standard of care, nor is it intended to dictate an exclusive course of management. It presents recognized methods and techniques of clinical practice for obstetrician–gynecologists to consider incorporating in their practices. Variations of practice that take into account the needs of the individual patient, resources, and the limitations that are special to the institution or type of practice may be appropriate.

Each unit of PROLOG is presented as a two-part set, with performance information and cognate credit available to those who choose to submit their answer sheets for confidential scoring. The first part of the PROLOG set is the Question Book, which contains educational objectives for the unit and multiple-choice questions, and an answer sheet with return mailing envelope. Participants can work through the questions at their own pace, choosing to use PROLOG as a closed- or open-book assessment. Return of the answer sheet for scoring is encouraged but voluntary.

The second part of PROLOG is the Critique Book, which reviews the educational objectives and questions set forth in the Question Book and contains a discussion, or critique, of each question. The critique provides the rationale for correct and incorrect options. Current, accessible references are listed for each question.

## Continuing Medical Education Credit

The American College of Obstetricians and Gynecologists (ACOG) is accredited by the Accreditation Council for Continuing Medical Education (ACCME) to provide continuing medical education for physicians. The American College of Obstetricians and Gynecologists designates this educational activity for a maximum of 25 *AMA PRA Category 1 Credits*™ or up to a maximum of 25 Category 1 ACOG cognate credits. Physicians should claim credit only if commensurate with the extent of their participation in the activity.

Fellows who submit their answer sheets for scoring will be credited with the number of hours they designate in the appropriate box on the answer sheet. (Important: Unless hours are noted, CME credit cannot be awarded and the test sheet will be returned.) Participants who return their answer sheets for CME credit will receive a Performance Report that provides a comparison of their scores with the scores of a sample group of physicians who have taken the unit as an examination. An individual may request credit only once for each unit. *Please allow 1 month to process answer sheets.*

Credit for PROLOG *Patient Management in the Office*, Fifth Edition, is initially available through December 2009. During that year, the unit will be reevaluated. If the content remains current, credit is extended for an additional 3 years, with credit for the unit automatically withdrawn after December 2012.

**Conclusion**

PROLOG was developed specifically as a personal study resource for the practicing obstetrician–gynecologist. It is presented as a self-assessment mechanism that, with its accompanying performance information, should assist the physician in designing a personal, self-directed learning program. The many quality resources developed by the College, as detailed each year in the ACOG *Publications and Educational Materials Catalog*, are available to help fulfill the educational interests and needs that have been identified. PROLOG is not intended as a substitute for the certification or recertification programs of the American Board of Obstetrics and Gynecology.

# PROLOG Objectives

PROLOG is a voluntary, strictly confidential, personal continuing education resource that is designed to be both stimulating and enjoyable. By participating in PROLOG, obstetrician–gynecologists will be able to do the following:

- Review and update clinical knowledge
- Recognize areas of knowledge and practice in which they excel, be stimulated to explore other areas of the specialty, and identify areas requiring further study
- Plan continuing education activities in light of identified strengths and deficiencies
- Compare and relate current knowledge and skills with those of other participants
- Obtain continuing medical education credit, if desired
- Have complete personal control of the setting and the pace of the experience

The obstetrician–gynecologist who completes *Patient Management in the Office*, Fifth Edition, will be able to do the following:
- Identify epidemiologic factors that contribute to women's health problems encountered in office practice and determine appropriate screening approaches to identify health issues in women.
- Correlate presenting signs and symptoms with appropriate diagnostic tools in making diagnoses of a variety of women's health care needs encountered in office practice.
- Describe appropriate traditional and alternative management strategies for select conditions encountered in office practice.
- Counsel patients about the impact of health and illness throughout their lives and about risks and benefits of treatment.
- Apply professional medical ethics to the practice of obstetrics and gynecology.
- Incorporate appropriate legal, risk management, and office management guidelines and techniques in clinical practice.

*Patient Management in the Office*, Fifth Edition, includes the following topics:

## SCREENING AND DIAGNOSIS
Anal incontinence
Apathetic hypothyroidism in the elderly
Appendectomy in the third trimester of pregnancy
Arthritis
Association of anal and urinary incontinence
Atypical gastroesophageal reflux disease
Bacterial vaginosis
Bloody nipple discharge
Breast cancer screening
Cancer screening in postmenopausal women
Cervical cytology screening
Cervical length screening
Chronic cough caused by drug therapy
Colon cancer screening
Complex adnexal masses
Cornual pregnancy
Coronary heart disease
Diagnosis of insulin resistance
Diagnosis of skin condition
Diverticulitis
Evaluation of hematuria

Evaluation of skin rash in pregnancy
Fetal cardiovascular malformations and inheritance patterns
Fetal Down syndrome
Headache
Health maintenance choices
*Helicobacter pylori* and peptic ulcer disease
Home evaluation of asthma in the pregnant patient
Human papillomavirus testing
Interstitial cystitis
Mammography in patient with no family history of breast cancer
New cytologic screening guidelines
Palpable breast lump with negative mammography test result
Pigmented vulvar lesion
Postpartum depression
Rhinosinusitis
Role of saline infusion sonohysterography in postmenopausal bleeding
Screening interval for cholesterol
Skin cancer screening
Testing for chlamydia
Thrombophilia and warfarin use
Ultrasonographic findings in adnexal torsion
Urge incontinence
Vertebral fractures

**MEDICAL MANAGEMENT**
Abnormal bleeding
Abnormal cervical cytology
Allergies to heparin
Adnexal cyst in postmenopausal women
Asthma
Blood pressure in type 2 diabetes mellitus
Body weight as a factor in contraceptive method failure
Breast cancer prophylaxis
Care of a patient treated for syphilis
Chronic bronchitis
Condylomata in the pregnant patient
Depot medroxyprogesterone acetate and bone density
Depression in adolescents
Depression in pregnancy
Diet and blood pressure
Domestic violence
Dysmenorrhea
Early pregnancy loss
Emergency contraception
Extended cycle contraception
Gastrointestinal illness
Graves' disease
Hepatitis C virus
Herpes simplex virus in pregnancy
Hirsutism in polycystic ovary syndrome patient
Hormone therapy in patients with breast cancer
Hormone therapy options
Indications for varicella vaccination
Iron-deficiency anemia in postmenopausal women
Low back pain

Methods to increase lactation
Methotrexate and tubal ectopic pregnancy
Management of prehypertension
Neuropathic pain
Nonsteroidal antiinflammatory drug use in the elderly
Outpatient therapy for venous thrombosis
Parvovirus exposure during pregnancy
Pessary fitting and choice
Polycystic ovary syndrome
Positive tuberculin skin test in pregnancy
Premenstrual disorder
Pyelonephritis in pregnancy
Salpingitis
Severe osteopenia
Suppressive herpes simplex virus therapy
Syphilis in a pregnant patient with penicillin allergy
Tamoxifen use and adverse effects
Thyroid disease
Treatment of insulin resistance
Unruptured ectopic pregnancy
Vaginitis
Vulvar lichen planus
Vulvodynia
Weight-bearing exercise in the elderly

## SURGICAL MANAGEMENT
Delivery method for a patient infected with human immunodeficiency virus
Preoperative evaluation for hypertension
Surgery to correct stress urinary incontinence
Surgery for uterine leiomyomata
Transcervical hysteroscopic sterilization
Tubal sterilization

## EPIDEMIOLOGY
Blood transfusion risks
Case–control vs prospective study design
Date rape
Indications for influenza vaccination
In vitro fertilization and pregnancy outcome
Mortality data in adolescents
Relationship between prevalence and positive predictive value
Risk of colon cancer
Risks of deep vein thrombosis

## COUNSELING
Benefits of glycemic control in microvascular disease
Calcium and vitamin D supplements in postmenopausal women
Cardioprotective effects of hormone therapy
Cardiovascular disease during menopause
Contraception advice for patient with systemic lupus
Contraception following thrombosis
Contraception in epilepsy
Contraception use by adolescents
Family history of mental retardation
Grieving after stillbirth

Indications for hepatitis B vaccine
Risk of failed vaginal birth after cesarean delivery
Risks of untreated asymptomatic bacteriuria in pregnancy
Safety of breastfeeding with hepatitis C viremia
Smoking cessation strategies
Therapy to decrease risk of colon cancer
Unplanned or unwanted pregnancy
Use of antiviral treatment
Use of intrauterine device

**ETHICAL AND LEGAL ISSUES**
Elective cesarean delivery
Full disclosure
Informed consent
Medical ethics
Patient advocacy
Practice patterns to decrease legal risk

**OFFICE PROCEDURES**
Coding for a counseling visit
Collection procedures
Determining the correct coding for a short office visit
Diagnosis in office practice
Health Insurance Portability and Accountability Act
Office infertility workup
Office testing for fetal fibronectin

A subject matter index appears at the end of the Critique Book.

# 1

## Treatment of depression in pregnancy

A 34-year-old woman, gravida 4, para 3, comes to the office at 10 weeks of gestation for her first prenatal visit. She has a history of major depression diagnosed 2 years ago when she was hospitalized for 4 weeks. She was treated with tricyclic antidepressants, but was changed to paroxetine, a selective serotonin reuptake inhibitor (SSRI), with improvement. She has done well, except for a minor exacerbation of depression 6 months ago, but stopped her medicine 2 weeks ago because of the pregnancy. She denies being depressed at present, but notes some anxiousness despite sleeping 12–14 hours per day. She is caring for her three children at home, but has struggled with behavioral issues and parenting during the past few weeks. She has a follow-up appointment with her psychiatrist in 6 weeks. The best pharmacologic recommendation for the patient is to start

      (A) nortriptyline hydrochloride
\*   (B) fluoxetine
      (C) clonazepam
      (D) diazepam (Valium)

A number of clinical situations involve the use of antidepressants during pregnancy, including the following:

- Depression in women who are planning to get pregnant
- Women who conceive while taking antidepressants
- New or recurrent episodes of depression during pregnancy
- Postpartum depression

Each of these issues is fraught with complexities and dilemmas regarding outcomes for mother and infant. Physicians have to balance the risk of untreated depression and the likelihood of relapse if the drug is discontinued with the potential for harm to the fetus from drug exposure.

Although pregnancy is traditionally considered a time of emotional well-being, recent data indicate that 7–13% of pregnant women experience significant depressive symptoms. Confusion in the diagnosis of depression can occur because many of the neurovegetative signs and symptoms characteristic of major depression also can be seen in nondepressed women during early pregnancy. Sleep disturbances, changes in appetite, decreased libido, poor concentration, and low energy can occur in major depression and in normal pregnancy. Obstetricians need to take a comprehensive history to elicit features that help confirm a diagnosis of major depression (eg, anhedonia, feelings of guilt or hopelessness, and suicidal thoughts). Women with a history of major depression are particularly vulnerable to a recurrent episode during pregnancy. Some studies report a risk of first-trimester recurrence in up to 70% of patients who discontinue antidepressants before conception.

It is common for women to choose or be advised to discontinue antidepressant treatment during pregnancy even when indicated in cases of significant depression. The clinician faces certain challenges in prescribing medication for the depressed patient. When clinicians make recommendations to patients, the focus is often on the risks of fetal exposure to medications, but it is clear that untreated psychiatric illness carries significant risks when it occurs during pregnancy.

Depression may lead to poor self-care, poor nutrition, and poor compliance with prenatal care. Pregnant women with depression are more likely to smoke, use alcohol, use drugs, and engage in behaviors that increase risks to the fetus. In addition, studies indicate that major depression in pregnancy is associated with adverse fetal outcomes, such as preterm delivery, preeclampsia, small for gestational age, neurodevelopmental sequela, and emotional or behavioral problems. Depression during pregnancy also significantly increases a patient's risk for postpartum depression.

When clinicians are consulted about the use of psychiatric medications during pregnancy, concerns for the fetus include the following risks:

- Teratogenesis
- Neonatal toxicity or withdrawal syndromes
- Long-term sequelae

All decisions regarding the continuation or initiation of treatment during pregnancy must not only reflect risks of fetal exposure to medication, but also maternal risks, including the risk of untreated illness in the mother and the risk of relapse associated with discontinuation of maintenance treatment.

\* Indicates correct answer.
Note: See Appendix A for a table of normal values for laboratory tests.

1

This patient has a clear history of major depression within the past 2 years and a milder recurrence 6 months ago. She currently experiences symptoms that are likely to be related to her depression and she is at high risk for recurrence. Early detection of illness may significantly reduce morbidity and facilitate treatment. The best option would be to restart an antidepressant.

Because all antidepressants cross the placenta, some degree of fetal exposure will occur. The exposure to the fetus will be influenced by the drug, dose, and gestational age. Among the SSRIs, fluoxetine has been most widely studied, and the literature supports its reproductive safety and its use even in the first and second trimesters. Literature also is accumulating to support use of the newer SSRIs, including paroxetine, sertraline hydrochloride, fluvoxamine maleate, and citalopram hydrochloride.

Although this patient most likely is experiencing an exacerbation of her depression, paroxetine has a short half-life (21 hours) and has been associated with a discontinuation syndrome much more frequently than other SSRIs. The symptoms described could be consistent with a discontinuation syndrome (ie, disequilibrium, gastrointestinal symptoms, influenzalike symptoms, sensory disturbances, sleep disturbances, anxiety, and irritability) that typically occur 1–3 days after treatment cessation and can last for an average of 10 days. Fluoxetine, on the other hand, has a longer half-life and much less risk of discontinuation syndrome. In addition, the U.S. Food and Drug Administration (FDA) recently reported that paroxetine, taken in the first 3 months of pregnancy, may increase a woman's risk of having a baby born with a heart defect. Considering the patient's pregnancy and her history of self-discontinuation of her medicine, the best choice for her would be an SSRI with a longer half-life and no known teratogenicity such as fluoxetine.

Tricyclic antidepressants also can be used in pregnancy. Amitriptyline hydrochloride and clomipramine hydrochloride are listed as FDA pregnancy category C, and nortriptyline hydrochloride, imipramine hydrochloride, and desipramine hydrochloride are listed as "safety in pregnancy not known." Overall, studies have not shown significant associations between fetal exposure to tricyclic antidepressants and the risk for any major congenital anomaly. If using a tricyclic antidepressant in pregnancy, nortriptyline hydrochloride and desipramine hydrochloride would be preferred because they are less anticholinergic and less likely to exacerbate orthostatic hypotension that occurs in pregnancy. Because this patient was changed from a tricyclic antidepressant to an SSRI 1 year ago, there seems no clear indication to start nortriptyline hydrochloride.

Benzodiazepines (eg, clonazepam, diazepam) are FDA pregnancy category D drugs and are avoided in pregnancy because of concerns over possibly causing a fetal benzodiazepine syndrome. Although reports of their teratogenicity are conflicting and no risks of anomalies have been confirmed in prospective studies, the risk–benefit ratio does not justify their use in pregnancy. In addition, benzodiazepines are not typically prescribed for treatment of depression.

Follow-up with the psychiatrist for ongoing psychotherapy is recommended, and an immediate psychiatric consultation can be done if needed. Psychiatric assistance also can be helpful as a pregnant patient on an SSRI approaches her due date. Reports of neonatal withdrawal from SSRIs have prompted clinicians to taper the SSRI to the lowest acceptable dose before delivery to avoid this complication. Following delivery, the SSRI should be restarted at the therapeutic dose.

Bennett HA, Einarson A, Taddio A, Koren G, Einarson TR. Prevalence of depression during pregnancy: systematic review. Obstet Gynecol 2004;103:698–709.

Gentile S. The safety of newer antidepressants in pregnancy and breast-feeding. Drug Saf 2005;28:137–52.

Henry AL, Beach AJ, Stowe ZN, Newport DJ. The fetus and maternal depression: implications for antenatal treatment guidelines. Clin Obstet Gynecol 2004;47:535–46.

Nonacs R, Cohen LS. Depression during pregnancy: diagnosis and treatment options. J Clin Psychiatry 2002;63(suppl 7):24–30.

Patkar AA, Bilal L, Masand PS. Pharmacotherapy of depression in pregnancy. Ann Clin Psychiatry 2004;16:87–100.

# 2

## Colon cancer screening

A 48-year-old woman tells you she has intermittent rectal bleeding with small amounts of bright red blood on the toilet tissue after bowel movements. She reports formed stools every 1–2 days. She denies any change in the frequency, consistency, or size of her bowel movements. Her family history is significant for a first cousin with Crohn's disease, and her paternal grandfather died from colon cancer at age 60 years. The patient's abdominal examination is unremarkable. Inspection of her anus reveals a small fissure at the 12 o'clock position. The rectal examination is normal. The next step in care is to

       (A) begin annual Hemoccult testing
\*   (B) refer for colonoscopy
       (C) order a barium enema
       (D) cauterize the fissure
       (E) order fecal DNA analysis

Colon cancer poses a significant risk for women. Worldwide, an estimated 1 million new cases of carcinoma of the colon and rectum occur each year, with a male to female ratio of 1.2:1. In terms of incidence, colorectal cancer ranks third among cancers in women by prevalence. Dietary and environmental factors play an important role in the development of colorectal malignancy with highest incidence rates in North America, Australia, New Zealand, Western Europe, and Japan. Other risk factors include excess body weight and central obesity.

Screening for colorectal cancer in asymptomatic adults, both women and men, is recommended to begin at age 50 years. Annual fecal occult blood testing, consisting of an at-home collection of two samples from three consecutive bowel movements, is recommended. In-office digital rectal examination and collection of stool are not an adequate substitute. Future development of fecal immunochemical tests may be equally or more sensitive and more "patient-friendly."

There are several screening options:

- Colonoscopy every 10 years
- Screening by flexible sigmoidoscopy every 5 years plus annual fecal screening
- Double-contrast barium enema every 5 years
- Annual fecal occult testing, as recommended by some organizations (Table 2-1)

Colonoscopy would be the best choice for this patient. It allows for visualization of the entire large colon and enables immediate biopsy of polyps and suspicious lesions.

Risk factors, such as family history, rectal bleeding, or disturbances in bowel function, may prompt earlier testing. Systematic reviews suggest the effectiveness of screening as a means of reducing death from colorectal malignancy. Annual fecal occult blood testing has been shown to be effective in reducing mortality rates as have sigmoidoscopy or colonoscopy, especially through a combined strategy. Double-contrast barium enema has not been well studied.

Fecal DNA screening has been introduced recently as a screen for colorectal cancer. Oncogene mutations characteristic of colorectal neoplasia are detectable in exfoliated epithelial cells that are shed in the stool. Because this shedding occurs continuously (vs intermittent bleeding associated with colorectal malignancy), this test is potentially more sensitive. The test also may be more acceptable because it requires no dietary or medication restrictions before testing and testing is less frequent.

**TABLE 2-1.** Colorectal Cancer Screening Guidelines for Individuals at Average Risk

| Screening Test* | Recommended Interval (Beginning at Age 50 Years) |
|---|---|
| FOBT or FIT *or* | Annually |
| FS *or* | Every 5 years |
| FOBT or FIT and FS *or* | FOBT annually and FS every 5 years |
| Double-contrast barium enema *or* | Every 5 years |
| Colonoscopy | Every 10 years |

FOBT, fecal occult blood testing; FIT, fecal immunohistochemical testing; FS, flexible sigmoidoscopy

*Both FOBT and FS are preferred to FOBT or FS alone.

Routine cancer screening. ACOG Committee Opinion No. 356. American College of Obstetricians and Gynecologists. Obstet Gynecol 2006;108:1611–3.

However, some might find the requirement to collect and refrigerate an entire bowel movement to be unacceptable. Moreover, because at present the cost of fecal DNA screening is much greater than fecal occult blood testing, the test is not cost efficient.

Rectal fissures are common entities associated with constipation and straining. Management may be monitoring with addition of stool softeners, or the site may be cauterized and treated with a topical ointment. A severe

or prolonged course involving a rectal fissure may require surgical excision and closure.

Parkin DM, Bray F, Ferlay J, Pisani P. Global cancer statistics, 2002. CA Cancer J Clin 2005;55:74–108.

Screening for colorectal cancer: recommendations and rationale. U.S. Preventive Services Task Force. Ann Intern Med 2002;137:129–31.

Smith RA, Cokkinedes Z, Eyre HJ. American Cancer Society guidelines for the early detection of cancer, 2005. CA Cancer J Clin 2005; 55:31–44; quiz 55–6.

# 3

## Treatment of insulin resistance

A 30-year-old woman comes to your office for her postpartum visit and is found to have a fasting plasma glucose level of 115 mg/dL. She weighs 31.8 kg (70 lb) more than her prepregnancy weight. Her body mass index (weight in kilograms divided by height in meters squared [kg/m$^2$]) is 30.5, blood pressure reading is 135/85 mm Hg, and her waist circumference is 96 cm (38 in.). You recommend that the best nonpharmacologic sustainable approach to treat her glucose intolerance is

      (A) strenuous exercise 150 minutes per day
      (B) low-calorie diet, 800–1,500 kcal per day
      (C) very low-calorie diet, 250–800 kcal per day
\*    (D) modest reduction of 7% of body weight
      (E) liposuction of excess abdominal adipose tissue

The epidemic of diabetes mellitus needs to be addressed through primary prevention to modify the precursors to glucose intolerance. This patient meets the diagnostic criteria for metabolic syndrome (Appendix B). The first major therapeutic goal in patients with metabolic syndrome, recommended by the National Cholesterol Education Program Adult Treatment Panel III (ATP III) and the American Heart Association, is treatment of underlying causes (ie, overweight–obesity and physical inactivity) through weight management and increased physical activity. Prevention or reduction of obesity, particularly abdominal obesity, is the main therapeutic goal in patients with the metabolic syndrome.

Clinical trials have shown that lifestyle modifications can substantially reduce the risk of development of type 2 diabetes mellitus and risk of cardiovascular disease in patients at increased risk. The Diabetes Prevention Program showed that lifestyle changes aimed at modest weight reduction through a low-fat diet and increased exercise constituted a successful and sustainable strategy. The investigators recommended a low-fat diet and moderate exercise for 150 minutes per week. Removal of abdominal adipose tissue with liposuction does not

improve insulin sensitivity or eliminate risk factors for coronary heart disease because it does not remove visceral fat.

The centerpiece of dietary therapy is the low-calorie diet, 800–1,500 kcal per day. This diet is distinguished from the very low-calorie diet, 250–800 kcal per day, and diets of less than 250 kcal per day, termed starvation diets. Very low-calorie diets should be reserved for patients who require rapid weight loss for a specific purpose such as surgery. The basis for the starvation diet is that the lower the calorie intake, the more rapid the weight loss, because the energy withdrawn from body fat stores is a function of the energy deficit. Although the starvation diet is the ultimate very low-calorie diet and results in the most rapid weight loss, it is difficult to sustain. Likewise, although strenuous exercise 150 minutes per day may reduce weight, it is difficult to sustain on a long-term basis as a public health recommendation. Although once popular, very low-calorie diets are now rarely used to treat obesity. The weight gain when the diet is stopped is often rapid, and nutritional inadequacies will occur unless such diets are supplemented with vitamins and minerals. Thus, it is better to take a more sustainable approach.

The Mediterranean diet (less saturated fat and more fruits, vegetables, nuts, whole grains, and olive oil) may be particularly beneficial in patients with metabolic syndrome independent of weight loss. Compared to a standard low-fat diet, the Mediterranean diet may lead to improvements in blood pressure, endothelial function, markers of vascular inflammation, insulin action, and lipid profiles.

There are no data on glycemic control goals in nondiabetic patients with metabolic syndrome. Current recommendations for the treatment of impaired fasting glucose and impaired glucose tolerance are

- Moderate weight loss of approximately 7% of the baseline weight
- At least 30 minutes per day of moderately intense physical activity
- Dietary therapy with a low intake of saturated fats, trans fats, cholesterol, and simple sugars, and increased intake of fruits, vegetables, and whole grains

In the long run, however, sustained adherence to a diet, rather than diet type, was the key predictor of weight loss and cardiac risk factor reduction.

The second major therapeutic ATP III goal in patients with metabolic syndrome includes treatment of cardiovascular risk factors if they persist despite lifestyle modification. The general aspects of sustainable risk factor reduction include treatment of hypertension, cessation of smoking, glycemic control in patients with diabetes mellitus, administration of aspirin in patients with cardiovascular disease, and lowering of serum cholesterol according to recommended guidelines.

Esposito K, Marfella R, Ciotola M, Di Palo C, Giugliano F, Giugliano G, et al. Effect of a Mediterranean-style diet on endothelial dysfunction and markers of vascular inflammation in the metabolic syndrome: a randomized trial. JAMA 2004;292:1440–6.

Grundy SM, Cleeman JI, Daniels SR, Donato KA, Eckel RH, Franklin BA, et al. Diagnosis and management of the metabolic syndrome: an American Heart Association/National Heart, Lung, and Blood Institute Scientific Statement. American Heart Association; National Heart, Lung, and Blood Institute [published errata appear in Circulation 2005;112:e297; Circulation 2005;112:e298]. Circulation 2005;112: 2735–52.

Klein S, Fontana L, Young VL, Coggan AR, Kilo C, Patterson BW, et al. Absence of an effect of liposuction on insulin action and risk factors for coronary heart disease. N Engl J Med 2004;350:2549–57.

Knowler WC, Barrett-Connor E, Fowler SE, Hamman RF, Lachin JM, Walker EA, et al. Reduction in the incidence of type 2 diabetes with lifestyle intervention or metformin. N Engl J Med 2002;346:393–403.

National Institutes of Health, National Heart, Lung, and Blood Institute. Clinical guidelines on the identification, evaluation and treatment of overweight and obesity in adults, Publication no. 98-4083. Washington, DC: NIH; September 1998.

Obesity in pregnancy. ACOG Committee Opinion No. 315. American College of Obstetricians and Gynecologists. Obstet Gynecol 2005; 106:671–5.

The role of the obstetrician–gynecologist in the assessment and management of obesity. ACOG Committee Opinion No. 319. American College of Obstetricians and Gynecologists. Obstet Gynecol 2005; 106:895–9.

# 4

## Fetal Down syndrome

A 33-year-old woman, gravida 3, para 1, is seen at her first prenatal visit at 8 weeks of gestation. Her obstetric history includes a first-trimester loss at age 29 years followed by a full-term healthy neonate at age 30 years. The initial examination is unremarkable; a pelvic examination confirmed a uterine size compatible with 8–9 weeks of gestation. In her second pregnancy, an increased risk for Down syndrome based on biochemical screening at 15 weeks of gestation with the triple screen of alpha-fetoprotein, serum β-hCG, and unconjugated estriols, culminated in an amniocentesis with normal karyotype. This test caused her anxiety and is an experience that she would prefer not to repeat. However, she continues to be interested in screening for fetal Down syndrome. She would prefer a screening strategy that would maximize the detection of Down syndrome, but limit or minimize the risk of a false-positive result. The screening strategy that currently best accomplishes this goal is

      (A) first-trimester biochemical screening
      (B) first-trimester biochemical screening and nuchal translucency evaluation
      (C) second-trimester quadruple screening
      (D) second-trimester quadruple screening and genetic ultrasonography
*    (E) first-trimester screening and second-trimester screening

In 2001, the American College of Obstetricians and Gynecologists (ACOG) recommended invasive diagnostic procedures for prenatal diagnosis for women older than 35 years at the anticipated delivery date, as well as for other women at high risk of fetal aneuploidy. The latter category includes women who have had pregnancies affected by trisomy or sex aneuploidy (recurrence risk of 1% for both abnormalities) and women with a current fetus with structural anomaly, or in situations where the parents are carriers of balanced translocation, chromosome inversion, or aneuploidy.

In women younger than 35 years, strategies to determine whether the fetus is aneuploid include biochemical marker screening and ultrasonography. The triple screen includes evaluation of maternal serum, typically at 15–20 weeks of gestation, for alpha-fetoprotein, total β-hCG, and unconjugated estriol. Adjusted to a false-positive rate of 5%, the detection rate for Down syndrome is 60–70%, when a positive screening test is set to a risk of greater than 1 in 250. The addition of inhibin A to the triple screen increased the detection rate by 8% in one analysis of 46,193 screened pregnancies (with a positive test set at greater than 1:300 risk) (Table 4-1).

Second-trimester genetic ultrasonography currently is most often used to modify the probability risk in pregnancies with an elevated risk based on age, serum screening, or family history. Major structural abnormalities are present in 20–26% of cases of Down syndrome. In one study, with the addition of minor markers (eg, thickened nuchal fold, hyperechoic bowel, echogenic intracardiac focus, short upper and lower limbs, and renal pyelectasis), the

detection rate for Down syndrome was increased to 80% but with a false-positive rate of 12%. The absence of any major or minor dysmorphology, however, reduced the risk by 80% (Table 4-2). Perhaps the most useful aspect of second-trimester ultrasonography is to know that the probability of Down syndrome is reduced if no markers are identified. The presence of any marker based on the calculated likelihood ratio will not decrease risk. The risk remains the same or higher if the ultrasonographic findings include an anomaly, thickened nuchal fold, short humerus, or aggregate of multiple markers. When used alone, ultrasonography has a high false-positive rate, as suggested by the data.

Screening in the first trimester for Down syndrome has involved both biochemical marker testing (pregnancy-associated plasma protein A [PAPP-A] and free β-hCG) as well as ultrasonography (nuchal translucency). Studies

**TABLE 4-1.** Sensitivity and Positive Predictive Values for a Fixed 5% False-Positive Rate by Method of Screening in 88 Down Syndrome Pregnancies

| Screening Method | Setting the False-Positive Rate to 5% | |
| --- | --- | --- |
| | Sensitivity (Detection Rate) | Positive Predictive Value |
| Triple | 62% | 1.9% |
| Quadruple | 70% | 2.2% |

Modified from Wald NJ, Huttly WJ, Hackshaw AK. Antenatal screening for Down's syndrome with the quadruple test. Lancet 2003;361:835–6.

**TABLE 4-2.** Likelihood Ratios for Ultrasonographic Markers in Down Syndrome

| No. of Ultrasonographic Markers | Frequency of Marker | | Likelihood Ratio (95% Confidence Interval) |
|---|---|---|---|
| | Cases (n = 164) | Controls (n = 656) | |
| 0 | 32 | 575 | 0.2 (0.16–0.30) |
| 1 | 32 | 66 | 1.9 (1.3–2.5) |
| 2 | 20 | 13 | 6.2 (3.1–12.1) |
| 3 | 40 | 2 | 80 (19.5–327.6) |
| 4 | 28 | 0 | – |
| 5 | 9 | 0 | – |
| 6 | 3 | 0 | – |

Markers included nuchal fold of more than 6 mm, short humerus, short femur, echogenic intracardiac focus, pyelectasis, and hyperechoic bowel.

From Bromley B, Lieberman E, Shipp TD, Benacerraf BR. The genetic sonogram, a method of risk assessment for Down syndrome in the second trimester. J Ultrasound Med 2002;21:1090.

that use biochemical screening alone demonstrate a detection rate of approximately 60% with a false-positive rate of 5%. In the first trimester alone, nuchal translucency measurements are comparable to second-trimester biochemical screening with a detection rate of 77% and a false-positive rate of 5% as documented in a Swedish study of 16,295 women. It should be noted that in fetuses with increased nuchal translucency, but with a normal karyotype, there still remains a significant risk of adverse outcomes such as abortion, fetal death, and anomalies, including cardiac anomalies.

A multicenter study of 8,514 pregnancies, PAPP-A, and free β-hCG, combined with nuchal translucency evaluation, yielded a higher detection rate of 75.7% with a false-positive rate of 5% set to a risk threshold of 1:270. Ninety-one percent of patients with trisomy 18 were also detected with a false-positive rate of 2%.

The most effective strategy, with higher detection rate and lower false-positive rate, may be integrated testing that involves a combination of first-trimester screening (nuchal translucency, PAPP-A) and second-trimester biochemical screening (alpha-fetoprotein, total β-hCG, dimeric inhibin A, unconjugated estriol). The risk of Down syndrome is not revealed until testing in both the first and second trimester is completed. Two recent studies, one in England of 47,053 pregnancies (101 or 0.21% affected by Down syndrome), and one in the United States of 38,167 pregnancies (117 or 0.3% affected by Down syndrome) demonstrated that with the false-positive rate set to 5%, detection rates are 94% and 96%, respectively. Practical difficulties of the strategy include

that the patient must wait between the first-trimester evaluation and the subsequent second-trimester evaluation before the risk assessment is revealed.

American College of Obstetricians and Gynecologists. Prenatal diagnosis of fetal chromosomal abnormalities. ACOG Practice Bulletin 27. Washington, DC: ACOG; 2001.

Bromley B, Lieberman E, Shipp TD, Benacerraf BR. The genetic sonogram, a method of risk assessment for Down syndrome in the second trimester. J Ultrasound Med 2002;21:1087–96; quiz 1097–8.

DeVore GR, Romero R. Combined use of genetic sonography and maternal serum triple-marker screening: an effective method for increasing the detection of trisomy 21 in women younger than 35 years. J Ultrasound Med 2001;20:645–54.

First-trimester screening for fetal aneuploidy. ACOG Committee Opinion No. 296. American College of Obstetricians and Gynecologists. Obstet Gynecol 2004;104:215–7.

Malone FD, Canick JA, Ball RH, Nyberg DA, Comstock CH, Bukowski R, et al. First-trimester or second-trimester screening, or both, for Down's syndrome. N Engl J Med 2005;353:2001–11.

Souka AP, Krampl E, Bakalis S, Heath V, Nicolaides KH. Outcome of pregnancy in chromosomally normal fetuses with increased nuchal translucency in the first trimester. Ultrasound Obstet Gynecol 2001; 18:9–17.

Wald NJ, Huttly WJ, Hackshaw AK. Antenatal screening for Down's syndrome with the quadruple test. Lancet 2003;361:835–6.

Wald NJ, Rodeck C, Hackshaw A, Walters J, Chitty L, Mackinson AM. First and second trimester antenatal screening for Down's syndrome: the results of the Serum, Urine and Ultrasound Screening Study (SURUSS). J Med Screen 2003;10:56–104.

Wald NJ, Watt HC, Hackshaw AK. Integrated screening for Down's syndrome based on tests performed during the first and second trimester. N Engl J Med 1999;341:461–7.

Wapner R, Thom E, Simpson JL, Pergament E, Silver R, Filkins K, et al. First-trimester screening for trisomies 21 and 18. N Engl J Med 2003;349:1405–13.

# 5

## Evaluation of anal incontinence

A 37-year-old woman, gravida 2, para 2, soils her underclothes with loose stools approximately twice a week. She had a fourth-degree laceration with her last vaginal delivery. She also has abdominal bloating and rectal urgency that alternates with constipation. She has slightly decreased rectal sphincter tone on examination and an intact perineal body. The next step in the evaluation of this patient should be

      (A) anal manometry
      (B) barium enema
\*    (C) endoanal ultrasonography
      (D) defecography
      (E) pudendal nerve terminal motor latency

Fecal incontinence is the involuntary loss of rectal contents through the anal canal. Population-based studies provide widely varying prevalence estimates from 0.004% to 18%. Part of the problem in identifying its prevalence is the lack of definition in terms of flatus vs stools, severity, and frequency, as well as underreporting by patients and variation in patient populations being surveyed. Symptomatic fecal incontinence occurs in 21% of women with urinary incontinence, pelvic organ prolapse, or both.

The anal sphincter complex consists of the internal and external anal sphincters and the puborectalis muscles. The smooth muscle of the internal sphincter contributes 55% of the resting tone; the external sphincter, which is continuously active, contributes about 30%. The pudendal nerve is responsible for innervation. Acquired incontinence is most commonly caused by sphincter disruption from vaginal delivery; rates as determined by ultrasonography are as high as 35%. Trauma from accidents or pelvic fracture, and surgical procedures such as sphincterotomy, fistulotomy, hemorrhoidectomy, and anal dilation can result in incontinence.

It is believed that the incidence of postpartum sphincter disruption is underestimated. Rates of postpartum incontinence are variable and have been reported up to 23%, depending on the definition. Muscle disruption is associated with incontinence and operative vaginal delivery. Neuropathy from stretching of the pudendal nerve during the second stage of labor also may lead to muscle degeneration. The descent of the perineal floor that results in traction on the nerve as it emerges from Alcock's canal also can be caused by straining at stool and rectal prolapse.

Fecal impaction and resultant overflow incontinence have been attributed to inhibition of the internal sphincter and decreased sensation. The rectal anal inhibitory reflex involves coordination of external sphincter contraction and internal sphincter relaxation in response to rectal distention. An intact rectal anal inhibitory reflex in the absence of normal sensation can cause failure to evacuate the rectal contents and result in overflow incontinence.

Decreased sensation may be caused by diabetic neuropathy, multiple sclerosis, and spinal cord conditions. Dementia can result in functional incontinence and lack of motivation to use the toilet in a timely fashion. Altered stool consistency and diarrhea from irritable bowel syndrome, infection, inflammation, malabsorption, and radiation therapy can contribute to urgency and loss of liquid stools. Inadequate colonic reservoir or decreased compliance also may contribute to urgency and liquid stools.

Evaluation consists of taking a comprehensive medical history and performing a physical examination, with attention to pelvic floor support, rectal tone, perineal body, and neurologic evaluation, including perineal sensation and bulbocavernosus reflex (anal wink). Other indicated studies include sigmoidoscopy or colonoscopy if the patient has unexplained diarrhea or bleeding. Endoanal ultrasonography is the criterion standard for evaluating the anatomy of the sphincter. The hypoechoic internal sphincter and hyperechoic external sphincter can be evaluated with a sensitivity and specificity of 98–100%. Disruption of both muscles correlates with decreased squeeze and resting pressures by manometry.

Anorectal manometry assesses muscle function, rectal anal inhibitory reflex, and rectal sensation. Usually, the procedure is done only if ultrasonography is normal. Defecography has limited use in incontinent patients, but may reveal occult rectal prolapse or rectocele. It is more useful in the evaluation of obstruction. Pudendal nerve terminal motor latency is a measure of denervation by assessment of conduction times in the remaining nerve fibers. Consensus is lacking about accuracy and predictive value of pudendal nerve terminal motor latency for outcomes after surgery such as sphincteroplasty. A barium enema can give information about space-occupying lesions but is not generally helpful in the evaluation of incontinence.

Figure 5-1 illustrates the anatomy of the anal canal and rectum showing the physiologic mechanisms important to continence and defecation. Figures 5-2 and 5-3 show, respectively, an ultrasonogram of the mid-anal canal in a normal volunteer and an ultrasonogram of the mid-anal canal indicating a defect in the anal sphincter due to an obstetric injury.

Madoff RD, Parker SC, Varma MG, Lowry AC. Faecal incontinence in adults. Lancet 2004;364:621–32.

Nichols CM, Gill EJ, Nguyen T, Barber MD, Hurt WG. Anal sphincter injury in women with pelvic floor disorders. Obstet Gynecol 2004;104:690–6.

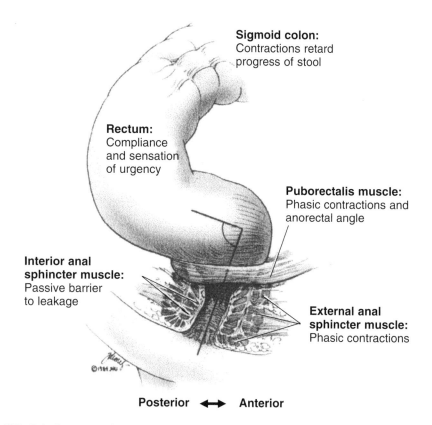

**Sigmoid colon:**
Contractions retard progress of stool

**Rectum:**
Compliance and sensation of urgency

**Puborectalis muscle:**
Phasic contractions and anorectal angle

**Interior anal sphincter muscle:**
Passive barrier to leakage

**External anal sphincter muscle:**
Phasic contractions

**Posterior ⟷ Anterior**

**FIG. 5-1.** Anatomy of the anal canal and rectum showing the physiologic mechanisms important to continence and defecation. (Reprinted from Gastrointestinal disorders: behavioral and physiological basis for treatment. Whitehead WE, Schuster MM. p. 233. Copyright © 1985, with permission from Elsevier.)

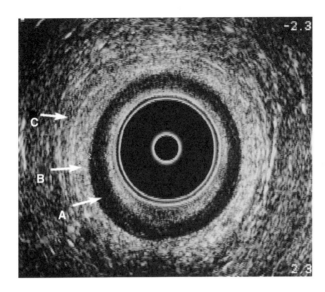

**FIG. 5-2.** Ultrasonogram of the mid-anal canal: normal sphincter appearance in an adult female volunteer. **A.** Internal anal sphincter. **B.** Longitudinal muscle. **C.** External anal sphincter. (Reproduced with permission from Rottenberg GT, Williams AB. Pictorial review: endoanal ultrasound. Br J Radiol 2002;75:484.)

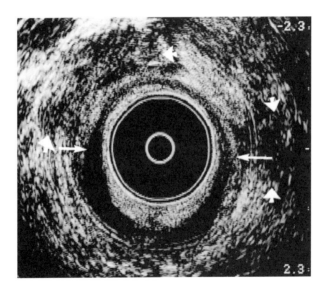

**FIG. 5-3.** Ultrasonogram of the mid-anal canal indicating a defect in the external anal sphincter due to an obstetric injury. The defect appears between the 9 o'clock and 12 o'clock positions and between the 2 o'clock and 3 o'clock positions (arrowheads). There is also a disruption of the internal anal sphincter (arrows). (Reproduced with permission from Rottenberg GT, Williams AB. Pictorial review: endoanal ultrasound. Br J Radiol 2002;75:486.)

# 6

## Evaluation of skin rash in pregnancy

A 26-year-old primigravid woman comes to your office at 37 weeks of gestation with a 1-week history of an intensely pruritic rash that began on her abdomen "in my stretch marks" and has since spread to her buttocks, chest, and upper arms. On examination, you note that she has a generalized erythematous skin eruption characterized by discrete raised lesions with areas of confluence as well as larger raised geographic lesions with pale pink coloration. Linear excoriations and periumbilical haloing are noted (Fig. 6-1; see color plate). The most appropriate next step is

* (A) no further diagnostic testing is necessary
  (B) punch biopsy of an affected area
  (C) antinuclear antibody (ANA) titer measurement
  (D) liver function tests
  (E) Wood's lamp examination

Polymorphic eruption of pregnancy (also known as pruritic urticarial papules and plaques of pregnancy) is the most common of the pregnancy-specific dermatoses; it occurs in approximately 1 in 300 pregnancies. It is a self-limited condition that may last up to 6 weeks and typically presents in primigravid women beginning late in the third trimester. The condition is common among women with multiple gestations. The rash has a classic appearance and initially appears in the striae of the abdomen as discrete urticarial lesions that coalesce into larger plaques and patchy erythema. Vesicles and target lesions may occasionally be seen. Within a few days, the rash may spread to the chest, back, thighs, buttocks, and extremities but typically spares the face, palms, and soles. Commonly, a clear area around the umbilicus is noted. The eruption is pruritic and at times may be intensely uncomfortable. In most cases, the condition is diagnosed easily by a combination of history and physical findings without further diagnostic testing.

The etiology of the condition is unknown and findings from biopsy with histology and direct immunofluorescence tend to be nonspecific. Punch biopsy with direct immunofluorescence may occasionally be necessary to differentiate it from pemphigus gestationis; however, this usually is not necessary. Many patients with autoimmune diseases may present with cutaneous manifestations. In the absence of other findings suggestive of autoimmune disease, antinuclear antibody testing would not be warranted. Intrahepatic cholestasis of pregnancy presents with intense pruritus but usually no cutaneous findings. Serum liver function tests would, therefore, be of little benefit. A Wood's lamp examination is helpful in differentiating epidermal melasma from the more-difficult-to-treat dermal melasma and is consequently of limited use in this situation. The diagnosis of polymorphic eruption of pregnancy is evident from physical findings in most cases, and therefore, an expensive diagnostic workup is neither cost-effective nor warranted. The next step for this patient should be treatment. The treatment is symptomatic and should focus on local measures to aid with the pruritus and the use of low potency topical steroids, such as hydrocortisone.

Aronson IK, Bond S, Fiedler VC, Vomvouras S, Gruber D, Ruiz C. Pruritic urticarial papules and plaques of pregnancy: clinical and immunopathologic observations in 57 patients. J Am Acad Dermatol 1998;39:933–9.

Kroumpouzos G, Cohen LM. Dermatoses of pregnancy. J Am Acad Dermatol 2001;45:1–19; quiz 19–22.

Kroumpouzos G, Cohen LM. Specific dermatoses of pregnancy: an evidence-based systematic review. Am J Obstet Gynecol 2003;188: 1083–92.

# 7

## Vertebral fractures

A 70-year-old woman tells you she is "getting fat" without any change in weight. Her abdomen has become larger, her clothes no longer fit, and she no longer appears to have a waist. She has had no recent trauma, but she has lost 4 cm (1.6 in.) in height since age 25 years. The patient describes a pain that often radiates bilaterally into the anterior abdomen in a "girdle of pain." Physical examination shows height 165 cm (65 in.), weight 49.9 kg (110 lb). Her body mass index (weight in kilograms divided by height in meters squared [kg/m²]) is 18.3. Your presumptive diagnosis of vertebral compression fracture is confirmed by spinal radiography. The physical finding that most often correlates with vertebral compression fractures is

* (A) loss of height
  (B) pain on spinal percussion
  (C) body mass index greater than 25
  (D) evidence of recent trauma
  (E) hirsutism

Two out of three vertebral compression fractures are asymptomatic. Most are diagnosed as an incidental finding on chest or abdominal X-ray. In many cases, there are known risk factors (Box 7-1). Although osteoporosis is associated with hypoestrogenemia and hypogonadism, it

---

**BOX 7-1**

### Osteoporotic Vertebral Fracture Risk Factors

Loss of height, 2.5–4.0 cm
Body mass index less than 19
History of previous low-trauma fracture, eg, falling
  from standing height
Low calcium intake
Maternal history of hip fracture, or fragility fracture
  in a first-degree relative
Chronic disorders, eg, hyperthyroidism and
  hyperparathyroidism
Prolonged corticosteroid use
Radiologic evidence of osteopenia
Current cigarette smoking
Low body weight, less than 58 kg (less than
  127 lb)
Female sex
White race
Advanced age
Alcoholism
Inadequate physical activity
Recurring falls
Dementia
Impaired eyesight despite adequate correction
Poor health/frailty
Estrogen deficiency (menopause age younger than
  45 years or bilateral oophorectomy, prolonged
  premenopausal amenorrhea greater than 1 year)

---

is not associated with hirsutism. Vertebral compression fractures are the most common type of osteoporotic fracture. Fractures commonly occur at the thoracolumbar junction (T12–L1) because a change in the facets provides less resistance to anteroposterior displacement at this level. Midthoracic fractures (T7–T8) are also common. In some women, the presence of vertebral fractures may become apparent only because of height loss or kyphosis. Compression fracture may be the first symptom of osteoporosis, although limb fracture or periodontal disease often precedes spinal complaints (Box 7-2).

Approximately 19% of patients who have a vertebral compression fracture will have another fracture in the next year. It has been reported that women with preexisting vertebral fractures have a fourfold greater risk of subsequent vertebral fractures than women without prior fractures. The presence of vertebral fractures also predicts future nonvertebral fractures, particularly hip fracture, and this risk increases with the number and severity of prior fractures.

Functional impairment from vertebral fractures can be as severe as impairment due to hip fracture, including difficulty bending, lifting, walking down stairs, or cooking. In addition, approximately 75% of patients who present with a symptomatic vertebral fracture complain of chronic pain. The small numbers of women who have a symptomatic vertebral fracture usually have no history of preceding trauma. If symptomatic, a patient may present with acute back pain after sudden bending, coughing, or lifting. The pain from a vertebral compression fracture is variable in quality and may be sharp or dull. Sitting and movement often aggravate the discomfort, and muscle spasms may disturb sleep.

---

**BOX 7-2**

**Physical Examination Maneuvers Suggesting Osteoporosis or Spinal Fracture**

*Wall–occiput distance*: Inability to touch occiput to the wall when standing with back and heels to the wall

*Weight*: Less than 51 kg (less than 112.4 lb)

*Rib–pelvis distance*: Less than two finger-breadths between the inferior margin of the ribs and the superior surface of the pelvis in the midaxillary line

*Tooth count*: Less than 20 teeth

*Self-reported humped back*: Patient reports that back has become humped

---

Green AD, Colon-Emeric CS, Bastian L, Drake MT, Lyles KW. Does this woman have osteoporosis? JAMA 2004;292:2898. Copyright © 2004. American Medical Association. All rights reserved.

---

Two out of three compression fractures are asymptomatic; the remaining symptomatic fractures are associated with pain that usually resolves after 4–6 weeks. Severe back pain that persists longer should raise the question of more fractures or another diagnosis. The pain often radiates bilaterally into the anterior abdomen in the distribution of contiguous nerve routes, the so-called "girdle of pain" observed with the patient described. Osteoporosis may lead to several types of vertebral fractures, including wedge fractures, biconcave or "codfish" deformities, and compression fractures. Radiographic characteristics of compression fractures include anterior wedging of one or more vertebra with vertebral collapse, vertebral end-plate irregularity, and general demineralization. Posterior wedging is uncommon and may indicate an underlying destructive lesion.

It is important to appreciate certain clues that suggest that vertebral fractures might be due to causes other than uncomplicated osteoporosis, such as a fracture that occurs in a woman who is neither elderly nor postmenopausal and solitary vertebral fractures due to osteoporosis in vertebrae higher than T7. In either instance, a contributing diagnosis should be considered. In these settings, other causes of osteopenia (eg, osteomalacia, hyperparathyroidism, granulomatous diseases, hematologic diseases) should be excluded.

Kyphosis ("dowager hump") is an indicator of multiple vertebral compression fractures, especially wedge fractures. Each complete compression fracture causes approximately 1 cm or more loss in height; loss of more than 4 cm in height is associated with 15 degrees of kyphosis. No simple clinical measures of kyphosis exist, and measures of height may be inconsistent due to variabilities in measurement technique and posture. Some potentially useful clinical tools include the distance from the occiput to the wall (normally 0 cm) and the size of the gap between the costal margin and the iliac crest, less than two finger-breadths (Fig. 7-1; see color plate).

Patients with kyphosis may describe themselves as "getting fat" without any change in weight. They note that their abdomen has become larger, that their clothes do not fit, or that they no longer have a waist. These symptoms are a reflection of the loss of height; the abdominal contents are compressed into less vertical space, causing them to bulge anteriorly.

Genant HK, Cooper C, Poor G, Reid I, Ehrlich G, Kanis J, et al. Interim report and recommendations of the World Health Organization Task Force for Osteoporosis. Osteoporos Int 1999;10:259–64.

Genant HK, Wu CY, van Kuijk C, Nevitt MC. Vertebral fracture assessment using a semiquantitative technique. J Bone Miner Res 1993;8:1137–48.

Green AD, Colon-Emeric CS, Bastian L, Drake MT, Lyles KW. Does this woman have osteoporosis? JAMA 2004;292:2890–900.

Lindsay R, Silverman SL, Cooper C, Hanley DA, Barton I, Broy SB, et al. Risk of new vertebral fracture in the year following a fracture. JAMA 2001;285:320–3.

Vogt TM, Ross PD, Palermo L, Musliner T, Genant HK, Black D, et al. Vertebral fracture prevalence among women screened for the Fracture Intervention Trial and a simple clinical tool to screen for undiagnosed vertebral fractures. Fracture Intervention Trial Research Group. Mayo Clin Proc 2000;75:888–96.

# 8

## Physician–patient relationship

An established patient has a habit of being disruptive to your practice by failing to keep appointments, being rude to staff, and demanding treatments and prescription medications that in your professional opinion are unnecessary. On several occasions in the past, you have personally discussed these problems with her and indicated that unless her behavior changes, she will be discharged from your practice. During her next visit, she continues to be disruptive and you inform her verbally that the physician–patient relationship is being terminated. You follow-up by sending a termination letter by certified mail, listing other sources of care. Three weeks later, the patient calls the office for a prescription refill. After you decline to refill the prescription, she states that she has a valid claim for abandonment because you failed to provide

        (A) enough medication to last her 3 months
*   (B) a reasonable amount of time to find another source of care
        (C) a valid reason for termination
        (D) transfer of care to another physician
        (E) copies of her medical records

The physician–patient relationship, once established, creates both legal and ethical obligations on the part of the physician that must be met before any change in that relationship is made. Physicians have a fiduciary responsibility to continue to provide care as long as treatment is medically indicated. The physician may decide to terminate the relationship for a variety of reasons (eg, noncompliance, disruptive behavior, unreasonably demanding attitude, or any behavior that negates the trust involved in the physician–patient relationship). Physicians also may terminate the relationship because of practical considerations such as relocation and retirement or contractual obligations required by managed care contracts. Physicians may not terminate care for any discriminatory reason, such as the patient's sex, race, age, sexual orientation, or disability. Although it is legal to end a physician–patient relationship because of nonpayment for services, this may be considered only when there is no acute need for care and after all other possible remedies have been explored.

Termination of care can occur only after the patient has received reasonable notice and sufficient time to make other arrangements. Written notice is recommended, preferably by certified mail with a return receipt required. This allows the physician to document notification. If the relationship is terminated by verbal notification in person, the physician should ask the patient to sign a statement acknowledging the conversation and written notice should still be sent. Thirty days is traditionally accepted

as a reasonable time to find other care. During that time, the physician should be prepared to provide emergency services and any needed ongoing care. In the case scenario, the patient had had only 3 weeks' notice and thus the physician failed to provide her a reasonable amount of time to find another source of care.

The physician is obligated to provide resources to aid the patient in finding a new care provider. This may be as simple as providing the patient with the number for the local hospital or medical board. The physician is not required to transfer the patient directly to another physician. The patient should be advised that her records are available for transfer on receipt of written authorization. The physician may charge a reasonable fee for copying and mailing the information.

Although it is sometimes in the best interest of both the patient and physician to terminate a professional relationship, good practice and ethical standards demand that physicians make every effort to meet the medical needs of their patients. Termination of the physician–patient relationship should always be a last resort. The physician should be aware of local, state, and medical regulations governing this process.

American Medical Association. Code of medical ethics. Chicago (IL): AMA; 2004.

American Medical Association. Ending the patient–physician relationship. Prepared by the AMA, Office of the General Counsel, Division of Health Law.

American College of Obstetricians and Gynecologists. Ethics in obstetrics and gynecology. 2nd ed. Washington, DC: ACOG; 2004.

# 9

## Hepatitis C virus therapy

A 45-year-old woman with hepatitis C, genotype I, and a twice normal serum alanine aminotransferase (ALT) takes pegylated interferon and ribavirin. She is seen in your office for her periodic health maintenance examination and requests your advice about continuing this treatment. She has just completed the first 3 months of therapy. She has a decrease in serum 2 log hepatitis C virus (HCV) RNA from 1 million to 10,000 copies/mL. She does not feel well on the pegylated interferon and ribavirin regimen. She has influenzalike symptoms, mild anemia, and fatigue. The best advice with regard to treatment is

*   (A) continue current therapy
     (B) stop all therapy
     (C) stop pegylated interferon and continue ribavirin
     (D) stop ribavirin and continue pegylated interferon
     (E) change to standard interferon alone

Hepatitis C virus (HCV) is a single-stranded RNA virus in the family *Flaviviridae*, with its own genus Hepacivirus. It is found worldwide, with at least six major genotypes and multiple subtypes. Genotypes differ by 30% of their amino acid sequence and subtypes differ by 5–10% of their amino acid sequence within genotypes. Quasispecies are additional variants that may be present in an individual as a result of mutations during replication and immune selection pressure. Genotypes 1a and 1b are the most common in the United States; approximately 25% of infections in North America are genotypes 2 and 3. In Europe and Japan, genotype 1b is the most common. In Egypt, genotype 4 is the most prevalent and infects approximately 10–30% of individuals. Genotype 6 is most common in Southeast Asia.

In the United States, the prevalence is 1.8%. Approximately 2.7 million people have persistent infection. Hepatitis C infection is most commonly chronic. Long-term infection is the most common underlying cause of end-stage liver disease and thus is the leading indication for liver transplants in the United States.

Hepatitis C is detected with anti-HCV enzyme immunoassays (EIAs) with sensitivity of 98–100%. The EIAs are less sensitive in dialysis patients, immunocompromised patients, and patients with HCV-associated mixed cryoglobulinemia. A supplemental recombinant immunoblot assay may be used to confirm infection. Qualitative HCV polymerase chain reaction (PCR) or transcription-mediated amplification RNA testing also is performed to confirm infection. Quantitative HCV RNA levels are measured to monitor ongoing infection and treatment; this is commonly referred to as "viral load" testing. The World Health Organization has defined an international standard for HCV RNA quantification. When patients are being treated, the same units, the same

test, and the same laboratory should be used to follow serial viral loads to monitor response to treatment. Hepatitis C genotyping is necessary for infected individuals, primarily to predict response to therapy.

Therapy is indicated in patients with chronic HCV infection with detectable viral load and elevated ALT levels. Cirrhosis, liver fibrosis, or moderate inflammation on liver biopsy all support intervention, but liver biopsy is not required before treatment. The goal of therapy is to achieve a sustained virologic response with negative HCV RNA quantitative testing. Patients with a sustained viral response may have favorable histologic and clinical outcomes, including halting progression of cirrhosis. The genotype is the most important factor in predicting the response to treatment with antivirals. Genotype 1 responds less well to all current therapies than do genotypes 2 and 3. Women respond better than men. However, the combination pegylated interferon and ribavirin is U.S. Food and Drug Administration category X in pregnancy. Therefore, treatment in women should be avoided in pregnancy. This combination is also contraindicated in men whose female partners are pregnant. Two contraceptive methods are recommended for women of childbearing potential during treatment and for 6 months after treatment conclusion. Lower body surface area, age younger than 40 years, and absence of significant fibrosis of the liver all enhance response. Laboratory values of HCV RNA less than 2 million copies/mL and ALT more than three times the upper limit of normal also predict a favorable response to antivirals. The most effective therapy currently available combines pegylated interferon $\alpha$-2a or pegylated interferon $\alpha$-2b with ribavirin. Patients with genotypes 2 or 3 are treated for 4 weeks then the HCV RNA level is determined. If the HCV RNA is undetectable, they are treated for 12 weeks. If virus is still detectable, they are treated for 24 weeks and then the viral load is again assessed. They have a high (61–76%) likelihood of response.

Patients with genotype 1 should be treated for 12 weeks, then an HCV viral load should be determined. An early virologic response is defined as undetectable HCV RNA or a 2-log decrease in HCV RNA. Those with an early virologic response should continue therapy for 48 weeks with the expectation that 65% will achieve a sustained virologic response. Patients without an early virologic response should have therapy stopped because less than 3% will achieve a sustained virologic response (Fig. 9-1). Individualization of treatment is necessary. Some practitioners continue to treat patients that have a significant decline in HCV RNA but not the full 2 log response at 12 weeks, and reevaluate the HCV RNA levels at 24 weeks. The most common side effects of pegylated interferon and ribavirin include influenzalike symptoms of myalgias, fevers, and rigors. Other side effects include thrombocytopenia, neutropenia, anemia, depression, weight loss, nausea, and alopecia. Uncommon (1%) but serious adverse reactions include autoimmune disease, diabetes mellitus, seizures, cardiovascular disease, and thyroid disease. Some patients who achieve an early virologic response but who have bothersome side effects may need decreased doses of pegylated interferon and rib-

avirin. There is a good sustained virologic response if patients can tolerate at least 80% of their original dose. Therapy with standard interferon alone has a lower response rate than a reduced dose of pegylated interferon and ribavirin combination therapy. Use of pegylated interferon or ribavirin alone is also not as effective as combination therapy. In this case, where the patient had an appropriate early virologic response, therapy should be continued. Side effects occur as expected and may be managed by counseling and medical support. A slight reduction in dosage, so that her therapy is continued at a level at least 80% of her original dose, might also decrease her side effects, but still give her a sustained virologic response.

Berger A, Preiser W. Viral genome quantification as a tool for improving patient management: the example of HIV, HBV, HCV, and CMV. J Antimicrob Chemother 2002;49:713–21.

Dal Molin G, Tiribelli C, Campello C. A rational use of laboratory tests in the diagnosis and management of hepatitis C virus infection. Ann Hepatol 2002;2:76–83.

Fried MW. Viral factors affecting the outcome of therapy for chronic hepatitis C. Rev Gastroenterol Dis 2004;4(suppl 1):S8–S13.

Mangia A, Santoro R, Minerva N, Ricci GL, Carette V, Persico M, et al. Peginterferon alfa-2b and ribavirin for 12 vs 24 weeks in HCV genotype 2 or 3. N Engl J Med 2005;352:2609–17.

McHutchison JG, Fried MW. Current therapy for hepatitis C: pegylated interferon and ribavirin. Clin Liver Dis 2003;7:149–61.

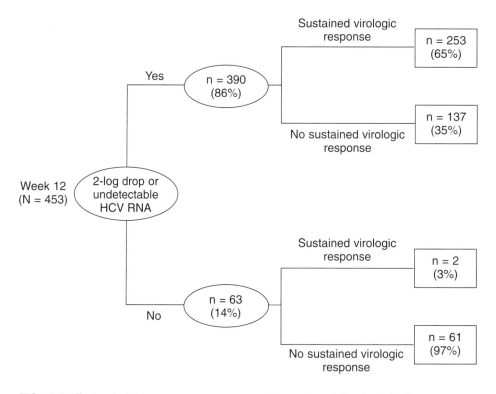

**FIG. 9-1.** Early virologic response as a predictor of sustained virologic response. Pegylated interferon α-2a in combination therapy: implications of early virologic response. HCV, hepatitis C virus; RNA, ribonucleic acid; SVR, sustained virologic response. (Fried MW, Shiffman ML, Reddy KR, Smith C, Marinos G, Goncales FL Jr, et al. Combination peginterferon α-2a plus ribavirin in patients with chronic hepatitis C virus infection. N Engl J Med 2002;347:980. Copyright © 2002 Massachusetts Medical Society. All rights reserved.)

# 10

## Depot medroxyprogesterone acetate and bone density

During an annual gynecology visit, a 17-year-old adolescent asks you about contraception. She has used depot medroxyprogesterone acetate injections for 2 years and has received all of her injections on time. Although she has repeatedly been counseled regarding the importance of consistent condom use in preventing sexually transmitted diseases, she uses condoms inconsistently, has had three sex partners in the past 2 years, and indicates that becoming pregnant now would disrupt her plans to go to college. She has heard that depot medroxyprogesterone acetate may cause low bone density. She indicates that she is a poor pill taker and that she is not interested in using the birth control patch or vaginal ring. The most appropriate contraceptive recommendation for her is

  (A) condoms
  (B) combination oral contraceptives
  (C) progestin-only oral contraceptives
* (D) continue depot medroxyprogesterone acetate injections
  (E) intrauterine device (IUD)

In a 2002 survey, among U.S. female adolescents aged 15–19 years who had ever been sexually active, more than 20% reported current or prior use of depot medroxyprogesterone acetate. This convenient, effective, and long-acting birth control method has played an important role in reducing adolescent pregnancies and abortions. As with other progestational contraceptives, depot medroxyprogesterone acetate not only suppresses ovulation but also reduces ovarian estradiol production. This leads to declines in bone mineral density (BMD) at the hip and spine in current users of depot medroxyprogesterone acetate that approximate 1–2% annually. After depot medroxyprogesterone acetate is discontinued in adults as well as in adolescents, BMD recovers. Within 3 years of discontinuing depot medroxyprogesterone acetate injections, BMD was noted to be as high (or higher) in teens who had previously used depot medroxyprogesterone acetate as in those who had never used it.

In late 2004, the U.S. Food and Drug Administration added a black box warning to the labeling of depot medroxyprogesterone acetate recommending that in women who have used the product for 2 years, as with the patient in this case, alternate contraceptive options be considered because of the effect of depot medroxyprogesterone acetate on BMD. It should be noted that in postmenopausal women, BMD is equivalent in former and never users of depot medroxyprogesterone acetate. Its use has not been linked to the occurrence of osteoporosis or fractures. As with depot medroxyprogesterone acetate use, lactation represents a hypoestrogenic state during which spinal BMD decreases approximately 4% at 6 months then returns to prepregnant levels when lactation is discontinued.

Recommending to this 17-year-old adolescent who reports previous inconsistent use of condoms that she discontinue depot medroxyprogesterone acetate and rely on condom contraception may result in unintended pregnancy. Many women and particularly teenagers, such as this adolescent, are poor pill takers. Accordingly, prescribing combination or progestin-only oral contraceptives to this patient may not provide her adequate contraceptive protection. Given her multiple sexual partners and inconsistent use of condoms, recommending an IUD is not advisable.

World Health Organization criteria to assess BMD apply only to postmenopausal women. Assessment of BMD of this 17-year-old adolescent with dual energy X-ray absorptiometry would not provide clinically useful information. Given that depot medroxyprogesterone acetate represents a safe contraceptive option more likely to prevent unintended pregnancy than alternate methods of birth control, it would be appropriate for this young woman to continue depot medroxyprogesterone acetate injections. No data indicate the optimal duration of its use. However, clinicians should balance the real risks of unintended pregnancy in an adolescent vs the theoretic increased risks of skeletal health problems with depot medroxyprogesterone acetate use.

Abma JC, Martinez GM, Mosher WD, Dawson BS. Teenagers in the United States: sexual activity, contraceptive use, and childbearing, 2002. Vital Health Stat 23. 2004;(24):1–48.

Grimes DA, Schultz KF. Surrogate end points in clinical research: hazardous to your health. Obstet Gynecol 2005;105:1114–8.

Kalkwarf HJ, Specker BL. Bone mineral loss during lactation and recovery after weaning. Obstet Gynecol 1995;86:26–32.

Kaunitz AM. Depo-Provera's black box: time to reconsider? Contraception 2005;72:165–7.

Orr-Walker BJ, Evans MC, Ames RW, Clearwater JM, Cundy T, Reid IR. The effect of past use of the injectable contraceptive depot medroxyprogesterone acetate on bone mineral density in normal postmenopausal women. Clin Endocrinol (Oxf) 1998;49:615–8.

Scholes D, LaCroix AZ, Ichikawa LE, Barlow WE, Ott SM. Change in bone mineral density among adolescent women using and discontinuing

depot medroxyprogesterone acetate contraception. Arch Pediatr Adolesc Med 2005;159:139–44.

Scholes D, LaCroix AZ, Ichikawa LE, Barlow WE, Ott SM. Injectable hormone contraception and bone density: results from a prospective study [published erratum appears in Epidemiology 2002;13:749]. Epidemiology 2002;13:581–7.

# 11

## In vitro fertilization and pregnancy outcome

A 38-year-old woman became pregnant by means of in vitro fertilization (IVF), developed preterm labor, and had a cesarean delivery secondary to breech presentation at 28 weeks of gestation. Her infant has spina bifida and suffered intraventricular hemorrhage. The outcome encountered that is associated with in vitro fertilization is

* (A) preterm delivery
  (B) cesarean delivery
  (C) spina bifida
  (D) breech presentation
  (E) intraventricular hemorrhage

Assisted reproductive technology (ART) is now responsible for 1 in 100 live births in the United States. Since the first IVF pregnancy more than 20 years ago, IVF has become a standard treatment in the United States for women with infertility. Although multiple gestation has long been associated with ART, other potentially adverse effects on the resultant offspring are less well understood. There is an increasing awareness, based on recently published data, that IVF may lead to adverse pregnancy outcomes not explained by baseline maternal risk factors.

Preterm birth occurs in 11% of pregnancies in the United States. Complications related to prematurity account for most of the perinatal morbidity and mortality in otherwise normal neonates. The risk for both preterm birth and infertility increase with maternal age, thus the population undergoing IVF has an increased risk of prematurity that is not necessarily related to the mode of conception. A recent study compared the outcome of 62,551 IVF-conceived pregnancies from 1996 to 2000 with the outcomes for all pregnancies in the United States during the same time period. The risk for low birth weight and premature delivery remained elevated after controlling for maternal age, parity, and ethnicity. The standardized risk ratio for preterm delivery was 1.4 (95% confidence interval 1.3–1.5). The mechanisms for these effects are unknown. Awareness of these risks may aid in early identification and treatment to mitigate the effects of preterm delivery.

The relative risk or risk ratio is the ratio of incidence of disease in exposed individuals compared to the incidence

in unexposed individuals. This ratio is determined by either a cohort study or clinical trial where groups of individuals are identified that are either exposed or unexposed to a given risk factor. Risk ratios less than 1.0 indicate that the exposure reduced the chance that the outcome would occur, whereas risk ratios greater than 1.0 indicate that the exposure increased the chance of the outcome.

The risk for cesarean delivery is not independently increased by IVF. Other factors may increase the risk for cesarean delivery:

- Previous cesarean delivery
- Malpresentation
- Abnormalities of placentation
- Medical complications of pregnancy
- Oligohydramnios

Some of these conditions are more common in older women regardless of whether they undergo IVF.

Studies have suggested increased risks for certain birth defects with IVF, including genitourinary, neural tube, gastrointestinal, musculoskeletal, cardiovascular, and chromosomal abnormalities. The association of birth defects with IVF is neither consistent nor conclusive and further study is needed.

Malpresentation, although associated with prematurity, has not been specifically linked to pregnancies conceived by IVF. The risk for malpresentation is increased with conditions such as abnormal placentation, oligohydramnios or polyhydramnios, uterine malformations, and fetal hydrocephalus. Intraventricular hemorrhage is associated with prematurity and intrauterine growth restriction, but not directly with IVF.

Hansen M, Kurinczuk JJ, Bower C, Webb S. The risk of major birth defects after intracytoplasmic sperm injection and in vitro fertilization. N Engl J Med 2002;346:725–30.

Schieve LA, Ferre C, Peterson HB, Macaluso M, Reynolds MA, Wright VC. Perinatal outcome among singleton infants conceived through assisted reproductive technology in the United States. Obstet Gynecol 2004;103:1144–53.

Schieve LA, Meikle SF, Ferre C, Peterson HB, Jeng G, Wilcox LS. Low and very low birth weight in infants conceived with use of assisted reproductive technology. N Engl J Med 2002;346:731–7.

Schieve LA, Rasmussen SA, Buck GM, Schendel DE, Reynolds MA, Wright VC. Are children born after assisted reproductive technology at increased risk for adverse health outcomes? Obstet Gynecol 2004; 103:1154–63.

# 12

## Asthma

A 28-year-old primigravid woman with no major health problems comes to your office for a prenatal visit at 10 weeks of gestation. She has a history of asthma since childhood that is treated with an albuterol metered-dose inhaler on most days. She has had six visits to the emergency room over the last few years and one hospitalization for 2 days at which time she was treated with inhalers and an oral corticosteroid taper. She is comfortable managing her asthma and knows it is triggered by environmental agents and cold weather. On examination, the patient has good breath sounds with scattered wheezes. The best treatment for this patient is to continue the albuterol metered-dose inhaler and to add

      (A) acetylcysteine nebulized solution
      (B) pulse doses of systemic corticosteroids
\*   (C) an inhaled corticosteroid
      (D) sustained-release theophylline
      (E) a leukotriene modifier

Up to 7% of pregnant women are affected by asthma, one of the most common medical conditions that can complicate pregnancy. Maintaining control of asthma during pregnancy is important for the health and well-being of mother and fetus. Maternal asthma increases the risk of perinatal mortality, preeclampsia, preterm birth, and low birth weight. The National Asthma Education Program Working Group on Asthma and Pregnancy has concluded that medications used to control asthma during pregnancy are generally safer for both the mother and fetus compared with the risks of uncontrolled asthma. All asthma control medications fall within the U.S. Food and Drug Administration pregnancy categories B and C.

Asthma severity is classified according to features present before treatment or adequate control. Depending on the severity, a stepwise treatment approach is advocated with clear guidelines to assist clinical decision making (Appendix C). The patient described has almost daily symptoms despite frequent use of an albuterol metered dose inhaler. Additional objective measurements, such as forced expiratory volume in 1 second ($FEV_1$) and peak expiratory flow rate (PEFR), are excellent aids to determine the extent of airway obstruction or the response to prescribed treatment.

This patient would fall into a category of moderate persistent asthma and would benefit from inhaled corticosteroids and possibly the addition of long-acting inhaled $\beta_2$-agonist therapy. Inhaled corticosteroids are the most effective class of asthma control medications and are the preferred long-term treatment for persistent asthma. Studies show that inhaled corticosteroids used throughout pregnancy significantly reduce the risk of an acute asthma exacerbation and improve lung function. Considering safety in pregnancy, no studies to date have related inhaled corticosteroid use to any increases in congenital malformations or other adverse perinatal outcomes. Most of the inhaled corticosteroid data on safety come from budesonide, which has recently been changed to a pregnancy category B rating. All other inhaled corticosteroids carry a pregnancy category C rating based on the lack of adequate and well-controlled human pregnancy studies. Inhaled corticosteroids other than budesonide may be continued in patients whose asthma was well controlled with these agents before they became pregnant.

Albuterol is the preferred drug for short-acting bronchodilators because it has an excellent safety profile and it has been studied most extensively for safety in pregnancy. When short-acting $\beta_2$-agonists are used more than twice a week, initiating or increasing long-term therapy should be considered. Good evidence exists that better control is provided by a longer acting inhaled $\beta_2$-agonist added to an inhaled corticosteroid. Although limited safety data are available on the two long-acting inhaled $\beta_2$-agonists, salmeterol and formoterol, there is justification for expecting that the long-acting $\beta_2$-agonists have a similar profile to that of albuterol.

Oral corticosteroids may be necessary to treat pregnant patients with severe asthma or with moderate to severe exacerbations (Appendix D). Some data show an association between the general use of oral corticosteroids in the first trimester and an increased risk of cleft lip or palate. Not many asthmatic pregnant women have been included in these studies, and oral corticosteroids are not linked to these malformations if used in the second or third trimester. When a pregnant woman needs oral corticosteroids, efforts should be made to reduce systemic doses and maintain control with higher doses of inhaled corticosteroids.

Theophylline, leukotriene receptor antagonists, and cromolyn sodium can be used in pregnancy, but in general these are listed as alternatives to inhaled corticosteroids and are not preferred therapies. Theophylline is now infrequently used in pregnancy due to availability of other agents. Leukotriene modifiers are antiinflammatory agents that protect against bronchoconstriction, reduce asthma symptoms and exacerbations, and improve pulmonary function in mild to moderate asthma. There are some reassuring animal data on their safety, but minimal data on safety with human pregnancy. The leukotriene modifiers, montelukast and zafirlukast, show no teratogenicity in animals and are listed as pregnancy category B, whereas zileuton is listed as pregnancy category C due to an increase in cleft palate in laboratory rabbits.

Boushey HA, Sorkness CA, King TS, Sullivan SD, Fahy JV, Lazarus SC, et al. Daily versus as-needed corticosteroids for mild persistent asthma. National Heart, Lung, and Blood Institute's Asthma Clinical Research Network. N Engl J Med 2005;352:1519–28.

Gluck JC, Gluck PA. Asthma controller therapy during pregnancy. Am J Obstet Gynecol 2005;192:369–80.

NAEPP expert panel report. Managing asthma during pregnancy: recommendations for pharmacologic treatment—2004 update. National Heart, Lung, and Blood Institute; National Asthma Education and Prevention Program Asthma and Pregnancy Working Group. J Allergy Clin Immunol 2005;115:34–46.

# 13

## Care of patient with history of early pregnancy loss

A 32-year-old woman, gravida 3, para 1, is seen at 7 weeks of gestation by last menstrual period for antenatal care. Her history is significant for a first-trimester loss followed by a 22-week spontaneous loss. She denies any history of sexually transmitted diseases or gynecologic procedures. In-office ultrasonography reveals a crown–rump length consistent with the estimated gestational age. Her cervix is closed and 4 cm long. In addition to her routine new obstetric intake protocol, you would recommend that based on her history she should have

     (A) serial cervical ultrasonography weekly through the end of the second trimester

\*   (B) ultrasonographic measurement of cervical length at 16–20 weeks

     (C) no further evaluation

     (D) bedrest from 12 weeks through the end of the second trimester

     (E) cerclage placement at 16 weeks

Cervical insufficiency is defined as the inability of the uterine cervix to retain a pregnancy to term in the absence of preterm labor. Typically, cervical insufficiency presents as painless cervical dilation with ultimate expulsion of the pregnancy in the early second trimester. Recent studies using ultrasonographic measurement have demonstrated the function of the cervix by its closed length to be a continuum with varying degrees of competency. Cervical length is a marker for function or competence. Cervical insufficiency can result from trauma to the cervix during excision or overdilation of the cervix during termination, which can lead to removal or destruction of some length of cervical collagen and elastin that support it. Alternatively, congenital deficiencies in collagen or müllerian anomalies have been proposed as possible etiologies.

Cervical shortening and any associated funneling, ie, wedge-shaped separation of the cervix at the internal os (Fig. 13-1; see color plate), demonstrable by ultrasonography has been studied as a predictive factor for cervical insufficiency. However, standard objective ranges of length outside those at which a patient is believed at risk have been difficult to define. In normal pregnancies, cervical length measurements have shown a wide range of normal up to 20 weeks. In early gestation, because it is difficult to distinguish between the cervix and the lower uterine segment, measurements are not always accurate.

Researchers have made a major effort to find a more objective and thus reliable measure of cervical competency. Women with normal pregnancies have been shown to have an average cervical length of 4 cm (4.16 plus or minus 1.02 cm standard deviation [SD]) between 14 and 28 weeks of gestation. This average length steadily decreased between 28 and 40 weeks (3.23 plus or minus 1.16 cm SD). There is some evidence, however, that decreased cervical length between 24 and 28 weeks of gestation is correlated with preterm delivery. One study showed that 12.3% of women with a high risk for preterm delivery by history had cervical shortening with or without funneling at or before 24 weeks of gestation. A prospective but nonrandomized study found that 37% of women with a cervical length less than 2.5 cm with or without funneling of 25% before 24 weeks of gestation had preterm deliveries (relative risk = 4.8; 95% confidence interval, 2.3–10.1). The presence of funneling in addition to a shortened cervical length (2.5 cm or less) has been shown to be a significant risk factor for earlier preterm delivery and neonatal morbidity. These data suggest that serial ultrasonography is useful in patients with a history of births in the second or early third trimester. However, because the lower uterine segment is difficult to assess before 16–20 weeks of gestation, serial ultrasonographic screening examinations should not begin prior to that time.

The patient described has a history consistent with a second-trimester loss. Thus, given that she is at high risk of recurrent loss, and even though her current cervical length is normal, a repeat ultrasonographic examination of the cervical length at 16–20 weeks of gestation is warranted. No evidence exists to support starting serial examinations in the first trimester. Placing a patient on bedrest without objective data that this pregnancy is abnormal is not supported by the literature. Although this patient is at increased risk for preterm delivery because of her history of a prior loss, no data support a cerclage at 16 weeks of gestation without confirmation of the presence of cervical insufficiency because of shortened cervical length between 16–20 weeks. There is some evidence that cerclage may reduce preterm delivery in women with a short cervical length and a history of preterm delivery, but this issue needs further study to resolve some conflicting data.

Berghella V, Daly SF, Tolosa JE, DiVito MM, Chalmers R, Garg N, et al. Prediction of preterm delivery with transvaginal ultrasonography of the cervix in patients with high-risk pregnancies: does cerclage prevent prematurity? Am J Obstet Gynecol 1999;181:809–15.

Berghella V, Odibo AO, To MS, Rust OA, Althuisius SM. Cerclage for short cervix on ultrasonography: meta-analysis of trials using individual patient-level data. Obstet Gynecol 2005;106:181–9.

Botsis D, Papagianni V, Vitoratos N, Makrakis E, Aravantinos L, Creatsas G. Prediction of preterm delivery by sonographic estimation of cervical length. Biol Neonate 2005;88:42–5.

Cervical insufficiency. ACOG Practice Bulletin No. 48. American College of Obstetrics and Gynecologists. Obstet Gynecol 2003;102: 1091–9.

Macdonald R, Smith P, Vyas S. Cervical incompetence: the use of transvaginal sonography to provide an objective diagnosis. Ultrasound Obstet Gynecol 2001;18:211–6.

Rust OA, Atlas RO, Kimmel S, Roberts WE, Hess LW. Does the presence of a funnel increase the risk of adverse perinatal outcome in a patient with a short cervix? Am J Obstet Gynecol 2005;192:1060–6.

# 14

## Ultrasonographic findings of cornual pregnancies

A 34-year-old woman at 12 weeks of gestation presents with acute onset of right-sided pelvic pain and vomiting. On examination, the cervix is closed and a small of amount of vaginal bleeding is noted. The uterus is tender with marked right adnexal tenderness. Pelvic ultrasonography is performed (Fig. 14-1). The most likely diagnosis is

*   (A) cornual pregnancy
    (B) ruptured corpus luteum cyst
    (C) intrauterine pregnancy
    (D) tubal pregnancy

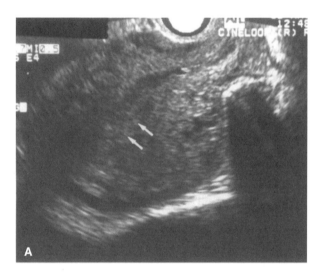

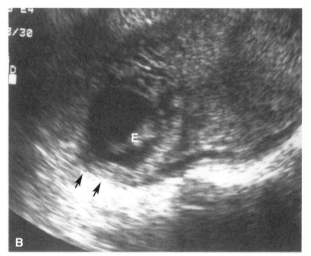

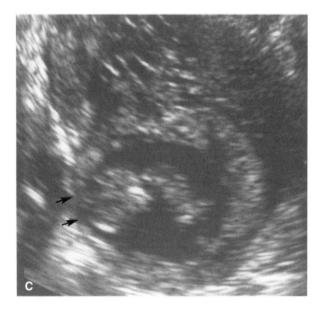

**FIG. 14-1**. Pelvic ultrasonograms.

Interstitial or cornual pregnancies account for 2–4% of all ectopic pregnancies. In general, cornual pregnancies present later and are difficult to diagnose. Access to the myometrial blood supply can lead to massive hemorrhage when cornual pregnancies rupture, which accounts for greater morbidity and mortality risk. Because cornual pregnancies are relatively rare, the clinician's index of suspicion for the diagnosis is low. Consequently, cornual pregnancies tend to be misdiagnosed as intrauterine pregnancies, leading to an increase in the chance of rupture.

The ultrasonographic criteria for diagnosis of cornual pregnancies have been variably described and are not universally present. Such criteria include an empty uterine cavity, a gestational sac seen separately and more than 1 cm from the most lateral edge of the uterine cavity, and a thinner-than-normal layer of myometrium surrounding the sac. Additionally, the endometrial echo may be seen. The interstitial line sign has been described as useful in the diagnosis of cornual pregnancies. An echogenic line is seen extending right up to the gestational sac, which may represent the intramural portion of the fallopian tube or the endometrial canal. Magnetic resonance imaging (MRI) may be useful in cases where ultrasonographic findings are equivocal or nondiagnostic.

The corpus luteum forms within the ovarian cortex at the site of ovulation and produces progesterone to sustain implantation until later in the first trimester. The corpus luteum may rupture through the surface of the ovary, which can lead to intraperitoneal hemorrhage. The presence of free fluid and a cystic structure in the ovary on transvaginal ultrasonography should raise the possibility of a bleeding corpus luteum. Use of Doppler imaging can help to distinguish a corpus luteum from an ectopic gestation. With Doppler, the corpus luteum often has a ringlike vascular pattern in the periphery of the mass. In most cases, the bleeding from a corpus luteum is self-limited, and intervention by means of laparoscopy rarely is required.

The diagnosis of an intrauterine pregnancy by ultrasonography requires visualization of a gestational sac. If the serum human chorionic gonadotropin (hCG) titer is greater than 2,000 mIU/mL, most normal intrauterine pregnancies will be visualized by transvaginal ultrasonography. This discriminatory threshold for hCG has been variably reported to be in the region of 1,000–2,000 mIU/mL depending on the resolution of the ultrasonographic equipment and the skill of the technician. The double decidual sign, created by the layers of the chorion, confirms the presence of an intrauterine pregnancy, excluding the "pseudo sac" sign seen occasionally with ectopic gestations. Further confirmation of an intrauterine pregnancy is provided by visualization of a yolk sac or embryonic pole within the gestational sac. By the time the gestational sac reaches 10 mm, a yolk sac should be seen in all normal intrauterine pregnancies. If the embryonic pole is 5 mm or greater, cardiac activity should be seen if the pregnancy is viable.

Ectopic pregnancies usually are diagnosed by excluding the presence of an intrauterine pregnancy. Only 20% of ectopic pregnancies are seen by ultrasonography. Definitive evidence for a tubal gestation includes visualization of cardiac activity outside the uterus within the adnexa. Other than imaging an extrauterine gestational sac, the presence of a moderate to large amount of fluid in the posterior cul-de-sac is also highly suggestive of ectopic pregnancy.

Ackerman TE, Levi CS, Dashefsky SM, Holt SC, Lindsay DJ. Interstitial line: sonographic finding in interstitial (cornual) ectopic pregnancy. Radiology 1993;189:83–7.

Takeuchi K, Yamada T, Oomori S, Ideta K, Moriyama T, Maruo T. Comparison of magnetic resonance imaging and ultrasonography in the early diagnosis of interstitial pregnancy. J Reprod Med 1999;44:265–8.

Timor-Tritsch IE, Monteagudo A, Matera C, Veit CR. Sonographic evolution of cornual pregnancies treated without surgery. Obstet Gynecol 1992;79:1044–9.

# 15
## Arthritis

A 58-year-old postmenopausal woman comes to the office for an annual examination. She reports deep aches in her joints, particularly in her knees, her hands, and her left hip. She is stiff in the morning for approximately 15 minutes, then improves, but notes that the pain often worsens with more activity. She has noticed occasional swelling in the left knee that gets better when she takes ibuprofen. Her family history is significant for her mother who has arthritis. She weighs 80.7 kg (178 lb), is 1.7 m (5 ft 7 in.) tall, and is afebrile. The physical examination is significant for nodules in her distal interphalangeal joints and normal range of motion in her knees with mild tenderness and crepitus in her left knee. The most likely diagnosis is

      (A) rheumatoid arthritis
      (B) gout
      (C) systemic lupus erythematosus
\*   (D) osteoarthritis
      (E) psoriatic arthritis

Osteoarthritis is the most common joint disorder and a leading cause of disability that affects women more than men. The incidence of joint findings increases from less than 2% in women younger than 45 years to 68% in women older than 65 years. Patients with osteoarthritis seek pain relief and improved physical function. Pain is the predominant symptom; it commonly begins in one joint with others subsequently becoming painful. Typically, pain is described as a deep ache accompanied by joint stiffness lasting less than 30 minutes following periods of inactivity. Pain is aggravated by using the involved joints and is commonly relieved by rest. Osteoarthritis affects large weight-bearing joints (hips, knees, lumbar and lower cervical spine), joints in the hands (the distal interphalangeal, proximal interphalangeal, and the first carpometacarpal joint), and the first metatarsophalangeal joint in the feet. The shoulders, elbows, wrists, and ankles are seldom affected in primary osteoarthritis, an important distinguishing feature from the inflammatory arthropathies including rheumatoid arthritis (Fig. 15-1; see color plate).

On physical examination, the joints may demonstrate tenderness, crepitus, and a limited range of motion. Joint swelling may be due to an effusion or to bony enlargement and the presence of osteophytes. Slowly progressive bony enlargements of the distal interphalangeal joints are called *Heberden's nodes* and enlargements of the proximal interphalangeal joints are called *Bouchard's nodes* (Fig. 15-2; see color plate). Systemic manifestations, such as fever, weight loss, anemia, and an elevated erythrocyte sedimentation rate, are not present even with severe disease. Although correlation between the clinical symptoms and radiographic findings is poor, pathognomonic findings on plain film X-ray of involved joints include the presence of osteophytes at the margins of the joints, associated joint space narrowing, and evidence of bony reaction with more severe disease.

The American College of Rheumatology has formulated guidelines for progressive stepwise treatment of patients with knee and hip osteoarthritis. Nonpharmacologic therapies include patient education, weight loss if needed, and exercise programs (eg, strengthening and range of motion). Physical therapy and exercise programs, although frequently overlooked, provide important benefits and should be used as baseline therapy for all patients to improve muscle strength and range of motion. Walking aids (eg, a cane or shoe wedges) may improve biomechanics. Additional treatments for symptomatic relief include heat and cold therapies, periods of rest, and acupuncture.

Pharmacologic therapy should be considered as additions to nonpharmacologic therapy. For patients with mild to moderate osteoarthritis, symptomatic relief usually can be achieved with acetaminophen, which is comparable to nonsteroidal antiinflammatory drugs (NSAIDs) with a lower cost and lower toxicity profile. The daily dose of acetaminophen should not exceed 4 g. In patients who have inadequate pain relief or signs of joint inflammation, a trial of NSAIDs is merited. Appendix E shows classes of NSAIDs. Other treatment options include intraarticular therapy with glucocorticoids or hyaluronic acid, topical analgesics (eg, capsaicin or methyl salicylate cream), tramadol hydrochloride (Ultram), or opioids. Glucosamine and chondroitin sulfate have been shown to be effective in a number of studies, but without further evidence it is premature to make specific recommendations about their use. Patients with severe symptomatic osteoarthritis who have failed to respond to medical therapy are candidates for orthopedic surgery.

Rheumatoid arthritis is a systemic disease with such features as fatigue, low-grade fevers, anemia, and elevations of acute phase reactants (eg, erythrocyte sedimentation rate and C-reactive protein). The joints involved at presentation are variable, but symptoms typically start in small joints of the hands (proximal interphalangeal and metacarpophalangeal) and toes (metatarsophalangeal). Rheumatoid arthritis spares distal interphalangeal and small joints of the toes. Later, rheumatoid arthritis moves to larger joints such as the wrists, knees, elbows, ankles, hips, and shoulders. Morning stiffness lasting more than 1 hour is a hallmark of inflammatory arthritis and a prominent feature in rheumatoid arthritis. In addition, the diagnosis requires the presence of inflammation (swelling or warmth) on examination of the joints.

Gout, which results from tissue deposition of monosodium urate crystals, classically presents as recurrent attacks of acute arthritis and inflammation in one or a few joints. It is twice as common in men as in women. The presentation can be associated with systemic leukocytosis, and the synovial fluid demonstrates urate crystals and leukocytosis. Acute treatment consists primarily of NSAIDs or colchicine.

Musculoskeletal manifestations of arthralgias and arthritis are present in 95% of patients with systemic lupus erythematosus. Symptoms tend to be asymmetric and migratory with complaints of pain in a particular joint lasting 1–3 days. The fingers, hands, wrists, and knees are more commonly affected than ankles, elbows, shoulders, and hips. The diagnosis is made when 4 of 11 criteria are present (Table 15-1).

**TABLE 15-1.** Criteria for Classification of Systemic Lupus Erythematosus

| Criterion | Definition |
| --- | --- |
| 1. Malar rash | Fixed erythema, flat or raised, over the malar eminences, tending to spare the nasolabial folds |
| 2. Discoid rash | Erythematous raised patches with adherent keratotic scaling and follicular plugging; atrophic scarring may occur in older lesions |
| 3. Photosensitivity | Skin rash as a result of unusual reaction to sunlight, determined by patient history or physician observation |
| 4. Oral ulcers | Oral or nasopharyngeal ulceration, usually painless, observed by a physician |
| 5. Arthritis | Nonerosive arthritis involving two or more peripheral joints and characterized by tenderness, swelling, or effusion |
| 6. Serositis | a. Pleuritis—convincing history of pleuritic pain or rub heard by a physician or evidence of pleural effusion *or* |
| | b. Pericarditis—documented by electrocardiogram or rub or by evidence of pericardial effusion |
| 7. Renal disorder | a. Persistent proteinuria more than 0.5 g/day or more than 3+ if quantitation is not performed *or* |
| | b. Cellular casts—may be red blood cell, hemoglobin, granular, tabular, or mixed |
| 8. Neurologic disorder | Seizures—in the absence of offending drugs or known metabolic derangements, eg, uremia, ketoacidosis, or electrolyte imbalance |
| 9. Hematologic disorder | a. Hemolytic anemia with reticulocytosis *or* |
| | b. Leukopenia less than 4,000/mm on two or more occasions |
| | c. Lymphopenia less than 1,500/mm on two or more occasions |
| | d. Thrombocytopenia less than 100,000/mm in the absence of offending drugs |
| 10. Immunologic disorder | a. Anti-DNA: antibody to native DNA in abnormal titer *or* |
| | b. Anti-Sm: presence of antibody to Sm nuclear antigen *or* |
| | c. Positive findings of antiphospholipid antibodies based on 1) an abnormal serum level of immunoglobulin (Ig) G or Ig M anticardiolipin antibodies, 2) a positive test result for lupus anticoagulant with the use of a standard method, or 3) a false-positive result on serologic test for syphilis known to be positive for at least 6 months and confirmed by *Treponema pallidum* immobilization or fluorescent treponemal antibody absorption test |
| 11. Antinuclear antibody | An abnormal titer of antinuclear antibody by immunofluorescence or an equivalent assay at any point and in the absence of drugs known to be associated with "drug-induced lupus" syndrome |

The classification is based on 11 criteria. For the purpose of identifying patients in clinical studies, a person shall be said to have systemic lupus erythematosus if any 4 or more of the 11 criteria are present, serially or simultaneously, during any interval of observation. Reprinted from Schur PH. Systemic lupus erythematosus. In: Goldman L, Ausiello D, editors. Cecil textbook of medicine. 22nd ed. Philadelphia (PA): WB Saunders; 2004. p. 1661. Copyright © 2004, with permission from Elsevier.

Psoriatic arthritis develops in 5–7% of patients with psoriasis. The presentation is variable, but typically is an asymmetric arthritis involving both small and large joints. The diagnosis frequently depends on finding articular changes in association with psoriatic changes in the skin or nails.

Mies Richie A, Francis ML. Diagnostic approach to polyarticular joint pain. Am Fam Physician 2003;68:1151–60.

O'Dell JR. Rheumatoid arthritis. In: Goldman L, Ausiello D, editors. Cecil textbook of medicine. 22nd ed. Philadelphia (PA): WB Saunders; 2004. p. 1644–54.

Recommendations for the medical management of osteoarthritis of the hip and knee: 2000 update. American College of Rheumatology Subcommittee on Osteoarthritis Guidelines. Arthritis Rheum 2000;43: 1905–15.

Schnitzer TJ, Lane NE. Osteoarthritis. In: Goldman L, Ausiello D, editors. Cecil textbook of medicine. 22nd ed. Philadelphia (PA): WB Saunders; 2004. p. 1698–702.

Schur PH. Systemic lupus erythematosus. In: Goldman L, Ausiello D, editors. Cecil textbook of medicine. 22nd ed. Philadelphia (PA): WB Saunders; 2004. p. 1660–70.

# 16

## Full disclosure

While you are performing a hysterectomy on a 49-year-old woman for leiomyoma, a bowel injury occurs and the resultant repair requires a temporary diverting colostomy. You desire to tell the patient that you are "sorry" that the injury occurred, but are advised by the risk management office not to do so. The most likely result of telling the patient that you are "sorry" for this complication is to

      (A) increase her anger
      (B) motivate her to initiate a medical professional liability suit
*    (C) improve the patient–physician relationship
      (D) void your medical professional liability insurance coverage

Among other contributing factors in the current medical professional liability crisis are patient safety issues, preventable medical errors, an inefficient tort system, and unqualified practitioners. The health care industry must focus on the elimination of avoidable medical injuries, improvement of patient safety, development of alternative methods of dispute resolution, and identification of practitioners who will benefit from further training. During surgical procedures, complications will occur and the patient must be made aware of everything that has happened to her. All medical errors must be identified early and fully acknowledged to the patient and her family.

Evidence exists to support the importance and positive impact of early full disclosure to the patient of any adverse outcome. Most patients are angry about the "wall of silence" that exists surrounding any adverse outcome. Full disclosure is difficult for many physicians and institutions to accept, but its benefits include removing the wall of silence and improving the patient–physician relationship. Telling the patient that you are "sorry" for the adverse outcome or apologizing for something that did

not go as planned has been demonstrated to decrease both patient anger and the risk of a professional liability suit. Disclosure to the patient of any adverse outcome should be done by someone trained in proper communication skills. The risk management office at the physician's institution should be involved in the process.

An excellent example of full disclosure and its benefits is the 3Rs ("Recognize, Respond, Resolve") program of the Colorado Physicians Insurance Company (COPIC). During the initial 18 months of the pilot program, 592 adverse patient outcomes were reported by physicians. In 360 cases, discussion by a trained team resolved the issue and in 232 cases, some financial compensation (maximum $30,000) was offered at a level less than the cost of a legal defense. No lawsuits were filed, even though patients were not asked to waive their rights to initiate a suit. Physicians in the 3Rs program must agree to report adverse events promptly, fully disclose all patient injuries, participate in education programs on effective physician–patient communication, and make changes to prevent future medical errors. By this process, physicians accrue points used to obtain preferred premium rate status. Resolution of the event with financial compensation is not reported to the state or to the National Practitioner Data Bank. The program has been so successful that COPIC now requires participation by all their policyholders.

It is important that the medical professional liability insurance carrier be notified of any adverse outcome so that early investigation can be initiated. The physician should determine whether his or her carrier has guidelines regarding disclosure or unexpected outcomes or events. Currently, there is no evidence that telling the patient that you are "sorry" for the adverse outcome will affect your liability insurance coverage.

Gibson R, Prasad Singh J. Wall of silence. Washington, DC: Regency Publishing Co; 2003.

Levenson W. Physician–patient communication: a key to malpractice prevention. JAMA 1994;272:1619–20.

Schmidek JM, Weeks WB. Relationship between tort claims and patient incident reports in the Veterans Health Administration. Qual Saf Health Care 2005;14:117–22.

Weinstein L. A multifaceted approach to improve patient safety, prevent medical errors and resolve the professional liability crisis. Am J Obstet Gynecol 2006;194:1160–5; discussion 1165–7.

Zimmerman R. Doctors' new tool to fight lawsuits: saying "I'm sorry." Malpractice insurers find owning up to errors soothes patient anger. "The risks are extraordinary." J Oklahoma State Med Assoc 2004; 97(6):245–7.

# 17

## Ultrasonography for complex adnexal masses

A 40-year-old woman with a history of endometriosis and pelvic pain is found to have a complex adnexal mass on transvaginal ultrasonography. You inform her that the ultrasonographic characteristic most predictive of malignancy is

       (A) free fluid in the cul-de-sac
\*   (B) papillary areas inside a cyst
       (C) septations
       (D) size greater than 6 cm
       (E) wall thickness of 2 mm

Ovarian cysts are a common finding in women in all age groups, particularly in those of reproductive age. It is not uncommon for postmenopausal women to have benign cysts, although the risk of cancer rises with age. The increase in use of transvaginal ultrasonography has led to an increase in the diagnosis of cysts. It is important to differentiate between benign and malignant conditions in order to avoid unnecessary surgery without missing any cancers. Criteria developed in the 1980s noted the low chance of malignancy in patients with unilocular simple cysts less than 6 cm in diameter that were unaccompanied by ascites or matted bowel. Ultrasonographic findings of solid or papillary areas in simple cysts have been associated with 3–6 times higher rates of malignancy. Solid or complex characteristics of masses, especially if bilateral, increase the risk of cancer. Cysts greater than 6 cm also have an increased chance of cancer.

Scoring systems to predict malignancy have been hampered by complex benign masses that give the ultrasonographic appearance of malignancy (Table 17-1). Characteristics that have been examined include irregularities in wall structure, including papillary areas greater than 3 mm, thick septae greater than 3 mm, and mixed or high echogenicity rather than sonolucent areas. In general, the negative predictive value of ultrasonography for malignancy is 90% or greater, whereas the positive predictive value ranges from 30% to 73%. Ultrasonography appears to be more specific but less sensitive than magnetic resonance imaging or computed tomography using the criteria of septae 2 mm thick, walls 3 mm, wall nodularity, solid components, and complex mass greater than 5 cm. Doppler indices are unproven at this time as a predictor of malignancy, because results overlap between benign and malignant cysts. An algorithm that could be used for management is included in Figure 17-1.

**TABLE 17-1.** Ultrasonographic Morphology Index for Ovarian Tumors

| | Category by Volume (cm³)* | | | | | |
|---|---|---|---|---|---|---|
| | **0** | **1** | **2** | **3** | **4** | **5** |
| | Less than 10 | 10–50 | More than 50–100 | More than 100–200 | More than 200–500 | More than 500 |
| Structure | Smooth wall, sonolucent | Smooth wall, diffuse echogenicity | Wall thickening, less than 3 mm fine septa | Papillary projection 3 mm or more | Complex, predominantly solid | Complex, solid and cystic areas with extratumoral fluid |

*Calculated using prolate ellipsoid formula (L × H × W × 0.523)
Van Nagell JR, DePriest PD. Management of adnexal masses in postmenopausal women. Am J Obstet Gynecol 2005;193:31.

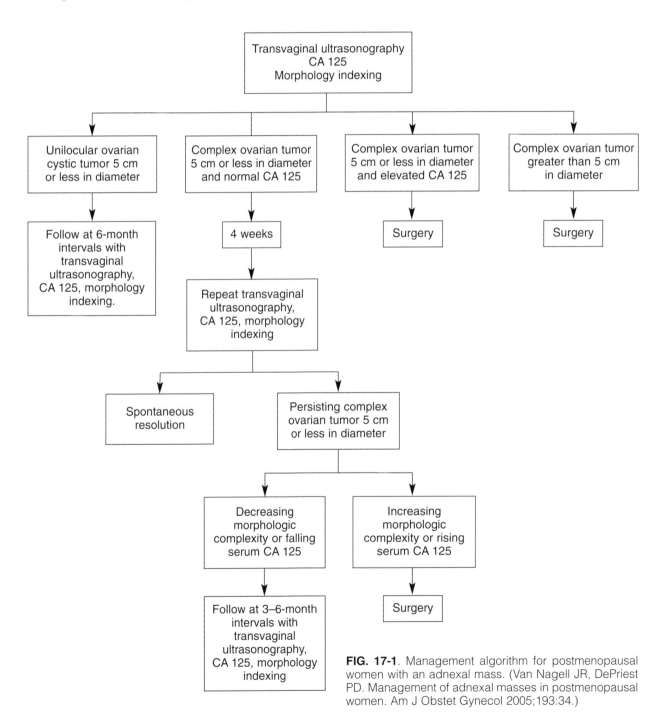

**FIG. 17-1.** Management algorithm for postmenopausal women with an adnexal mass. (Van Nagell JR, DePriest PD. Management of adnexal masses in postmenopausal women. Am J Obstet Gynecol 2005;193:34.)

Ekerhovd D, Wienerroith H, Staudach A, Granberg S. Preoperative assessment of unilocular adnexal cysts by transvaginal ultrasonography: a comparison between ultrasonographic morphologic imaging and histopathologic diagnosis. Am J Obstet Gynecol 2001;184:48–54.

Herrmann UJ, Gottfried LW, Goldhirsch A. Sonographic patterns of ovarian tumors: prediction of malignancy. Obstet Gynecol 1987;69:777–81.

Kurtz AB, Tsimikas JV, Tempany CM, Hamper UM, Arger PH, Bree RL, et al. Diagnosis and staging of ovarian cancer: comparative values of Doppler and conventional ultrasound, CT and MR imaging correlated with surgery and histopathologic analysis—report of the Radiology Diagnostic Oncology Group. Radiology 1999;212:19–27.

Lerner JP, Timor-Tritsch IE, Federman A, Abramovich G. Transvaginal ultrasonographic characterization of ovarian masses with an improved, weighted scoring system. Am J Obstet Gynecol 1994;170:81–5.

Sassone AM, Timor-Tritsch IE, Artner A, Westhoff C, Warren WB. Transvaginal sonographic characterization of ovarian disease: evaluation of a new scoring system to predict ovarian malignancy. Obstet Gynecol 1991;78:70–6.

Van Nagell JR, Ueland FR. Ultrasound evaluation of pelvic masses: predictors of malignancy for the general gynecologist. Curr Opin Obstet Gynecol 1999;11:45–49.

Van Nagell JR, DePriest PD. Management of adnexal masses in postmenopausal women. Am J Obstet Gynecol 2005;193:30–5.

# 18

## Vaginitis

A 35-year-old woman has had six documented yeast infections in the past 10 months. Wet mount again reveals hyphae with no evidence of trichomonas or clue cells. Prior vaginal culture documented yeast sensitivity to fluconazole. She is given fluconazole every 3 days for four doses, which resolves the current episode. As the best strategy to reduce her risk of future recurrences, you recommend

       (A) daily antifungal vaginal cream for 2 weeks
       (B) vaginal lactobacillus
\*    (C) weekly fluconazole for 6 months
       (D) hygiene and dietary changes
       (E) treating her sexual partner with fluconazole

Vulvovaginal candidiasis is common: 75% of women experience at least one episode and up to 45% have two or more infections in their lifetime. Less than 5% of women will have recurrent vulvovaginal candidiasis defined as four or more infections in 12 months. Most patients have no predisposing risk factors (eg, diabetes mellitus). Measures such as decreasing sugar in the diet, wearing cotton underwear, blow drying the genital area, and wiping away from the genital area have been recommended, but none have been proved to reduce rates of infections. Treating the sexual partner also has not been shown to be effective. Adding a daily antifungal cream to an effective oral regimen also has not been shown to be more effective than adequate oral therapy as in this case. Products containing lactobacillus species to prevent vaginal candidiasis have been studied. In one randomized, placebo-controlled trial of lactobacillus orally or vaginally, there was no difference in the rate of cultures positive for vaginal candidiasis in women who received one or both forms of the lactobacillus compared to placebo.

Maintenance oral therapy for several months has been shown to reduce recurrence of vaginitis. In a large prospective trial, 387 women with recurrent vulvovaginal candidiasis were initially treated with fluconazole 150 mg every 3 days for four doses, then randomized to placebo vs fluconazole 150 mg weekly for 6 months. There were significant reductions in the fluconazole group compared to the placebo group at 6 months (91% vs 36%), 9 months (73% vs 28%), and 12 months (43% vs 22%). Vaginal culture should confirm a negative result in order to determine efficacy of the treatment.

Pirotta M, Gunn J, Chondros P, Grover S, O'Malley P, Hurley S, et al. Effect of lactobacillus in preventing post-antibiotic vulvovaginal candidiasis: a randomised controlled trial. BMJ 2004;329:548–51.

Sobel JD, Wiesenfeld HC, Martens M, Danna P, Hooton TM, Rompalo A, et al. Maintenance fluconazole therapy for recurrent vulvovaginal candidiasis. N Engl J Med 2004;351:876–83.

# 19

## Patient demand for elective cesarean delivery

A 28-year-old woman, gravida 1, at 32 weeks of gestation requests an elective cesarean delivery. She has had a normal pregnancy to date, but continues to be concerned about a "tear" at term and incontinence in the future. During this visit and follow-up in 2 weeks, you review known maternal and fetal risks of vaginal delivery and elective cesarean delivery. You give support, provide education, and offer counseling. Despite your recommendation for a trial of labor, she persists in her request for an elective cesarean delivery. You are uncomfortable in complying due to your judgment and assessment. Your best approach is to

(A) recognize her autonomy and go along with her request
(B) consult your urogynecologist for further discussion
* (C) explain your position and assist her in finding another provider
(D) notify risk management of the issue

The question of offering or performing an elective cesarean delivery has received considerable attention. Increasingly, patients may ask about the possibility or make requests for an elective cesarean delivery. Many arguments can be made on both sides about maternal and fetal risks and benefits. In the current era of evidence-based medicine, physicians must understand the scientific arguments, but it is just as important that they understand how to ethically assess the benefits and burdens of elective primary cesarean delivery.

To address a request for an elective cesarean delivery, a substantial amount of time is needed. In trying to communicate the risks and benefits to herself and the fetus, the clinician must try to provide a qualitative and quantitative assessment from data that are incomplete. The clinician also must attempt to understand the reason for the woman's request. Her request may be motivated by anxiety and the many fears or uncertainties of childbirth (eg, fears of pain, pelvic floor damage, the unknown).

Professionally, doctors have an ethical and legal duty of care. This includes an assessment of the ethical principles of justice, beneficence, nonmaleficence, and autonomy. The principle of justice is a population-based ethical principle. Justice obligates the physician not to exploit a population of patients. It requires a fair process of allocating benefits and burdens. Given current data, a large number of elective cesarean deliveries would be required to prevent each instance of morbidity related to vaginal deliveries.

The physician is obligated to beneficence, the ethical principle that obligates physicians to take actions that benefit patients or to seek a greater balance of clinical good over clinical harm for patients. As embodied in the Hippocratic Oath, the principle of nonmaleficence states, "Above all, do no harm." This forbids physicians from providing ineffective interventions or acting without due

care. Although there are arguments for elective cesarean deliveries and individual exceptions can be made, current evidence does not support a judgment that elective cesarean delivery is necessarily beneficial to both the mother and infant.

The physician's ethical principle of respect for autonomy is often the basis for considering the request for an elective cesarean delivery. The pregnant patient has a right to bodily self-determination, and her ability to make an informed decision should be respected. Hence, informed consent is vital. Proper informed consent requires the disclosure of adequate information about the pregnancy and its management; an understanding of the information by the patient; and a voluntary decision to authorize or refuse the treatment. After these discussions, the patient may still request or demand a cesarean delivery. In this case, a physician may conclude that this request for a cesarean delivery should be implemented. However, such conclusion is not inevitable because it fails to make a distinction between negative and positive rights. Negative rights involve claims to noninterference in one's decisions and actions as they affect oneself. Positive rights involve claims on the resources of others to achieve one's goals and intentions. Negative rights have few limits because respecting them requires little sacrifice on the part of others. Positive rights have limits because they involve a sacrifice of resources of other individuals. Basing the decision on positive rights devalues expert clinical judgment.

Physicians must be prepared and willing to make recommendations based on the available evidence, their judgment, and their experience. Physicians using expert, professional clinical judgment that is beneficence-based are not obligated to perform an elective cesarean delivery if the procedure is felt to be contrary to good medical practice or against deeply held values. Therefore, in the face of pressure to perform a procedure not judged to be warranted, the obstetrician can then inform the patient that he or she is unable to honor the patient's request and help arrange transfer to another physician who might be willing to comply with the request.

An additional consultation with a urogynecologist or other colleague may be helpful to gain additional knowledge or insight, but still does not answer the question of whether to perform a procedure that a clinician feels is unwarranted. Notification of risk management personnel is important in certain situations, but it would be premature to notify them in this situation.

American College of Obstetricians and Gynecologists. Surgery and patient choice. In: Ethics in obstetrics and gynecology. 2nd ed. Washington, DC: ACOG; 2004. p. 21–5.

Bewley S, Cockburn J. I. The unethics of "request" caesarean section. BJOG 2002;109:593–6.

Hale RW, Harer WB Jr. Elective prophylactic cesarean delivery. ACOG Clin Rev 2005;10(2):1, 15.

Minkoff H, Chervenak FA. Elective primary cesarean delivery. N Engl J Med 2003;348:946–50.

Minkoff H, Powderly KR, Chervenak F, McCullough LB. Ethical dimensions of elective primary cesarean delivery. Obstet Gynecol 2004;103:387–92.

Nygaard I, Cruikshank DP. Should all women be offered elective cesarean delivery? Obstet Gynecol 2003;102:217–9.

# 20

## Oncogenes that increase the risk of colon cancer

A 35-year-old woman tells you that colorectal cancer has been newly diagnosed in her 55-year-old mother. She has no other family history of colorectal cancer. You inform her that the percentage of colorectal cancer attributable to family history in a first-degree relative is approximately

       (A) 1%
*    (B) 10%
       (C) 30%
       (D) 50%
       (E) 70%

Colorectal cancer is a common and lethal disease, but it generally can be prevented with proven effective screening techniques due to its long premalignant stage. In the United States, colon cancer is diagnosed annually in nearly 140,000 women and men and leads to the death of nearly 60,000 individuals, making it the second leading cause of cancer deaths. The risk factors for colorectal cancer are both environmental and genetic. The mode of presentation of colorectal cancer follows one of three patterns that are reflective of these different risk factors:

1. Sporadic
2. Inherited
3. Familial

Environmental and genetic factors can increase the likelihood of development of the disease. Although inherited susceptibility results in increases in risk, most colorectal cancers are sporadic rather than familial or inherited.

Approximately 10% of colorectal cancer cases are attributable to a family history in a first-degree relative. These cases are subdivided according to whether or not colonic polyps are a major disease manifestation.

Autosomal dominant diseases with polyposis include familial adenomatous polyposis and the hamartomatous polyposis syndromes (Peutz-Jeghers syndrome, juvenile polyposis). Autosomal dominant diseases without polyposis include hereditary nonpolyposis colorectal cancer (HNPCC), Lynch syndrome I, and the cancer family syndrome (Lynch syndrome II). These conditions are associated with a high risk of developing colorectal cancer, and many of the underlying genetic mutations have been identified. Familial adenomatous polyposis and its variants, Turcot's syndrome (familial adenomatous polyposis associated with brain tumors), Gardner's syndrome (familial adenomatous polyposis associated with extraintestinal manifestations), and attenuated familial adenomatous polyposis, are autosomal dominant diseases caused by mutations in the adenomatous polyposis coli gene.

Approximately 70% of all colorectal cancers occur as sporadic cases with no family history. Dietary and environmental factors have been etiologically implicated and age is a major risk factor. Before age 40 years, colorectal cancer is a rare diagnosis; incidence rates increase significantly between ages 40 and 50 years and in each succeeding decade thereafter. The lifetime incidence of colorectal cancer in patients at average risk is approximately 5%, with 90% of cases in patients older than 50 years.

A family history of either adenomatous polyps or colorectal cancer constitutes a risk factor for colon cancer. Siblings and parents of patients with adenomatous polyps are at increased risk for colorectal cancer, particularly when the adenoma is diagnosed before age 60 years or, in the case of siblings, when a parent has had colorectal cancer. Likewise, a single affected first-degree relative (parent, sibling, or child) with colorectal cancer increases the risk 1.7-fold compared with the general population. Risk is further increased if two first-degree relatives have colon cancer or if the index case is diagnosed in a relative younger than 55 years. The presence of a family history of a colonic adenoma appears to carry the same significance as a positive family history of colorectal cancer.

Colonoscopic surveillance should be considered in the latter two situations, beginning at age 40 years, or 10 years earlier than the youngest family member to have cancer. Figure 20-1 shows an algorithm for screening for colorectal cancer with recommendations in regard to family history of colorectal cancer.

Most colorectal carcinomas arise from adenomatous polyps over an average of 7 years. Furthermore, adenoma removal by colonoscopic polypectomy decreases colon cancer incidence and mortality. For a mean of 6 years, the National Polyp Study Work Group followed patients after a complete colonoscopic examination had led to the removal of one or more adenomas in the colon or rectum. Compared to several historic reference groups, including those in which adenomas were not removed, it was estimated that the incidence of colon cancer was reduced by 76–90%.

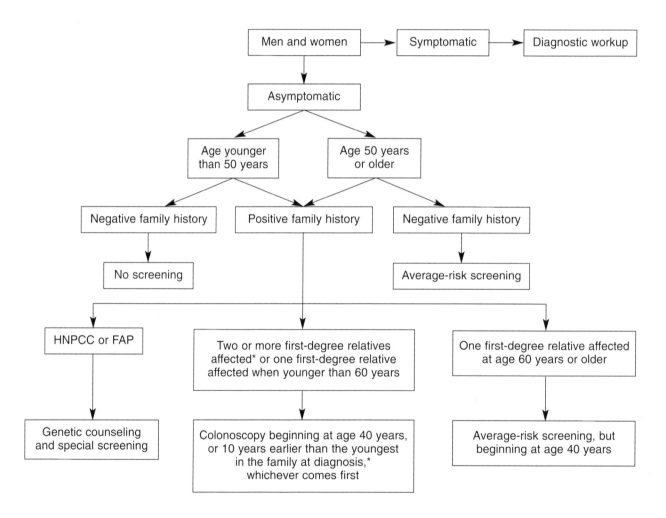

**FIG. 20-1.** Algorithm for screening for colorectal cancer with recommendations in regard to family history of colorectal cancer. FAP, familial adenomatous polyposis; HNPCC, hereditary nonpolyposis colorectal cancer. *Either colorectal cancer or adenomatous polyp. (Modified from Winawer S, Fletcher R, Rex D, Bond J, Burt R, Ferrucci J, et al. Colorectal cancer screening and surveillance: clinical guidelines and rationale—update based on new evidence. Gastroenterology 2003;124:546. Copyright © 2003 with permission from Elsevier.)

Burt RW, Bishop DT, Lynch HT, Rozen P, Winawer SJ. Risk and surveillance of individuals with heritable factors for colorectal cancer. WHO Collaborating Centre for the Prevention of Colorectal Cancer. Bull World Health Organ 1990;68:655–65.

Fuchs CS, Giovannucci EL, Colditz GA, Hunter DJ, Speizer FE, Willett WC. A prospective study of family history and the risk of colorectal cancer. N Engl J Med 1994;331:1669–74.

Lynch JP, Hoops TC. The genetic pathogenesis of colorectal cancer. Hematol Oncol Clin North Am 2002;16:775–810.

Schmeler KM, Lynch HT, Chen LM, Munsell MF, Soliman PT, Clark MB, et al. Prophylactic surgery to reduce the risk of gynecologic cancers in the Lynch syndrome. N Engl J Med 2006;354:261–9.

Winawer S, Fletcher R, Rex D, Bond J, Burt R, Ferrucci J, et al. Colorectal cancer screening and surveillance: clinical guidelines and rationale—update based on new evidence. Gastrointestinal Consortium Panel. Gastroenterology 2003;124:544–60.

Winawer SJ, Zauber AG, Ho MN, O'Brien MJ, Gottlieb LS, Sternberg SS, et al. Prevention of colorectal cancer by colonoscopic polypectomy. The National Polyp Study Workgroup. N Engl J Med 1993;329:1977–81.

# 21

## Risks of blood transfusion

A 33-year-old woman with a history of two cesarean deliveries is pregnant at 34 weeks of gestation with an anterior, low-lying placenta. She has been counseled about the risk of placenta accreta and the potential for her to receive blood transfusions. She asks about the risks of blood transfusions. You tell her that the most frequent serious complication associated with blood transfusion is

    (A) acute hemolytic transfusion reaction
\*   (B) transfusion-related lung injury
    (C) hepatitis C transmission
    (D) cytomegalovirus transmission
    (E) hepatitis B transmission

The risk of blood transfusion during pregnancy is generally low, but with this patient's history of two cesarean deliveries and anterior placentation, the possibility of accreta and postpartum hemorrhage exists. Awareness of the potential adverse consequences of transfusion of blood or its components constitutes an important part of the counseling of patients.

The most frequent severe morbidity encountered with blood transfusion is pulmonary distress. Since the mid-1980s, it has been recognized that transfusion-related lung injury is a distinct clinical entity. It is defined as acute respiratory distress syndrome, characterized by dyspnea, hypoxemia, and noncardiogenic pulmonary edema that occurs within 4 hours after transfusion. In Table 21-1, the estimated number of cases of transfusion-related lung injury, 125 in 1,000,000, is likely to be an underestimation because of underreporting.

Transfusion of plasma products appears most often associated with transfusion-related lung injury. This is compatible with the current hypothesized etiology of an immunologic reaction between donor antibodies targeted to recipient antigens on leukocytes. It is suggested that this is the predisposing condition that, in the face of a second insult such as surgery, activates neutrophils and results in lung injury. Although mortality and morbidity associated with this syndrome are increased, the studies published to date have included only studies of nonobstetric and nongynecologic populations such as cardiac surgery and liver dis-

**TABLE 21-1.** Estimated Risks of Blood Transfusion

| Condition | Frequency of Occurrence Per Million Units |
|---|---|
| Hepatitis C virus | 1 |
| Human immunodeficiency virus (HIV) | 1 |
| Hepatitis B virus | 4 |
| Acute hemolytic reaction | 1–4 |
| Transfusion-related lung injury | 125 |
| Cytomegalovirus (CMV) | Morbidity risk is low in healthy individuals |

Modified from Goodnough LT. Risks of blood transfusion. Crit Care Med 2003;31(suppl):S678–86.

ease patients. However, this remains the most common form of serious morbidity encountered with transfusion of blood products.

Acute hemolytic reaction is uncommon but the incidence varies in different reports. Such reactions can occur with the transfusion of incompatible blood; for example, as little as 10–15 mL of incompatible blood can trigger acute red cell hemolysis. Current blood bank practice is to determine recipient and donor blood compatibility by ABO blood grouping, Rh status, and antigen–antibody interactions. Transfusion of incompatible blood may be the result of administrative errors that can occur from the time of crossmatch to the point of transfusion. This reaction can be fatal, and the greatest urgency is not only prevention but rapid recognition and treatment. For an anesthetized patient, hematuria and evidence of disseminated intravascular coagulopathy may be the only signs. Treatment to maintain blood pressure and urine output is important.

The incidence of transfusion-related viral illness has decreased dramatically. The risk of human immunodeficiency virus (HIV) transmission has decreased due to the implementation of HIV antibody testing. Since implementation, five cases per year have been reported compared to 714 cases in the year before implementation.

Posttransfusion non-A, non-B hepatitis viral infection was greater than 20% in the 1960s. This rate decreased to 10% after exclusion of paid donor units. In 1988, hepatitis C was identified as the primary causative agent. With the implementation of screening for hepatitis C antibody, HIV, and alanine transaminase (ALT), the risk of transfusion-related hepatitis C infection is currently estimated at 1 in 1,000,000 units transfused. Today, hepatitis C infection is rarely the result of transfusion and is more likely the consequence of injection drug use.

Attention to exclusion of paid donor units, screening for ALT, and antibody to hepatitis B core antigen in donated units has decreased the risk of hepatitis B infection. Of patients who are infected with hepatitis B, approximately 35% of patients will develop a self-limited acute disease. Only 1–10% of patients will develop chronic disease. This is in contrast to hepatitis C infection, where 85% of patients develop chronic infection with 20% leading to cirrhosis and 5% to hepatocellular carcinoma.

Cytomegalovirus (CMV), a member of the herpesvirus family, can be transmitted via transfusion of blood products. It generally poses a threat to the health of only immunocompromised individuals such as the following:

- Bone marrow and solid organ transplant recipients
- Patients with a malignancy or acquired immunodeficiency syndrome (AIDS)
- Low-birth-weight premature infants

In immunosuppressed patients, transmitted CMV infection may result in pneumonia or hepatitis. The virus presumably remains in the leukocytes of infected patients because the risk of transmission is reduced both by evaluation of the donor for CMV antibodies and leukoreduction of donor units.

Goodnough LT. Risks of blood transfusion. Crit Care Med 2003;31 (suppl):S678–S686.

Kopko PM, Marshall CS, MacKenzie MR, Holland PV, Popovsky MA. Transfusion-related acute lung injury: report of a clinical look-back investigation. JAMA 2002;287:1968–71.

Recommendations for prevention and control of hepatitis C virus (HCV) infection and HCV-related chronic disease. Centers for Disease Control and Prevention. MMWR Recomm Rep 1998;47(RR-19):1–39.

# 22

## Treatment of bacterial vaginosis in pregnancy

A 28-year-old woman, gravida 2, para 1, comes to your office at 11 weeks of gestation for her first antenatal visit. She is otherwise healthy with a negative gynecologic history. For the past 6 weeks, she has experienced mild nausea that is improving slightly. In addition, she has noticed increased vaginal discharge, which she describes as malodorous. Examination reveals increased homogeneous white discharge with a vaginal pH of 5.0. Wet mount reveals the pattern shown in Figure 22-1 (see color plate). The most appropriate management of this patient's discharge is

|   | (A) | oral metronidazole in a single dose |
|---|-----|-------------------------------------|
| * | (B) | oral metronidazole for 7 days |
|   | (C) | vaginal metronidazole for 5 days |
|   | (D) | oral clindamycin for 3 days |
|   | (E) | vaginal clindamycin for 3 days |

Bacterial vaginosis is a condition characterized by an imbalance in the normal vaginal flora. This imbalance includes a decrease in the typically high levels of lactobacilli and an increase in anaerobes, *Gardnerella* and *Mycoplasma* species. Bacterial vaginosis has been linked to a number of adverse pregnancy outcomes, including preterm delivery, preterm rupture of membranes, spontaneous abortion, and postpartum endometritis. Antibiotics can return the flora to its natural baseline, but recurrence is common and true cure rates are variable. Up to 20% of pregnancies will be affected by bacterial vaginosis and 50% of all cases are asymptomatic. Therefore, an important consideration is when and how to treat the condition.

In nonpregnant women, bacterial vaginosis has a tendency to come and go on its own without treatment. In pregnancy, there is evidence that the spontaneous clearance often seen in nonpregnant women does not occur. Given its association with preterm delivery, any treatment strategy would be considered successful in pregnancy only if it decreases the rate of preterm delivery and other adverse pregnancy outcomes associated with bacterial vaginosis. Because 50% of cases are asymptomatic, research has focused on when screening is appropriate. Available data fail to fully support routine screening of asymptomatic pregnant women who do not have a history of preterm delivery. No demonstrated beneficial effect on adverse outcomes has been observed, and there is the possibility of adverse effects from the antibiotics. However, the Centers for Disease Control and Prevention (CDC) promotes screening women at high risk of preterm delivery (ie, those with a history of a preterm birth) because data indicate a reduction in adverse outcomes. The ideal time to screen and treat is unclear although the recommendation is to screen at the first prenatal visit. The optimal screening test is also uncertain.

To date, the most reliable screening tool is whether the patient has three of the following four clinical criteria:

1. Vaginal pH greater than 4.5
2. Amine odor with potassium hydroxide (KOH) application
3. Homogeneous vaginal discharge
4. Clue cells on wet mount

Treatment is thought to be appropriate for pregnant women who are symptomatic with bacterial vaginosis. These women may be at higher risk for adverse outcomes than those without symptoms and were excluded for the most part from the screening trials that have been performed to date. Early studies that examined effective therapy for bacterial vaginosis primarily looked at clindamycin because it was hypothesized that there was a teratogenic effect with oral metronidazole. However, no data demonstrated a teratogenic effect with oral metronidazole. Oral regimens of metronidazole for 7 days in duration are safe and highly effective in pregnant women. Furthermore, there is evidence that treatment of bacterial vaginosis with oral metronidazole in women at high risk for preterm delivery reduces the rate of preterm delivery. For treatment in pregnancy, oral antibiotics appear to be the best option. The medical literature does not support the use of any topical antibiotics in pregnancy. The recurrence risk in such cases is high. In addition, data from three trials suggest an increase in adverse events (prematurity and neonatal infections) after the use of clindamycin cream. The CDC consequently recommends a regimen of oral metronidazole for 7 days as first-line therapy for bacterial vaginosis in pregnant women and oral clindamycin for 7 days as a secondary regimen.

Overall, the evidence supports a treatment regimen for pregnant women of oral antibiotics for longer time frames than nonpregnant patients. Infections in pregnant women seem to be more tenacious. This could be due to more difficult elimination of offending bacteria in pregnancy or the presence of an ascending infection that is already in the cervix or uterus at the time of treatment and thus requires systemic therapy for elimination. This also explains why treatment earlier in pregnancy has a higher rate of success.

The patient described has symptomatic bacterial vaginosis as documented by three of the four clinical criteria required (pH greater than 4.5; homogeneous discharge; and clue cells on wet mount). Her condition puts her at a higher risk for adverse pregnancy outcomes, and she requires treatment for symptomatic relief. The data support oral metronidazole for 7 days for optimal relief, which is the initial regimen recommended by the CDC.

Oral antibiotics for less than 7 days in pregnancy are not effective in relief of symptoms (ie, recurrence is high) or in reduction of adverse pregnancy outcomes. A 7-day course of oral clindamycin also is included in the CDC recommended treatment regimens. Topical antibiotics of any kind are not recommended for treatment of bacterial vaginosis in pregnancy. The recurrence rate is high and there is no evidence of decreased rates of adverse pregnancy outcomes.

Leitich H, Brunbauer M, Bodner-Adler B, Kaider A, Egarter C, Husslein P. Antibiotic treatment of bacterial vaginosis in pregnancy: a meta-analysis. Am J Obstet Gynecol 2003;188:752–8.

Screening for bacterial vaginosis in pregnancy; recommendations and rationale. U.S. Preventive Services Task Force. Am J Prev Med 2001;20 suppl:59–61.

Sexually transmitted diseases treatment guidelines, 2006. Centers for Disease Control and Prevention [published erratum appears in MMWR Recomm Rep 2006;55(36):997]. MMWR Recomm Rep 2006;55 (RR-11):1–94.

# 23

## Case–control vs prospective study design

Several doctors from one clinic are concerned about the number of women who present with wound disruption following a cesarean delivery. The physicians want to know if there is a pattern of maternal characteristics that increases the likelihood of wound disruption in their patient population. They identify 50 consecutive women with wound disruption over the past 2 years and 50 consecutive women without wound disruption for comparison. Data on maternal characteristics, sociodemographic data, pregnancy history, and medical comorbidities are extracted from patient charts, and odds ratios are calculated. This type of study design is best described as a

(A) clinical trial
(B) prospective cohort study
(C) retrospective cohort study
* (D) case–control study
(E) case series

The scenario describes a case–control study. Subjects are enrolled based on presence or absence of a particular morbidity—in this case, wound disruption following cesarean delivery. In most case–control studies, the morbidity (cases) or lack thereof (controls) has already occurred. Patients or patient charts are examined retrospectively for characteristics (eg, family history, environmental exposure, etc.) that may correlate with the outcome. The frequency of these characteristics can then be compared between groups, and the odds of developing morbidity, given the presence or absence of the characteristic, can be calculated.

A clinical trial requires that patients be assigned, preferably by random assignment, to one of two or more treatments or exposures (eg, therapy A vs therapy B) and outcomes assessed after treatment or exposure. The goal of this design is to distribute patient characteristics randomly across the two groups to minimize or eliminate confounding variables. This study design allows a more direct assessment of the relationship between treatment and outcome rather than examining how patient characteristics might group together to influence outcome.

A prospective cohort study identifies patients' risk characteristics or treatments at enrollment, and patients naturally fall into different groups based on the presence or absence of those risk factors or based on the treatment option they choose. Patients are then monitored over time to see what morbidity develops, if any. In a retrospective cohort study, patient cohorts are identified retrospectively by the presence or absence of risk characteristics or treatment chosen and examined for subsequent development of morbidity. The difference between prospective and retrospective cohort study designs is the point in time at which risk factor identification and outcomes occur relative to enrollment.

A case series describes patients with a common morbidity. No controls are used in a case series. This type of study is used to call attention to an interesting or unusual finding or occurrence and frequently involves rare diseases or novel treatments.

Grimes DA, Schultz KF. An overview of clinical research: the lay of the land. Lancet 2002;359:57–61.

Guyatt G, Rennie D, editors. Users' guides to the medical literature: a manual for evidence-based clinical practice. Chicago (IL): American Medical Association; 2002. p. 88–9, 365–6.

Newman TB, Browner WS, Cummings SR, Hulley SB. Designing an observational study: cross-sectional and case–control studies. In: Hulley SB, Cummings SR, Browner WS, Grady D, Hearst N, Newman TB, editors. Designing clinical research: an epidemiologic approach. 2nd ed. Baltimore (MD): Lippincott Williams & Wilkins; 2001. p. 107–21.

Sackett DL, Straus SE, Richardson WS, Rosenberg W, Haynes RB. Evidence-based medicine: how to practice and teach EBM. 2nd ed. Edinburgh: Churchill Livingstone; 2000. p. 158–9, 245.

# 24

## Evaluation of patient with urge incontinence

A 72-year-old woman reports frequent urine loss that requires changing several large pads daily. She notes urine loss on arising as well as with daily activity. She also experiences urgency and loss of urine while trying to reach the restroom. Results of the pelvic organ prolapse quantification (POP-Q) assessment are shown in Table 24-1 and demonstrate stage 1 prolapse. The best method to diagnose the cause of her symptoms is

      (A) postvoid residual measurement
      (B) pad test
\*   (C) cystometrogram
      (D) voiding diary
      (E) urinalysis

**TABLE 24-1.** A 3 × 3 Grid Showing Pelvic Organ Prolapse Quantification (POP-Q) Evaluation of This Patient

| | | |
|---|---|---|
| –2 Aa<br>Anterior<br>vaginal wall | –2 Ba<br>Anterior vaginal<br>wall | –7 C<br>Cervix or cuff |
| 3 gh<br>Genital hiatus | 2 pb<br>Perineal body | 8 tvl<br>Total vaginal<br>length |
| –3 Ap<br>Posterior<br>vaginal wall | –3 Bp<br>Posterior<br>vaginal wall | –8 D<br>Posterior fornix |

Urge incontinence or detrusor overactivity is defined as the complaint of involuntary leakage accompanied by or immediately preceded by urgency. Stress incontinence is the complaint of involuntary leakage on effort or exertion, or on sneezing or coughing. Mixed incontinence involves both problems, that is, involuntary leakage associated with urgency and also with exertion, effort, sneezing, or coughing. Each type occurs in approximately 33% of all incontinent patients. No underlying cause is found for

90% of patients with diagnosed urge incontinence. Reversible causes to be ruled out include infections, stones, diuretics, bladder cancer, and psychologic issues. The remaining 10% of patients with diagnosed urge incontinence have neurologic abnormalities. Urge incontinence is more common in older patients.

Distinguishing between stress and urge incontinence can be difficult because the patient's symptoms do not always correlate with the underlying diagnosis made in the urodynamics laboratory. For example, coughing can trigger detrusor contractions and thus mimic stress incontinence. Patients with irritative symptoms, such as urgency, may be found to have no abnormality on urodynamic testing. For this reason, voiding diaries and other clinical evaluations short of urodynamic testing, although helpful, are not definitive. Mixed symptoms are reported in as many as 55% of women with stress incontinence in the laboratory. Approximately 38% of women with diagnosed urge incontinence on urodynamic testing report symptoms of stress as well as urgency.

Urodynamics is the observation of the changing function of the lower urinary tract over time. It provides the best method to differentiate stress, urge, and mixed incontinence. It may consist of several tests, including cystom-etry and measurement of urethral closure pressure or Valsalva leak point pressure. Cystometry measures the pressure and volume relationship of the bladder with fill-ing. A simple or complex subtracted cystometrogram may reveal detrusor contractions coincident with urine loss. Postvoid residual measurement would identify uri-nary retention but would not establish the diagnosis of stress or urge incontinence. Pad testing is a method to quantify urine loss by standardizing pad weight and quantifying the increase in weight due to leakage.

Urinalysis may rule out infection or hematuria but does not directly give the underlying diagnosis.

Abrams P, Cardozo L, Fall M, Griffiths D, Rosier P, Ulmsten U, et al. The standardisation of terminology in lower urinary tract function: report from the Standardisation Sub-committee of the International Continence Society. Standardisation Sub-committee of the International Continence Society. Urology 2003;61:37–49.

Bump RC, Norton PA, Zinner NR, Yalcin I. Mixed urinary incontinence symptoms: urodynamic findings, incontinence severity, and treatment response. Duloxetine Urinary Incontinence Study Group. Obstet Gynecol 2003;102:76–83.

Chaliha C, Khullar V. Mixed incontinence. Urology 2004;63(suppl 1): 51–7.

# 25

## Thrombophilia and warfarin use

A 25-year-old woman, gravida 1, para 0, is concerned that she might have a hereditary throm-bophilia because her sister recently had a pulmonary embolus 2 weeks postpartum. She brings you the sister's thrombophilia laboratory values, obtained from the sister while on warfarin. When a patient is taking warfarin, the only test that can accurately detect a thrombophilia is

* (A) DNA-based test
(B) protein C activity
(C) protein S activity
(D) factor X

The term *venous thromboembolism* encompasses both deep vein thrombosis and pulmonary embolism. Virchow's triad of hypercoagulability, stasis, and vascular damage occur to some degree in pregnancy and in the puerperium, thus placing patients at some risk for venous thromboembolism. Thrombophilias or prothrombotic dis-orders also contribute to hypercoagulability. The first inherited disorder described was antithrombin deficiency. Protein C and protein S deficiencies occur as the result of many different gene mutations. A single mutation in the factor V gene, the factor V Leiden mutation, and another point mutation in the prothrombin gene (G20210A) also are associated with hypercoagulable states. These throm-bophilias also may contribute to increased risk of preg-nancy loss and preeclampsia.

Screening asymptomatic family members after an index case of venous thromboembolism is controversial and is appropriate only if it will alter medical manage-ment. Homozygous or doubly heterozygous patients (ie, heterozygotes for two different thrombophilias) are at increased risk of thrombosis. Some inherited throm-bophilias increase the risk of thrombosis only modestly, whereas others, such as protein S deficiency and antithrombin deficiency, may increase the cumulative risk of thrombosis up to 50% by age 50 years.

Knowledge of an increased thrombosis risk associated with a thrombophilia would necessitate decisions on pro-phylaxis and therapy for a patient during pregnancy and for 6 weeks postpartum. Increased preeclampsia and increased pregnancy loss rate correlations with the throm-bophilias are controversial and their management is less clear.

Evaluation of thrombophilia is most accurate when performed in the nonpregnant patient. Pregnancy affects the levels of protein C activity and protein S activity. Oral contraceptives also may affect testing. Anticoagulation or a recent thrombosis also will affect functional assays. Anticoagulation with anti-thrombin III is not reliable dur-ing an acute thrombosis nor while a patient is taking heparin.

Interpretation of functional values requires knowledge of which factors are vitamin K–dependent regulatory fac-tors. Protein S and protein C will appear deficient in a patient who is on warfarin. Protein-based, functional assays should be obtained only after at least 2 weeks without anticoagulants, and in the nonpregnant state, at least 6 weeks postpartum. Tests that are based on DNA assays will not be affected by anticoagulants.

Factor X deficiency is an autosomal recessive condi-tion. Patients with this condition may bleed spontaneously following trauma. In women, it may be associated with menorrhagia. A specific factor X activity test may be ordered. Several mutations have been described in factor X deficiency, but this is not a thrombophilia. This test also is affected by warfarin.

For the patient described, who is taking warfarin, the tests that can accurately detect a thrombophilia are the prothrombin gene mutation and the factor V Leiden mutation polymerase chain reaction (PCR) tests.

Caprini JA, Glase CJ, Anderson CB, Hathaway K. Laboratory markers in the diagnosis of venous thromboembolism. Circulation 2004; 109(suppl 1):I4–8.

Jordaan DJ, Schoon MG, Badenhorst PN. Thrombophilia screening in pregnancy. Obstet Gynecol Surv 2005;60:394–404.

Lin J, August P. Genetic thrombophilias and preeclampsia: a meta-analysis. Obstet Gynecol 2005;105:182–92.

Reich LM, Bower M, Key NS. Role of the geneticist in testing and counseling for inherited thrombophilia. Genet Med 2003;5:133–43.

Turchetti D, Romeo G. Problems related to counseling in genetic thrombophilias. Pathophysiol Haemost Thromb 2002;32:254–7.

# 26

## Management of abnormal cervical cytology

A 23-year-old single nulligravid woman came to the office for her annual examination. She was sexually active on oral contraceptives and had no prior abnormal cytologic results. Her examination was normal. The cytopathology laboratory informs you that human papillomavirus (HPV) DNA typing is being performed because her cervical cytology is abnormal. Such typing is indicated when cervical cytology is consistent with

> (A) low-grade squamous intraepithelial lesion (LSIL)
> (B) atypical squamous cells, cannot exclude high-grade SIL (ASC-H)
> * (C) atypical squamous cells, undetermined significance (ASC-US)
> (D) high-grade squamous intraepithelial lesion (HSIL)
> (E) atypical glandular cells (AGC)

Genital HPV is easily sexually transmitted and is the cause of cervical cancer. Although HPV is a necessary factor in the development of cervical neoplasia, most infected women will clear the infection within 2 years and never develop significant cervical pathology. Studies have confirmed the presence of high-risk types of HPV in cervical cancer specimens. In a study of more than 500 patients with cervical cancer, high-risk HPV was found in every case. High-risk (oncogenic) types of HPV associated with cervical cancer include HPV subtypes 16, 18, 31, 33, 35, 39, 45, 51, 52, 56, 58, 59, 68, 73, and 82. Of these, HPV subtypes 16 and 18 account for 70% of cases of cervical cancer.

Cervical cytology screening at recommended intervals has been responsible for the continued decreasing rates of cervical cancer in the United States (Fig. 26-1). The addition of HPV testing has been proven beneficial in selected scenarios and of little use in others. For example, HPV DNA testing for oncogenic types is not useful in ASC-H, LSIL, and HSIL on cytologic evaluation. This is because high-risk HPV panels test positive in up to 100% of patients with HSIL, up to 83% with LSIL, and most

patients with ASC-H. In these cases, colposcopy is indicated. Because of the high association of these abnormal cervical cytology categories with high-risk types of HPV, it is only useful to perform HPV DNA typing in cases where uncertainty exists and results would affect the decision to perform colposcopy.

If cervical cytology reveals ASC-US, HPV DNA typing is recommended to assist with management. This is referred to as reflex HPV testing. If the test result is negative for oncogenic HPV, the patient is at extremely low risk of significant cervical pathology, and cervical cytologic screening can be repeated in 1 year. If the test result is positive, then colposcopy is indicated to rule out cervical neoplasia. Using reflex oncogenic HPV typing in cases of ASC-US can reduce the need for colposcopy significantly, by up to 56%, making it a convenient and cost-effective approach to management of this cytologic finding. This method of triage of ASC-US may not be beneficial in sexually active adolescents where the percentage of adolescents with HPV may be as high as 90% and most of these cases are the oncogenic types. In one study, 80% of ASC-US cytologic reports in adolescents

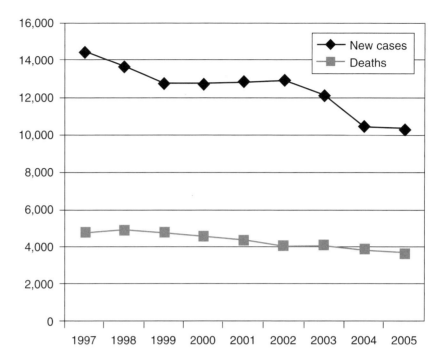

**FIG. 26-1.** Trends in cervical cancer, 1997–2005. (Data from the American Cancer Society.)

younger than 20 years were positive for oncogenic types. Despite this finding, colposcopy in young adolescents may not be warranted because most will clear the infection in 2 years, the rate of significant cervical pathology is extremely low, and cancer is almost never seen in adolescents. This accumulated information on the natural history of HPV in young women has lead to the recommendation by the American College of Obstetricians and Gynecologists and the American Cancer Society that cytologic screening not begin in adolescents until approximately 3 years after the onset of sexual activity or at age 21 years. This recommendation will greatly reduce unnecessary colposcopies and other procedures in this age group, which has a high rate of minimally abnormal cytologic abnormalities and a high rate of infection clearance, but negligible risk of cervical cancer.

Boardman LA, Stanko C, Weitzen S, Sung CJ. Atypical squamous cells of undetermined significance: human papillomavirus testing in adolescents. Obstet Gynecol 2005;105:741–6.

Bohmer G, van den Brule AJ, Brummer O, Meijer CL, Petry KU. No confirmed case of human papillomavirus DNA-negative cervical intraepithelial neoplasia grade 3 or invasive primary cancer of the uterine cervix among 511 patients. Am J Obstet Gynecol 2003;189:118–20.

Ho GY, Bierman R, Beardsley L, Chang CJ, Burk RD. Natural history of cervicovaginal papillomavirus infection in young women. N Engl J Med 1998;338:423–8.

Human papillomavirus testing for triage of women with cytologic evidence of low-grade squamous intraepithelial lesions: baseline data from a randomized trial. The Atypical Squamous Cells of Undetermined Significance/Low-Grade Squamous Intraepithelial Lesions Triage Study (ALTS) Group. J Natl Cancer Inst 2000;92:397–402.

Kim JJ, Wright TC, Goldie SJ. Cost-effectiveness of alternative triage strategies for atypical squamous cells of undetermined significance. JAMA 2002;287:2382–90.

Management of abnormal cervical cytology and histology. ACOG Practice Bulletin No. 66. American College of Obstetricians and Gynecologists. Obstet Gynecol 2005;106:645–64.

Munoz N, Bosch FX, de Sanjose S, Herrero R, Castellsague X, Shah KV, et al. Epidemiologic classification of human papillomavirus types associated with cervical cancer. International Agency for Research on Cancer Multicenter Cervical Cancer Study Group. N Engl J Med 2003; 348:518–27.

# 27

## Tubal sterilization

A 27-year-old woman at 32 weeks of gestation comes to your office for a routine prenatal visit with questions about tubal sterilization. You counsel her that the tubal sterilization method with lowest long-term rate of failure for her is

   \*   (A) postpartum partial salpingectomy
        (B) laparoscopic tubal occlusion with spring clips
        (C) laparoscopic bipolar tubal cautery
        (D) laparoscopic tubal banding with silastic rings
        (E) hysteroscopic placement of titanium intratubal coils

Tubal sterilization is one of the most common surgical procedures performed on women, and up to 28% of U.S. reproductive-aged women opt for it as a permanent method of contraception. A multitude of different techniques for tubal sterilization exist today. A number of factors must be considered when counseling women about sterilization. All of the currently available methods represent safe and effective forms of permanent contraception; however, in certain contexts, some methods have advantages over others.

It is especially important in women younger than 30 years to consider the long-term risk of tubal sterilization failure. The U.S. Collaborative Review of Sterilization (CREST) was the first study to look at the long-term effectiveness of various tubal sterilization techniques. In the study, 10,685 women were followed for 3, 5, 8, and 14 years after tubal sterilization. Of those women, 143 experienced a true tubal failure, resulting in an overall pregnancy rate of 18.5 per 1,000 women for all types of sterilization procedures. Postpartum partial salpingectomy had the lowest overall failure rate at 7.5 per 1,000 procedures, and laparoscopic spring clip had the highest overall failure rate at 36.5 per 1,000 procedures. Overall failure rates for laparoscopic bipolar cautery and laparoscopic tubal occlusion with silastic rings were 24.8 and 17.7, respectively. The CREST study also showed that the failure rate of tubal sterilization was closely tied not only to the method of the procedure but also to the age at which it was performed. Long-term follow-up indicated that women sterilized earlier in life have a greater probability of tubal failure especially if the procedure was performed in those younger than 34 years. When adjusted for age, the cumulative failure rates for bipolar cautery, spring clips, and silastic bands were statistically higher than that for postpartum partial salpingectomy. The CREST study showed also that these failure rates have other implications for pregnancy. When looked at in the long term, the risk of ectopic pregnancy was much higher for bipolar cautery than postpartum partial salpingectomy and other methods of tubal sterilization. Interval partial salpingectomy was not considered in the CREST study. It should be noted that the annual risk of tubal sterilization remains constant. Physicians should be aware that women who present even several years after the procedure should be taken seriously.

Newer methods of tubal sterilization show promise and offer women a greater diversity of choice when considering permanent sterilization. Hysteroscopic tubal occlusion with titanium coils (Essure) and newer modified spring clips (Filshie clips) have been shown to be effective methods for tubal occlusion and sterilization. To date, no studies have examined their long-term effectiveness in prevention of pregnancy. However, studies have shown that 5-year failure rates of Filshie clips compare favorably with the failure rates of other methods of occlusion and sterilization.

Baill IC, Cullins VE, Pati S. Counseling issues in tubal sterilization. Am Fam Physician 2003;67:1287–94.

Peterson HB, Xia Z, Hughes JM, Wilcox LS, Tylor LR, Trussell J. The risk of ectopic pregnancy after tubal sterilization. U.S. Collaborative Review of Sterilization Working Group. N Engl J Med 1997;336:762–7.

Peterson HB, Xia Z, Hughes JM, Wilcox LS, Tylor LR, Trussell J. The risk of pregnancy after tubal sterilization: findings from the U.S. Collaborative Review of Sterilization. Am J Obstet Gynecol 1996;174: 1161–8; discussion 1168–70.

# 28

## Role of saline infusion sonohysterography in postmenopausal bleeding

A 63-year-old menopausal woman has had vaginal bleeding for 3 weeks. An endometrial biopsy was performed by suction piston device, sounding to 6 cm. Insufficient tissue for diagnosis was obtained. Repeat endometrial biopsy yielded the same result. The endometrial stripe could not be imaged by transvaginal ultrasonography. The best next step in management is

      (A) pelvic magnetic resonance imaging (MRI)
\*   (B) sonohysterography
      (C) progestin withdrawal
      (D) dilation and curettage (D&C)

The situation described is a common clinical dilemma for the practitioner. Insufficient tissue is obtained in up to 30% of endometrial biopsies performed for postmenopausal bleeding. The finding may result from endometrial atrophy so that there is simply not enough tissue to biopsy, or from poor technique, with failure to enter the endometrial cavity itself with the biopsy device. The evaluation of postmenopausal bleeding has evolved to include ultrasonography-based triage schema to aid in solving this important clinical problem.

Transvaginal ultrasonographic imaging of the endometrial stripe has an excellent negative predictive value for excluding endometrial cancer and hyperplasia. A thickened stripe, however, may be secondary to cancer, polyps, leiomyomata, or simply ultrasonographic artifact. To further refine the accuracy of transvaginal ultrasonography, sonohysterography was developed. Sonohysterography uses intrauterine saline for contrast to outline the endometrial cavity. Saline is instilled via a transcervically placed catheter and the uterus is imaged using real-time transvaginal technique. Polyps, intracavitary leiomyomata, and focal endometrial thickening can be diagnosed with sonohysterography. Sonohysterography adds accuracy to unenhanced transvaginal ultrasonography. In the diagnostic workup of postmenopausal bleeding, sonohysterography is 95% sensitive for the diagnosis of intracavitary abnormalities.

For the patient described, sonohysterography would allow for visualization of the endometrial cavity. Because endometrial biopsy was unsuccessful in obtaining tissue for diagnosis, other diagnostic methods, including hysteroscopy, could be considered. Hysteroscopy and sono-hysterography are similar in diagnostic accuracy, and either would be acceptable to further evaluate a patient in which office endometrial sampling was nondiagnostic. Figure 28-1 shows a triage schema for evaluation of postmenopausal bleeding using sonohysterography. The sonohysterogram provides information that aids in the decision to proceed with operative or nonoperative management. It is easily performed in the outpatient setting with little additional equipment required beyond that typically available in most gynecologists' offices.

Pelvic MRI has not been well studied in the evaluation of postmenopausal bleeding. Cost and accessibility of MRI, along with the established accuracy of ultrasonography, have limited the experience with MRI for abnormal bleeding. Although MRI can produce high-resolution images of the endometrium, thickness of the endometrial stripe obtained by MRI has not been correlated with endometrial biopsy findings.

Progestin withdrawal would not be indicated given the patient's menopausal status. Use of progestins would be appropriate for bleeding thought to be secondary to anovulation in a premenopausal woman or for treatment of amenorrhea secondary to anovulation.

Blind D&C is not more accurate in the diagnosis of postmenopausal bleeding than office endometrial biopsy, although D&C may be of value when cervical stenosis precludes office sampling. In most cases, office endometrial biopsy offers the advantages of decreased cost and increased convenience without compromising diagnostic accuracy. After two biopsies without sufficient tissue, as in this case, D&C would be unlikely to have diagnostic value.

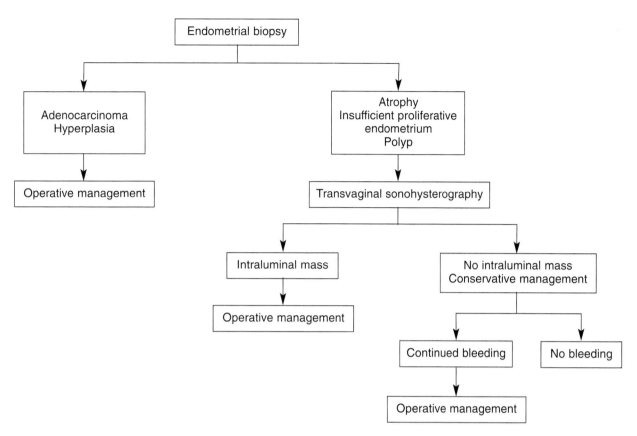

**FIG. 28-1.** Algorithm for triage of postmenopausal women with abnormal uterine bleeding. (Reprinted from O'Connell LP, Fries MH, Zeringue E, Brehm W. Triage of abnormal postmenopausal bleeding: a comparison of endometrial biopsy and transvaginal sonohysterography versus fractional curettage with hysteroscopy. Am J Obstet Gynecol 1998; 178:956–61. Copyright © 1998, with permission from Elsevier.)

Berridge DL, Winter TC. Saline infusion sonohysterography: technique, indications, and imaging findings. J Ultrasound Med 2004;23:97–112; quiz 114–5.

de Kroon CD, de Bock GH, Dieben SW, Jansen FW. Saline contrast hysterosonography in abnormal uterine bleeding: a systematic review and meta-analysis. BJOG 2003;110:938–47.

Good AE. Diagnostic options for assessment of postmenopausal bleeding. Mayo Clin Proc 1997;72:345–9.

Saline infusion sonohysterography. ACOG Technology Assessment in Obstetrics and Gynecology No. 3. American College of Obstetricians and Gynecologists. Obstet Gynecol 2003;102:659–62.

# 29

## Unplanned or unwanted pregnancy

A healthy 18-year-old single woman presents with signs and symptoms of early pregnancy. You determine that she has a 9-week intrauterine pregnancy. The patient indicates that, after discussions with her parents, she has rejected the option of raising or placing the baby for adoption and requests abortion. However, you have religious and moral objections to abortion. As her obstetrician–gynecologist, you are obligated to

(A) inform the patient that you cannot comply with her request
(B) counsel the patient regarding adoption
\* (C) refer the patient to a clinician who will counsel her on all reproductive options
(D) ensure that the patient is aware of risks associated with abortion

Unintended and unplanned pregnancies continue to be prevalent, constituting almost 50% of pregnancies in U.S. women. Because many women who face unintended pregnancies will choose to terminate them by abortion, the case described represents a patient that obstetrician–gynecologists commonly encounter.

As with the population in general, obstetrician–gynecologists vary as to their personal perspectives regarding abortion. The American College of Obstetricians and Gynecologists (ACOG) has stated that it respects the "…need and responsibility of its members to determine their individual positions based on personal values or beliefs."

The College also states, "A pregnant woman should be fully informed in a balanced manner about all options, including raising the child herself, placing the child for adoption, and abortion." The information conveyed should be appropriate to the duration of the pregnancy. The professional should make every effort to avoid introducing personal bias. The College supports access to care for all individuals, regardless of financial status, and supports the availability of all reproductive options. However, ACOG opposes unnecessary regulations that limit or delay access to care.

Accordingly, in the case of an obstetrician–gynecologist who cares for a woman who faces an unintended pregnancy, has rejected raising the child or placing it for adoption, and has chosen to terminate the pregnancy, the obstetrician–gynecologist has the obligation to personally provide the requested abortion or refer the patient to someone who is prepared to perform the abortion. State laws vary as to the obligation of the physician to provide counseling or referral. Thus, the physician is obligated to refer the patient to someone who will counsel her about all reproductive options, and, if appropriately counseled, she will presumably proceed with the requested abortion. Because this patient has decided to undergo an abortion, counseling regarding adoption would be unnecessary. Discussion about risks would not make sense if the physician does not intend to perform the procedure.

American College of Obstetricians and Gynecologists. Abortion policy. ACOG Statement of Policy. Washington, DC: ACOG, 2004.

Finer LB, Henshaw SK. Abortion incidence and services in the United States in 2000. Perspect Sex Reprod Health 2003;35:6–15.

Kaunitz AM, Grimes DA, Kaunitz KK. A physician's guide to adoption. JAMA 1987;258:3537–41.

Stubblefield PG, Carr-Ellis S, Borgatta L. Methods for induced abortion. Am J Obstet Gynecol 2004;104:174–85.

# 30

## Herpes simplex virus risk in pregnancy

A 32-year-old primigravid woman comes to your office for a routine antenatal visit at 20 weeks of gestation. Genital herpes was diagnosed in her current partner (and father of the baby) after he developed a painful penile ulcer 3 months ago. The patient has no known history of genital ulcers or other sexually transmitted diseases (STDs). She asks what she should do next to protect herself and her pregnancy. The most appropriate next step is

<blockquote>

(A) treat her sexual partner with suppressive therapy

(B) treat patient with suppressive therapy

(C) check partner's serology

   * (D) check patient's serology

(E) culture patient's cervico-vaginal secretions for viral shedding

</blockquote>

Genital herpes simplex virus (HSV) infection is a significant health concern for both the mother and the fetus. Perinatal HSV results in significant morbidity and even mortality in the infected newborn. Herpes simplex virus type 1 (HSV-1) causes most nongenital infections such as oral herpes and is typically contracted in childhood, whereas herpes simplex virus type 2 (HSV-2) is the major contributor to genital herpes. Although the two types are distinctly different in antigenic composition, their antibodies cross-react and result in some cross-coverage and immunity.

The peak incidence of HSV-2 in women is in the late teenage years through age 30 years. It is estimated that up to 30% of U.S. women have antibodies to HSV-2 although only 5% report a history of lesions. Because genital HSV is an STD, the risk factors for exposure are the same as those for other STDs (eg, multiple partners, early age of sexual intercourse). An estimated 1,500–2,000 U.S. newborns contract neonatal herpes each year. Most infections occur from contact with infected maternal secretions from asymptomatic mothers without identified lesions.

There are three stages of HSV infection based on serology and clinical presentation:

1. Primary infections, ie, presence of lesions but no antibodies to either HSV-1 or HSV-2

2. Nonprimary first episode, ie, presence of antibodies to either HSV-1 or HSV-2 when clinical presentation of the other type occurs

3. Recurrent HSV, ie, recurrent lesions with antibodies to the same type present

Primary infection with either HSV-1 or HSV-2 typically causes more severe symptoms than recurrent infection although some cases may be asymptomatic. Lesions occur 2–14 days after exposure. Subclinical viral shedding occurs at a rate of 2–3% in women with HSV-2 infection although there is an increase in subclinical viral shedding in the first 3 months after primary HSV-2 lesions have healed. Subclinical shedding with HSV-1 infection is approximately 0.65%. Patients are considered infectious during clinical and subclinical shedding.

A history of infection with HSV-1 only partially protects a patient from initial HSV-2 infection. Thus, in many cases, without serologic testing, it is difficult to discern primary lesions from nonprimary first episodes of the infection. Recurrent infection can be symptomatic or subclinical. Subclinical viral shedding occurs without symptoms or signs of lesions and lasts approximately 1–5 days. The overall viral load during subclinical shedding is less than when lesions are present but is still capable of infecting a susceptible patient. The annual risk of conversion in discordant couples is 31.9% in women who are both HSV-1- and HSV-2-negative vs only 9.1% in women who are HSV-1-positive. This demonstrates the protective effect of cross-reactive antibodies. In addition, most acquisition of new infection in discordant couples occurs when the partner has no signs or symptoms of active infection, which suggests that asymptomatic shedding is a common and important contributor to new cases of genital HSV. Data suggest that at least 10% of pregnant women are at risk of contracting HSV-2 from their seropositive partners.

Vertical transmission of genital HSV is related to gestational age at time of exposure and stage of infection (primary vs nonprimary first episode vs recurrent infection). Vertical transmission in women with recurrent infection is very low (0–3%); transmission after primary infection is approximately 50%. It is known that primary infection later in pregnancy (late second or third trimester) is much more likely to result in perinatal transmission.

Current serologic testing for HSV infections includes type-specific assays for immunoglobulin (Ig) G. Assays using glycoprotein-G–based tests have a very low false-positive rate for HSV-2 and should be used. The antibody is detectible 2–3 weeks after infection. Given the large difference in risk to both the patient and fetus based on stage of infection, it is recommended that serologic testing be used to manage sexual partners of individuals with genital HSV or to confirm a diagnosis of genital HSV where false-negative cultures are common.

The patient described has no history of symptomatic genital HSV. She could be serologically negative and be at significant risk of primary infection or she could be serologically positive, which would put her at worst at risk of a nonprimary first outbreak. It is possible that she has been previously exposed and thus already infected with HSV, because asymptomatic cases of genital HSV are common. The only way to confirm her status and thus to determine the level of risk to which she and her fetus are exposed is by serologic confirmation. If she has antibodies to neither HSV subtype, she is at significant risk of conversion and ultimate vertical transmission to her fetus. Thus, interventions such as avoiding intercourse during the remainder of her pregnancy could be instituted as a preventive and protective maneuver. It would also be important then to counsel the patient that, if she chooses to have sex, condoms would decrease but not eliminate her risk of conversion.

Suppressive therapy for the partner before confirming the patient's status is unnecessary because it is possible that the patient herself is already infected. The provider should focus attention on preventing outbreaks in the patient. No evidence exists that suppressive therapy completely eradicates subclinical viral shedding. Therefore, if the patient is at risk for conversion, suppression of disease in the partner would not necessarily protect her. Similarly,

suppressive therapy for the patient without knowing her serologic status is not necessary.

Suppressive therapy for recurrent infection is not necessary unless the patient is experiencing multiple symptomatic outbreaks and even then is not done until close to term. Checking the partner's serologic status is pointless because he already has genital herpes. The information gathered via this test would not help protect the patient or her fetus and, thus, is not helpful at this time. Without clinical symptoms or known seropositive status, checking the patient's cervico-vaginal secretions for HSV will likely show a high false-negative rate. It also does not confirm the patient's level of risk of conversion because it does not show whether she has previously been exposed.

American College of Obstetricians and Gynecologists. Management of herpes in pregnancy. Practice Bulletin 8. Washington, DC: ACOG; 1999.

Brown ZA, Benedetti J, Ashley R, Burchett S, Selke S, Berry S, et al. Neonatal herpes simplex virus infection in relation symptomatic maternal infection at the time of labor. N Engl J Med 1991;324: 1247–52.

Brown ZA, Selke S, Zeh J, Kopelman J, Maslow A, Ashley RL, et al. The acquisition of herpes simplex virus during pregnancy. N Engl J Med 1997;337:509–15.

Kulhanjian JA, Soroush V, Au DS, Bronzan RN, Yasukawa LL, Weylman LE, et al. Identification of women at unsuspected risk of primary infection with herpes simplex virus type 2 during pregnancy. N Engl J Med 1992;326:916–20.

Morrow RA, Brown ZA. Common use of inaccurate antibody assays to identify infection status with herpes simplex virus type 2. Am J Obstet Gynecol 2005;193:361–2.

Sexually transmitted diseases treatment guidelines, 2006. Centers for Disease Control and Prevention [published erratum appears in MMWR Recomm Rep 2006;55(36):997]. MMWR Recomm Rep 2006;55 (RR-11):1–94.

# 31

## Evaluation of bloody nipple discharge

A 45-year-old woman notes bloodstains on her brassiere and can express bloody fluid from one nipple. Physical examination reveals no breast mass. The most likely diagnosis is

    (A) ductal ectasia
    (B) ductal hyperplasia with atypia
    (C) intraductal carcinoma
    (D) fibrocystic change
\*   (E) intraductal papilloma

Nipple discharge is a frequent complaint of reproductive-aged women that occurs in 3–6% of patients who report to specialty breast clinics. The most serious underlying diagnosis is cancer, but this is less common than benign conditions. Only spontaneously occurring discharge mandates evaluation. The evaluation should proceed in a stepwise fashion because all cases not classified as galactorrhea will be

ductal in origin. Galactorrhea or nonbloody discharge often results from elevated prolactin levels. This can be caused by stress, lack of sleep, exercise, hypothyroidism, nipple stimulation, or recent breastfeeding as well as by prolactinomas. Medications, including oral contraceptives, opiates, tricyclic antidepressants, methyldopa, phenothiazine, risperidone, and other antipsychotic drugs can raise prolactin levels.

Ductal ectasia refers to dilation of the subaureolar ducts with inflammation and fibrosis around the ducts. It accounts for 17–36% of cases of nipple discharge. The resulting discharge is most commonly dark green or black although it can be bloody. Nonbloody discharge does not require surgical intervention.

Ductal hyperplasia with atypia is rarely seen as a cause of bloody discharge. Ductal carcinoma in situ or papillary carcinoma is also a rare cause of nipple discharge. It usually occurs in patients with a mass or an imaging abnormality. Fibrocystic change may produce serous or green multiductal discharge that is provoked rather than spontaneous. Mammography can supplement the physical examination and history of cyclic mastalgia. An intraductal papilloma is the most common cause of bloody unilateral discharge, and it accounts for 35–48%

of cases of nipple discharge. It is usually reproducible on palpation of a single duct orifice. Mammography is usually normal, and ultrasonography may show a dilated duct with an intraluminal lesion. Galactography can demonstrate the mass in the duct. Cytology of the discharge is not sensitive enough to exclude malignancy, with a 30% false-negative rate. Ductoscopy and ductal lavage as diagnostic techniques are still under investigation. Excision of the duct is indicated. Figure 31-1 shows an algorithm for the evaluation of nipple discharge.

Falkenberry SS. Nipple discharge. Obstet Gynecol Clin North Am 2002;29:21–9.

Vargas HI, Romero L, Chlebowski RT. Management of bloody nipple discharge. Curr Treat Options Oncol 2002;3:157–61.

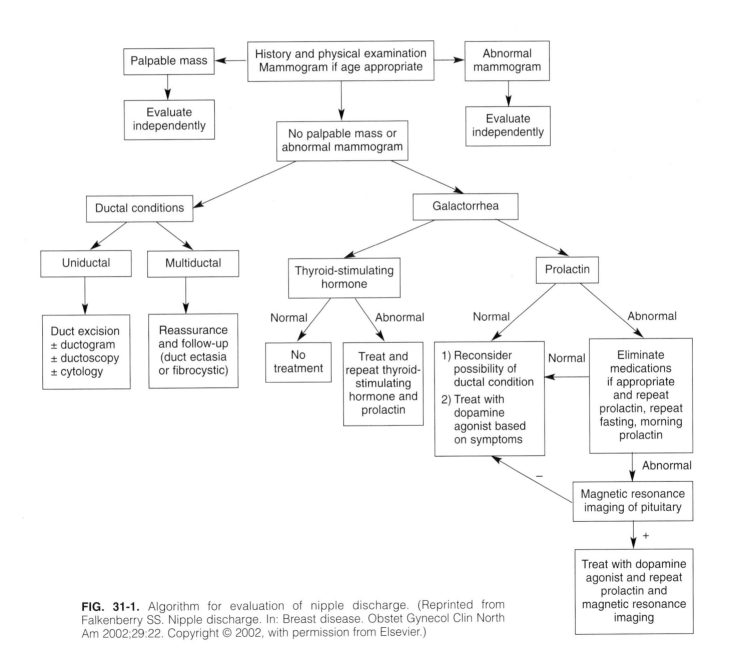

**FIG. 31-1.** Algorithm for evaluation of nipple discharge. (Reprinted from Falkenberry SS. Nipple discharge. In: Breast disease. Obstet Gynecol Clin North Am 2002;29:22. Copyright © 2002, with permission from Elsevier.)

# 32

## Iron-deficiency anemia in postmenopausal women

A 62-year-old postmenopausal woman whom you have cared for for years comes to the office for an annual examination and reports increased fatigue on her morning walks. She reports symptoms of heartburn and occasional constipation as well as an episode of vaginal spotting a few months ago. Physical examination is significant for a normal breast examination, vaginal atrophy, and a normal rectal examination with guaiac-negative stool. Laboratory findings show hemoglobin of 10.1 g/dL with a mean corpuscular volume (MCV) of 78 fL, platelets 400,000 mm³, creatinine 1.1 mg/dL, normal thyroid-stimulating hormone (TSH) level, and normal Pap test results. Endometrial biopsy shows atrophic endometrium. The most likely cause of her anemia is

      (A) dietary deficiency
      (B) celiac disease
\*    (C) upper intestinal disease
      (D) colonic disease
      (E) gynecologic pathology

Anemia is a common problem in gynecology with iron-deficiency anemia being the most frequent cause. Much has been written about premenopausal anemia, but postmenopausal iron-deficiency anemia and its causes are less well understood. Menstrual blood loss is the most common cause of anemia in premenopausal women; gastrointestinal blood loss is the most common cause in postmenopausal women.

Iron-deficiency anemia is characterized by fatigue that may be disproportionate to the severity of the anemia. Glossitis, atrophy of the lingual papillae, and angular stomatitis (erosions at the corners of the mouth) may occur but iron deficiency may present without physical findings. Early iron-deficiency anemia can present with normochromic, normocytic indices but later develops as a decrease in MCV with the classic hypochromic index. Findings of a low serum iron and an elevated transferrin level confirm the diagnosis. It also can be recognized if the serum ferritin level is less than 10 ng/mL. Fecal occult blood testing can be helpful but it shows poor sensitivity on a single stool sample obtained by digital rectal examination. In addition, fecal occult blood testing has a low detection rate for premalignant and early-stage lesions. The likelihood that a guaiac test will be positive is generally proportional to the quantity of fecal heme, which in turn is related to the size and location of the bleeding lesion. Additional tests for fecal blood, including the fecal immunochemical test, are increasingly being used because of improved sensitivity. However, a negative test should not be reassuring when clinical suspicion is high.

If a postmenopausal patient presents with an iron-deficiency anemia, the cause must be determined. Among patients who had been evaluated by upper and lower endoscopy, 36–56% were found to have upper gastrointestinal causes and 18–20% had lower intestinal etiologies. Therefore, upper gastrointestinal lesions (ie, peptic ulcers, esophagitis, gastritis, and gastric cancer) are more common, and upper endoscopy is needed to rule out potential causes. A history of aspirin or nonsteroidal anti-inflammatory drug use must be reviewed because use of such drugs increases the incidence and significance of these lesions. Although upper gastrointestinal lesions may be more common, malignancies are found more frequently in the colon. Colonoscopy is essential to rule out colon cancer, polyps, and angiodysplasia.

If no source of gastrointestinal bleeding is found, patients often are given iron supplementation and monitored. It is unusual to have a dietary deficiency as the cause of anemia in a postmenopausal woman who consumes a diet containing meat. Celiac disease can occasionally be a cause of iron deficiency and fecal blood loss in the population older than 60 years. Endoscopy of the small bowel can be helpful in diagnosing the disorder. Box 32-1 presents a comprehensive list of causes of occult gastrointestinal bleeding.

**BOX 32-1**

**Differential Diagnosis of Occult Gastrointestinal Bleeding***

Mass lesions
    Carcinoma (any site)[†]
    Large (more than 1.5 cm) adenoma (any site)
Inflammation
    Erosive esophagitis[†]
    Ulcer (any site)[†]
    Cameron lesions[‡]
    Erosive gastritis
    Celiac disease
    Ulcerative colitis
    Crohn's disease
    Colitis (nonspecific)
    Idiopathic cecal ulcer
Vascular disorders
    Vascular ectasia (any site)[†]
    Portal hypertensive gastropathy and colopathy
    Watermelon stomach
    Varices (any site)
    Hemangioma
    Dieulafoy's vascular malformation[§]
Infectious diseases
    Hookworm
    Whipworm
    Strongyloidiasis
    Ascariasis
    Tuberculosis enterocolitis
    Amebiasis
Surreptitious bleeding
    Hemoptysis
    Oropharyngeal bleeding (including epistaxis)
Other causes
    Hemosuccus pancreaticus
    Hemobilia
    Long-distance running
    Factitious cause

---

*Lesions that may lead to any form of occult gastrointestinal bleeding are listed here. Some lesions that may lead to recurrent obscure bleeding are not listed.

[†]These abnormalities are the most common.

[‡]These are linear erosions within a hiatus hernia.

[§]This is a large superficial artery underlying a small mucosal defect.

Rockey DC. Occult gastrointestinal bleeding. N Engl J Med 1999;341:40. Copyright ©1999 Massachusetts Medical Society. All rights reserved.

Collins JF, Lieberman DA, Durbin TE, Weiss DG. Accuracy of screening for fecal occult blood on a single stool sample obtained by digital rectal examination: a comparison with recommended sampling practice. Veterans Affairs Collaborative Study #380 Group. Ann Intern Med 2005;142:81–5.

Nahon S, Lahmek P, Lesgourgues B, Nahon-Uzan K, Tuszynski T, Traissac L, et al. Predictive factors of GI lesions in 241 women with iron deficiency anemia. Am J Gastroenterol 2002;97:590–3.

Rockey DC. Occult gastrointestinal bleeding. N Engl J Med 1999;341:38–46.

Zuckerman GR, Prakash C, Askin MP, Lewis BS. AGA technical review on the evaluation and management of occult and obscure gastrointestinal bleeding. Gastroenterology 2000;118:201–21.

# 33

## Diagnosis of postpartum depression

A 23-year-old woman at 6 weeks postpartum has had insomnia for 4 weeks. She had a medically uncomplicated pregnancy, labor, and delivery. She finds herself crying most of the day and lacks energy. She resents having to care for her newborn and feels overwhelmed by the responsibility. The most likely cause of her symptoms is

    (A) postpartum blues
    (B) postpartum psychosis
\*   (C) postpartum depression
    (D) bipolar disorder
    (E) posttraumatic stress disorder

Women are susceptible to a variety of psychiatric illnesses during the postpartum period. Because the obstetrician often sees the patient only 6 weeks after delivery, it is important to recognize the signs and symptoms of postpartum mood disorders and psychoses. Identification of risk factors can lead to earlier diagnosis and awareness. Many of these disorders also affect the mother–infant relationship significantly, giving further importance to early recognition and intervention.

Postpartum blues commonly occur in the first 4 days after delivery. Up to 75% of new mothers are affected by this transient mood disturbance. Common symptoms include mood lability and tearfulness. Other potential symptoms include anxiety, headache, and sleep disturbance. The condition is self-limited and most symptoms resolve by postpartum day 10. Treatment usually is supportive, with further intervention required if the symptoms extend beyond 2 weeks. Definitive diagnostic criteria or rating scales have not been developed for postpartum blues. The etiology is not understood, and risk factors have not been definitively identified. Postpartum blues do not appear to increase the risk of developing postpartum depression or other affective disorders. In the patient described, the duration of her symptoms excludes postpartum blues as an etiology.

Postpartum depression is characterized by a nonpsychotic depressive episode beginning in or extending into the postpartum period. The prevalence rate is 13%, making postpartum depression the most common psychiatric disorder of the puerperium. Criteria are identical to types of depression that occur at other time periods, which has sparked debate as to whether postpartum depression is a distinct entity. The *Diagnostic and Statistical Manual of Mental Disorders,* 4th edition (DSM-IV) criteria for depression are detailed in Box 33-1. Typically, the symptoms of postpartum depression begin within 4 weeks after delivery. The disease may have a more fluctuating course, and mood lability is often more common than for non-

postpartum depression. Other characteristics of postpartum depression can include severe anxiety, panic attacks, disinterest in the newborn, and insomnia. Guilt over feeling depressed during a time when most women are perceived to be happy is another feature observed in postpartum depression.

Pharmacologic therapies that have proven effective in the treatment of postpartum depression include sertraline hydrochloride (Zoloft), venlafaxine hydrochloride (Effexor), and fluoxetine hydrochloride (Prozac). Nonpharmacologic therapies useful to treat such depression include cognitive–behavioral therapy and interpersonal psychotherapy.

Postpartum psychosis occurs in 1–2 per 1,000 births. The risk of developing psychosis is highest in the first 30 days following delivery. Diagnostic criteria for psychosis

---

**BOX 33-1**

**Criteria for Major Depressive Episode**

Five or more of the following symptoms present during a 2-week period (at least two must include symptoms A and B below).

A. Depressed mood most of the day
B. Marked diminished interest or pleasure in daily activities
C. Significant weight loss or gain
D. Sleep disturbance
E. Psychomotor agitation or retardation
F. Fatigue
G. Feelings of worthlessness or excessive guilt
H. Diminished ability to think or concentrate
I. Recurrent thoughts of death or suicide

Modified from American Psychiatric Association. Diagnostic and statistical manual of mental disorders. 4th ed. Washington, DC: American Psychiatric Association; 1994. p. 327.

in the postpartum period do not differ from those during the rest of life, with the exception of time of onset. Women with postpartum psychosis often have associated manic symptoms including elation, mood lability, distractibility, and increased energy. The psychotic features include delusions and hallucinations. When compared to nonpostpartum psychosis, psychosis in the postpartum period is associated more frequently with features such as cognitive disorganization, bizarre behavior, and homicidal ideation. The disease may pose a risk to both mother and baby. In recent years, because of several high-profile tragic cases that have resulted in infanticide, considerable media attention has focused on the problem. Infanticide is a rare complication that occurs at a rate of 0.6–2.5 per 100,000 children. Treatment usually requires hospital admission; effective therapies include antipsychotic medication as well as mood stabilizers. The patient described in this question did not exhibit any psychotic features.

Bipolar disorder most commonly occurs in patients aged 20–30 years, with diagnosis occurring before age 50 years in more than 90% of those affected. The condition is defined by at least one manic episode, and most patients also will have a depressive episode. The manic episodes are characterized by heightened mood, flight of ideas, increased energy, pressured speech, and hyperactivity. Psychotic features commonly occur during manic episodes. The depressive episodes in bipolar disorder occur more acutely than in major depression. They tend to be heralded by psychomotor retardation, hyperphagia, and hypersomnolence. The depressive episode may be associated with delusions or hallucinations. The patient often will cycle between mania and depressive episodes over variable time courses. Acute treatment consists of use of mood stabilizing medications, such as lithium or carbamazepine often in combination with an antipsychotic drug. Although the patient described in this scenario did have symptoms consistent with depression, no manic features were described.

After a difficult delivery, posttraumatic stress disorder can manifest itself as a postpartum disorder that also can affect a subsequent pregnancy. The traumatic experience may result from pain, loss of control, or fear of death. The patient may develop a fear of labor, tension, nightmares, and flashbacks as labor approaches. Resultant sequelae include depression, an impaired mother–infant relationship, and sexual dysfunction. There was no evidence that the patient described had a traumatic birth experience or the resultant sequelae.

American Psychiatric Association. Diagnostic and statistical manual of mental disorders. 4th ed. Washington, DC: American Psychiatric Association; 1994. p. 320–7, 386–7.

Brockington I. Postpartum psychiatric disorders. Lancet 2004;363: 303–10.

Moore DP, Jefferson JW. Handbook of medical psychiatry. 2nd ed. Philadelphia (PA): Elsevier; 2004. p. 147–54.

Seyfried LS, Marcus SM. Postpartum mood disorders. Int Rev Psychiatry 2003;15:231–42.

# 34

## Treatment of chronic bronchitis

A 40-year-old woman with a history of smoking-related chronic bronchitis presents for the first time in 12 months with increased cough and dyspnea. She has no changes in her sputum production or sputum purulence. She has no other underlying health problems. In addition to reevaluation in 72 hours, the first step in therapy should be

* (A) observation
  (B) fluoroquinolone
  (C) amoxicillin/clavulanate
  (D) macrolide
  (E) extended spectrum cephalosporin

Chronic bronchitis is one of the manifestations of chronic obstructive pulmonary disease (COPD). It is a clinically diagnosed syndrome, defined as the presence of a productive cough on most days of the month for 3 months in each of the past 2 years. Chronic bronchitis occurs without other etiologies of chronic cough, such as lung cancer or tuberculosis. The most important causative factor is cigarette smoking. An acute exacerbation of chronic bronchitis is defined by patient-reported symptoms. These symptoms should reflect more than the day-to-day variation of chronic bronchitis symptoms. An acute exacerbation occurs when one or more of the following complaints are added to the chronic cough: increased dyspnea, increased sputum volume, increased sputum purulence. When all three symptoms are present, it is defined as a type 1 episode, with the worst prognosis. Type 2 has any two symptoms. Type 3 has only one symptom, and may be accompanied by other minor conditions, such as an upper respiratory tract infection.

The pathogenesis of an acute exacerbation of chronic bronchitis is varied. Anything that acutely increases airway inflammation can lead to bronchial wall edema, increased bronchial tone, and mucus production. Twenty percent of exacerbations are due to noninfectious stimuli, such as environmental pollutants, allergens, cigarette smoke, or noncompliance with medications. Fifty percent of exacerbations may be due to bacterial infections. The most common infecting aerobic bacteria include *Streptococcus pneumoniae, Haemophilus influenzae,* and *Moraxella catarrhalis. Pseudomonas aeruginosa* and other gram-negative bacilli occur with more severe exacerbations. Less than 10% of acute exacerbations are caused by atypical bacteria *(Chlamydophila pneumoniae, Mycoplasma pneumoniae,* and *Legionella pneumophila).* Up to 30% of exacerbations may be caused by viral infections, including influenza, parainfluenza, rhinovirus, respiratory syncytial virus, adenovirus, and meta pneumovirus.

The diagnosis is made clinically, with exclusion of pneumonia, congestive heart failure, pulmonary emboli, pneumothorax, drug interaction (such as tranquilizers), and upper respiratory infection. There are no characteristic physical findings of an exacerbation. Chest X-ray may be indicated to help exclude the diagnoses of congestive heart disease and pneumonia for patients seen in hospital emergency departments, and for hospitalized patients because physical findings exhibit significant interobserver disagreement. It is important to exclude pneumonia in the evaluation process.

Treatment is based on clinical severity of symptoms, comorbid conditions, and recent antibiotic use. Patients with mild acute exacerbations of chronic bronchitis (type 3) who have not had three or more exacerbations in the past year, have not been exposed to antibiotics in the past 3 months, and have no comorbidities can be observed without administering antibiotics. Antibiotics need to be added if there is worsening clinical status or inadequate response to supportive measures. Supportive treatments may include any combination of the following measures: removal of allergens, bronchodilator therapy, oxygen for hypoxemia, and oral or parenteral corticosteroids. There is no established role for mucolytics or leukotriene receptor antagonists. Patients with type 1 and 2 exacerbations (with two or more symptoms) should be treated with antibiotics. Patients with two or three of the cardinal symptoms (dyspnea, increased sputum volume, or increased sputum purulence) and simple COPD may be treated with a second-generation macrolide, ketolide, second- or third-generation cephalosporin, or doxycycline. Patients with complicated COPD (ie, forced expiratory volume in 1 second [$FEV_1$] of less than 50%), comorbid cardiac disease, three or more exacerbations in the previous 12 months, or antibiotics in the previous 3 months should be treated with a fluoroquinolone, or amoxicillin and clavulanate, or if the patient is at risk for pseudomonas, with ciprofloxacin. The choice of antibiotics is somewhat controversial, with patients exposed to antibiotics in the previous 3 months most likely to benefit from a fluoroquinolone. Knowledge of local susceptibility patterns may help to optimize antibacterial management. Older patients and immunocompromised patients require individualized evaluation and treatment because they are at higher risk for complications and failure of therapy. See Figure 34-1 for an algorithm of the risk-stratification approach to antibacterial therapy of acute exacerbations of COPD. In this patient with stable COPD, who is not elderly, not exposed to recent antibiotics, without increased sputum volume or purulence, and with only increased cough and dyspnea, antibiotics are not initially recommended. Rather, observation, removal of potential allergens, and symptomatic support are most appropriate initial treatments. She may require antibiotics if her condition worsens.

Acute bronchitis, in a patient without chronic bronchitis, also may be called acute tracheobronchitis, or a chest cold. It is usually viral in origin and does not respond to antibiotics. Acute tracheobronchitis may improve with inhaled β-agonist bronchodilators when wheezing is present. If acute, severe cough persists for more than 3 weeks, pertussis is found in approximately 20% of adults. A patient who coughs for 10–14 days may have *M pneumoniae* or *C pneumoniae* and may have improvement with a macrolide or doxycycline.

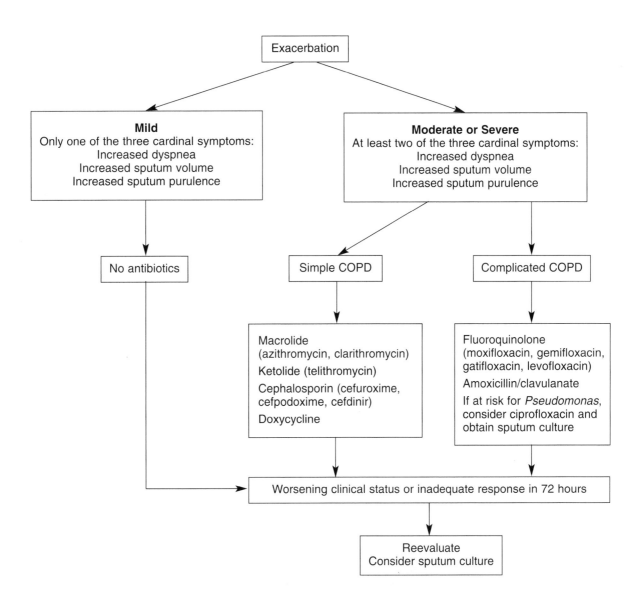

**FIG. 34-1**. Algorithm outlining a risk-stratification approach to antibacterial therapy of acute exacerbation of chronic obstructive pulmonary disease (COPD). (Modified from Sethi S, Murphy TF. Acute exacerbations of chronic bronchitis: new developments concerning microbiology and pathophysiology—impact on approaches to risk stratification and therapy. Infect Dis Clin North Am 2004;18:877. Copyright © 2004, with permission from Elsevier.)

Balter MS, La Forge J, Low DE, Mandell L, Grossman RF. Canadian guidelines for the management of acute exacerbations of chronic bronchitis. Canadian Thoracic Society, Canadian Infectious Disease Society. Can Respir J 2003;10(suppl B):3B–32B.

Brunton S, Carmichael BP, Colgan R, Feeney AS, Fendrick AM, Quintiliani R, et al. Acute exacerbation of chronic bronchitis: a primary care consensus guideline. Am J Manag Care 2004;10:689–96.

Dever LL, Shashikumar K, Johanson WG Jr. Antibiotics in the treatment of acute exacerbations of chronic bronchitis. Expert Opin Investig Drugs 2002;11:911–25.

Martinez FJ. Acute bronchitis: state of the art diagnosis and therapy. Compr Ther 2004;30:55–69.

Sethi S, Murphy TF. Acute exacerbations of chronic bronchitis: new developments concerning microbiology and pathophysiology—impact on approaches to risk stratification and therapy. Infect Dis Clin North Am 2004;18:861–82, ix.

Sethi S. Infectious etiology of acute exacerbations of chronic bronchitis. Chest 2000;117:380S–5S.

# 35

## New cytologic screening guidelines

A 65-year-old postmenopausal woman comes to the office for a health maintenance visit. Her last examination was 3 years ago. All three of her births were vaginal births. She had a hysterectomy for cervical carcinoma in situ at age 42 years. The pathology report from her hysterectomy was received and reviewed. Annual cytologic screening after her hysterectomy has been normal, including her most recent screening 3 years ago. Vasomotor symptoms indicate she went through menopause at age 53 years. She took combination hormone therapy for 3 years then discontinued. She complains of some vaginal dryness with sexual intercourse but reports no unusual vaginal discharge or bleeding. Based on her medical history, the most appropriate cytologic screening interval is

*    (A) no further screening necessary
      (B) annually
      (C) annually until negative three times then discontinue
      (D) every 3 years

Cervical cancer screening has been shown to be very effective. The rate of cervical cancer in the United States has steadily declined since the advent of the traditional Pap test in the 1950s. Although there are reasonably high rates of false-positive and false-negative results with cytologic screening, the relatively long premalignant stage of cervical cancer makes routine screening very effective; repeated screening over time diminishes the effect of false-negative tests. Ideal screening frequency is not clear although it has been demonstrated that annual screening does not offer an advantage in detecting high-grade dysplasia or worse conditions over screening every 2 or 3 years.

Cervical cancer develops in at-risk women who have been exposed to high-risk subtypes of human papillomavirus (HPV). The vulnerability of the cervix to this malignant change is highest during times of life where the transformation zone (area of squamous metaplasia) is most active, such as puberty. More frequent screening protocols should be implemented in younger women who are at higher risk and in women with significant risk factors (eg, multiple sexual partners and therefore higher risk of exposure to HPV, cigarette smoking, and immunocompromise).

A very low rate of cervical neoplasia is observed in postmenopausal women who have had normal regular screening before menopause. In the United States, the rate of cervical cancer plateaus at age 65 years. The American Cancer Society recommends discontinuation of screening at age 70 years in low-risk women. The U.S. Preventive Services Task Force recommends discontinuation at age 65 years. The American College of Obstetricians and Gynecologists (ACOG) has not stated a recommended upper limit for screening. The decision is left to physician discretion based on the risk factors.

Women in this older age group are believed to be at lower risk of neoplasia even when they are exposed to high-risk HPV due to the very low rate of metaplastic change on the menopausal cervix. The rate of vaginal cancer represents a very small fraction of gynecologic malignancies and occurs almost exclusively in patients who have had cervical neoplasia. Therefore, women who have had a hysterectomy and have no history of cervical neoplasia are at very low risk of a primary vaginal neoplasm. In this group, cytologic screening has a very low positive predictive value. A study of nearly 10,000 women who had had a hysterectomy for benign disease an average of 19 years earlier revealed a 1.1% rate of abnormal cytology, and none of the patients had vaginal intraepithelial neoplasia grade III or higher.

In women who have a history of cervical neoplasia and a hysterectomy, there is a possibility of developing vaginal neoplasia at the vaginal cuff, although this risk decreases over time. The recommendation of ACOG is that annual screening may be discontinued after three negative screens. The provider must be able to confirm, however, that there was no invasive disease at the time of hysterectomy, and cytopathology of the negative postoperative screening must be available to the provider to confirm negative status because patient recall of their status often is inaccurate. In addition, patients frequently underestimate the time interval since their last screening.

Given that this patient's hysterectomy was 23 years ago and she had normal cytology for many years postoperatively, it is safe to discontinue screening at this time. Due to the low positive predictive value of cytology in this clinical group, annual screening is not believed to be cost effective and may result in overtreatment and increased patient anxiety for its low yield.

American Cancer Society. Detailed guide: vaginal cancer. Can vaginal cancer be prevented. Available at: http://www.cancer.org/docroot/CRI/content/CRI_2_4_2X_Can_vaginal_cancer_be_prevented_55.asp. Retrieved August 27, 2005.

Cervical cytology screening. ACOG Practice Bulletin No. 45. American College of Obstetricians and Gynecologists. Obstet Gynecol 2003; 102:417–27.

Screening for cervical cancer. What's new from the USPSTF? AHRQ Publication No. APPIP03-0004. Rockville (MD): Agency for Healthcare Research and Quality; January 2003.

Sillman FH, Fruchter RG, Chen YS, Camilien L, Sedlis A, McTigue E. Vaginal intraepithelial neoplasia: risk factors for persistence, recurrence and invasion and its management. Am J Obstet Gynecol 1997;176:93–9.

U.S. Preventive Services Task Force. Screening for cervical cancer. Available at http://www.ahrq.gov/clinic/3rduspstf/cervcan/cervcanwh.htm. Retrieved August 27, 2005.

# 36

## Screening interval for cholesterol

A 50-year-old woman with type 2 diabetes mellitus undergoes serum cholesterol screening. She has no history of coronary heart disease (CHD) or hypertension and does not smoke. There is no family history of premature CHD. Her high-density lipoprotein (HDL) level is 50 mg/dL and her low-density lipoprotein (LDL) cholesterol level is 200 mg/dL. Optimal management involves decreasing her LDL cholesterol level, not to exceed

* (A) 100 mg/dL
  (B) 130 mg/dL
  (C) 160 mg/dL
  (D) 190 mg/dL

Hyperlipidemia is an important risk factor for the development of coronary artery disease in women. In 1996, the National Cholesterol Education Program provided screening guidelines for the detection of high cholesterol levels in adults (Adult Treatment Panel [ATP I]). These guidelines have twice been updated and modified. The ATP I outlined a strategy for primary prevention of CHD in individuals with LDL cholesterol higher than 160 mg/dL or borderline (130–159 mg/dL) LDL cholesterol with two risk factors. The second Adult Treatment Panel (ATP II) confirmed this and added intensive management of LDL cholesterol in persons with established CHD, establishing a lower goal of 100 mg/dL or less. The third Adult Treatment Panel guidelines (ATP III), published in 2001, has added diabetes mellitus as a CHD equivalent in terms of risk and approach to LDL cholesterol goals. The ATP III also identifies persons with metabolic syndrome as candidates for intensive lifestyle changes, recommends a complete lipoprotein panel as the preferred initial test rather than just HDL and total cholesterol, and encourages use of fiber and plant stanols and sterols to lower LDL cholesterol. The lower limit of normal HDL cholesterol was raised to 40 mg/dL and the triglyceride cutpoint was lowered.

Screening is recommended every 5 years for patients older than 20 years. The classifications for LDL, total, and HDL cholesterol are presented in Table 36-1. A total cholesterol level of less than 200 mg/dL is regarded as desirable, and levels higher than 240 mg/dL are high. An HDL cholesterol level below 40 mg/dL is considered a risk factor for CHD.

**TABLE 36-1.** ATP III Classification of Low-Density Lipoprotein (LDL), Total, and High-Density Lipoprotein (HDL) Cholesterol

| Cholesterol Level (mg/dL) | Classification |
|---|---|
| LDL cholesterol | |
| Less than 100 | Optimal |
| 100–129 | Near optimal/above optimal |
| 130–159 | Borderline high |
| 160–189 | High |
| 190 or higher | Very high |
| Total cholesterol | |
| Less than 200 | Desirable |
| 200–239 | Borderline high |
| 240 or higher | High |
| HDL cholesterol | |
| Less than 40 | Low |
| 60 or higher | High |

Executive Summary of the Third Report of the National Cholesterol Education Program (NCEP) Expert Panel on Detection, Evaluation, and Treatment of High Blood Cholesterol in Adults (Adult Treatment Panel III). JAMA 2001;285:2488.

Patient evaluation should begin with measurement of lipoprotein levels and assessment of risk factors. There are three general categories of risk:

1. The highest risk category includes individuals with CHD and its risk equivalents. Diabetes mellitus is listed as a CHD risk equivalent. Other CHD risk equivalents include other forms of atherosclerotic disease, abdominal aortic aneurysm, carotid artery disease, and peripheral arterial disease, as well as any combination of risk factors that confers a 10-year risk of CHD greater than 20% by Framingham Heart Disease Study risk scoring.

2. The second highest risk category includes patients with multiple risk factors in whom the 10-year risk is less than 20%. These risk factors are listed in Box 36-1. An HDL cholesterol level of 60 mg/dL or greater is a negative risk factor and removes one risk factor from the total count, decreasing the overall risk.

3. The third highest risk category are patients with one risk factor or less.

The treatment goals for each risk category are listed in Table 36-2.

The fact that the patient described has diabetes mellitus puts her at the same risk factor level as someone with coronary artery disease, even though she has none of the other major risk factors that modify LDL goals. She

---

**BOX 36-1**

**Major Risk Factors* That Modify Low-Density Lipoprotein [LDL] Goals**

Cigarette smoking

Hypertension (blood pressure 140/90 mm Hg or higher) or on antihypertensive medication

Low high-density lipoprotein (HDL) cholesterol (less than 40 mg/dL)[†]

Family history of premature coronary heart disease (CHD) (in male first-degree relative younger than 55 years; in female first-degree relative younger than 65 years)

Age (men 45 years or older; women 55 years or older)

*In ATP III, diabetes mellitus is regarded as a CHD risk equivalent.

[†]HDL cholesterol of 60 mg/dL or higher is regarded as a CHD risk equivalent.

Executive Summary of the Third Report of the National Cholesterol Education Program (NCEP) Expert Panel on Detection, Evaluation, and Treatment of High Blood Cholesterol in Adults (Adult Treatment Panel III). JAMA 2001;285:2488.

---

**TABLE 36-2.** Three Categories of Risk that Modify Low-Density Lipoprotein (LDL) Cholesterol Goals

| Risk Category | Goal (mg/dL) |
|---|---|
| Coronary heart disease (CHD) and CHD equivalents | Less than 100 |
| Two or more risk factors | Less than 130 |
| Zero to one risk factor | Less than 160 |

Executive Summary of the Third Report of the National Cholesterol Education Program (NCEP) Expert Panel on Detection, Evaluation, and Treatment of High Blood Cholesterol in Adults (Adult Treatment Panel III). JAMA 2001;285:2489.

should be treated aggressively with a goal of LDL cholesterol less than 100 mg/dL (Table 36-2). Treatment options for all patients should include lifestyle changes such as reduced intake of fat and cholesterol, increased physical activity, and weight control. Drug therapy can consist of 5-hydroxy-3-methylglutaryl-coenzyme A (HMG-CoA) reductase inhibitors or statins, bile acid sequestrants, nicotinic acid, and fibric acids.

Executive Summary of the Third Report of the National Cholesterol Education Program (NCEP) Expert Panel on Detection, Evaluation, and Treatment of High Blood Cholesterol in Adults (Adult Treatment Panel III). JAMA 2001;285:2486–97.

# 37

## Diagnosis of insulin resistance

A 45-year-old woman presents for a periodic health care maintenance visit. Her physical examination shows a blood pressure of 140/95 mm Hg. Her height is 165 cm and weight is 81.8 kg. Her waist circumference is 90 cm and her body mass index (BMI) (weight in kilograms divided by height in meters squared [kg/m²]) is 29.1. Her serum triglyceride level is 180 mg/dL, serum high-density lipoprotein (HDL) cholesterol level is 30 mg/dL, and fasting plasma glucose level is 120 mg/dL. The patient is at increased risk for

  (A) Addison's disease
\* (B) type 2 diabetes mellitus
  (C) hypothyroidism
  (D) Cushing's syndrome
  (E) hepatitis

The patient meets the five criteria for diagnosis of metabolic syndrome (Appendix B). A similar profile can be seen in individuals who have abdominal obesity but who do not have an excess of total body weight. Insulin resistance may lead to vascular endothelial dysfunction, an abnormal lipid profile, hypertension, and vascular inflammation, all of which promote the development of atherosclerotic cardiovascular (CV) disease. Other names applied to this constellation of findings have included syndrome X, the insulin resistance syndrome, or the obesity dyslipidemia syndrome. Genetic predisposition, lack of exercise, and body fat distribution all affect the likelihood that a given obese subject will become overtly diabetic or develop CV disease.

Other factors associated with an increased risk of metabolic syndrome in the third National Health and Nutrition Examination Survey (NHANES III) included postmenopausal status, smoking, high carbohydrate diet, no alcohol consumption, and physical inactivity. Data from NHANES III demonstrated that the prevalence of metabolic syndrome has continued to increase, particularly in women.

Metabolic syndrome results from the negative effects of abdominal obesity that acts essentially as a separate endocrine organ. It is associated with resistance to the effects of insulin on peripheral glucose and fatty acid utilization, and it often leads to diabetes mellitus type 2, especially among women. Metabolic syndrome increases the relative risk for incident diabetes by 2.1-fold according to the National Cholesterol Education Program (Adult Treatment Panel [ATP] III) definition of diabetes and by 3.6-fold using the World Health Organization (WHO) definition.

Metabolic syndrome is also a risk factor for incident CV disease and mortality. Among patients with metabolic syndrome at baseline in the ATP III, a 4.2-fold increased relative risk of mortality from coronary heart disease was observed and a 2.0-fold increased relative risk of all-cause mortality compared to those without the syndrome. In a report of 780 women from the Women's Ischemia Syndrome Evaluation (WISE) study, metabolic syndrome, but not BMI alone, was significantly associated with the subsequent 3-year risk of death or major adverse cardiovascular events. Many of these studies accounted for age, sex, smoking, and serum low-density lipoprotein (LDL) cholesterol in the analysis. However, it remains unresolved whether diagnosis of metabolic syndrome or measurement of insulin resistance adds to CV disease risk prediction beyond currently recommended CV disease risk calculators.

Metabolic syndrome has also been associated with several obesity-related disorders including polycystic ovary syndrome, fatty liver disease with steatosis, fibrosis, and cirrhosis; chronic kidney disease and microalbuminuria; and obstructive sleep apnea. Metabolic syndrome is not associated with Addison's disease, hypothyroidism, Cushing's syndrome, or hepatitis.

Conus F, Allison DB, Rabasa-Lhoret R, St-Onge M, St-Pierre DH, Tremblay-Lebeau A, et al. Metabolic and behavioral characteristics of metabolically obese but normal-weight women. J Clin Endocrinol Metab 2004;89:5013–20.

Ford ES, Giles WH, Mokdad AH. Increasing prevalence of the metabolic syndrome among U.S. adults. Diabetes Care 2004;27:2444–9.

Grundy SM, Cleeman JI, Daniels SR, Donato KA, Eckel RH, Franklin BA, et al. Diagnosis and management of the metabolic syndrome: an American Heart Association/National Heart, Lung, and Blood Institute Scientific Statement. American Heart Association; National Heart, Lung, and Blood Institute [published errata appear in Circulation 2005;112:e297; Circulation 2005;112:e298]. Circulation 2005;112:2735–52.

Kip KE, Marroquin OC, Kelley DE, Johnson BD, Kelsey SF, Shaw LJ, et al. Clinical importance of obesity versus the metabolic syndrome in cardiovascular risk in women: a report from the Women's Ischemia Syndrome Evaluation (WISE) study. Circulation 2004;109:706–13.

Park YW, Zhu S, Palaniappan L, Heshka S, Carnethon MR, Heymsfield SB. The metabolic syndrome: prevalence and associated risk factor findings in the US population from the Third National Health and Nutrition Examination Survey, 1988–1994. Arch Intern Med 2003;163:427–36.

# 38

## Methotrexate therapy and tubal ectopic pregnancy

A 33-year-old woman with an ectopic pregnancy was treated with a single intramuscular dose of methotrexate 7 days ago. Serum $\beta$-hCG titer on day 4 posttreatment was 4,086 mIU/mL, and the titer today is 3,603 mIU/mL. The best next step in management is

        (A) repeat $\beta$-hCG titer in 4 days
        (B) repeat $\beta$-hCG titer in 7 days
*    (C) repeat intramuscular injection of methotrexate
        (D) dilation and curettage (D&C)

Earlier detection of ectopic pregnancies has allowed for the emergence of medical treatment instead of surgery. Small unruptured ectopic pregnancies are effectively treated with intramuscular methotrexate. The doses used to treat ectopic pregnancy have few side effects, and success rates for single-dose regimens are approximately 84%. The potential for tubal rupture and hemorrhage exists with the use of methotrexate therapy. Thus, the patient must understand the need for close follow-up, and the clinician must be vigilant in the post-methotrexate surveillance to detect failures before tubal rupture occurs.

Criteria for the use of methotrexate include size of the adnexal or ectopic mass, presence of rupture, and desire for future fertility (Box 38-1). Gestational sac size greater than 3.5 cm is a relative contraindication to use of methotrexate as is presence of embryonic cardiac activity. High $\beta$-hCG titers, variably defined in the literature as from

**BOX 38-1**

**Criteria for Using Methotrexate to Treat Ectopic Pregnancy**

Absolute indications
* Patient is hemodynamically stable without active bleeding or signs of hemoperitoneum.
* Diagnosis is nonlaparoscopic.
* Patient desires future fertility.
* General anesthesia poses a significant risk.
* Patient is able to return for follow-up care.
* Patient has no contraindication to methotrexate.

Relative indications
* Unruptured mass is 3.5 cm or larger at its greatest dimension.
* No fetal cardiac motion is detected.
* Patient's $\beta$-hCG level does not exceed a predetermined value (6,000–15,000 mIU/mL).

American College of Obstetricians and Gynecologists. Medical management of tubal pregnancy. ACOG Practice Bulletin 3. Washington, DC: ACOG; 1998. p. 3.

6,000 to 15,000 mIU/mL, may increase the risk for methotrexate failure but are not an absolute contraindication to its use. Coexisting medical conditions, such as alcoholism, liver disease, blood dyscrasias, immunodeficiency, and peptic ulcer disease, represent absolute contraindications to use of medical therapy.

Methotrexate is administered intramuscularly after ensuring that renal, liver, and bone marrow functions are normal. Dosing usually is calculated based on body surface area. A dose of 50 mg/m$^2$ of methotrexate is given if the single-dose regimen is used. Another successful regimen uses alternating doses of methotrexate with leucovorin calcium over the course of 8 days. Conflicting data in regard to the comparative effectiveness of these two regimens exist in the published literature.

Follow-up after the single-dose regimen requires $\beta$-hCG titers to be drawn 4 days postinjection and 7 days postinjection. The patient's $\beta$-hCG titers increase following methotrexate injection and peak after 4 days (Fig. 38-1). Her $\beta$-hCG titer should decline by 7 days postinjection. If a decline of 15% is not seen between day 4 and day 7, further treatment is required. The treatment options are to repeat the single dose of intramuscular methotrexate with the same follow-up surveillance as with the first dose, or to perform surgery. If there is an appropriate decrease in $\beta$-hCG titers between day 4 and day 7, the $\beta$-hCG titers should be followed weekly until undetectable. In the case described, the patient's $\beta$-hCG titer decreased by 11%. Thus, repeat dosing with methotrexate is indicated. Surgical management would provide another viable treatment option.

Patients who receive medical therapy should be monitored for signs and symptoms of treatment failure. Such signs or symptoms include significantly worsening abdominal pain, hemodynamic instability, or lack of an appropriate $\beta$-hCG response. Up to two thirds of patients will experience abdominal pain but show no signs of tubal rupture. Worsening abdominal pain may be investigated by pelvic ultrasonography specifically looking for free fluid in the pelvis or an expanding complex mass in

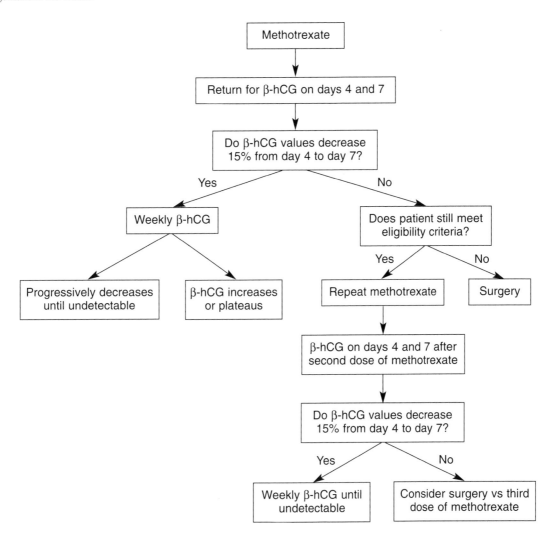

**FIG. 38-1.** Flow diagram of the follow-up after single-dose methotrexate therapy for ectopic pregnancy. (Adapted from University of Texas Medical Branch, Department of Obstetrics and Gynecology. Ectopic pregnancy clinical practice guideline/critical pathway. Galveston (TX): University of Texas Medical Branch, Galveston, Texas; 1997.)

the adnexa. Measurement of hemoglobin and hematocrit also would be indicated in the evaluation of a patient with abdominal pain after methotrexate treatment.

Dilation and curettage (D&C) often is indicated in the evaluation of ectopic pregnancy. When the β-hCG titer is above the discriminatory zone for detection of a viable intrauterine pregnancy by ultrasonography and no such pregnancy is identified, D&C is useful to discriminate between a nonviable intrauterine pregnancy and an ectopic gestation. The discriminatory zone is the range of serum β-hCG concentrations above which a normal intrauterine pregnancy can be visualized by ultrasonography. An intrauterine gestational sac in a normal uterus can be visualized when the β-hCG titer exceeds 1,000–2,000 mIU/mL. When the β-hCG titer exceeds the discriminatory zone, the absence of an intrauterine gestational sac is suggestive of

ectopic pregnancy, but this can occur with multiple gestation or failed intrauterine pregnancy.

American College of Obstetricians and Gynecologists. Medical management of tubal pregnancy. ACOG Practice Bulletin 3. Washington, DC: ACOG; 1998.

Barnhart KT, Gosman G, Ashby R, Sammel M. The medical management of ectopic pregnancy: a meta-analysis comparing "single dose" and "multidose" regimens. Obstet Gynecol 2003;101:778–84.

Lipscomb GH, Givens VM, Meyer NL, Bran D. Comparison of multidose and single-dose methotrexate protocols for the treatment of ectopic pregnancy. Am J Obstet Gynecol 2005;192:1844–7; discussion 1847–8.

Lipscomb GH, McCord ML, Stovall TG, Huff G, Portera SG, Ling FW. Predictors of success of methotrexate treatment in women with tubal ectopic pregnancies. N Engl J Med 1999;341:1974–8.

Tawfiq A, Agameya AF, Claman P. Predictors of treatment failure for ectopic pregnancy treated with single-dose methotrexate. Fertil Steril 2000;74:877–80.

# 39

## Coding for a counseling visit

A patient returns to your office to discuss her longstanding oligomenorrhea and infertility. You discuss the results of the laboratory studies obtained at the last visit, including thyroid-stimulating hormone, prolactin, follicle-stimulating hormone, luteinizing hormone, and fasting glucose to insulin ratio. You also discuss the results of a pelvic ultrasound examination. You tell the patient that her diagnosis is polycystic ovary syndrome with insulin resistance and discuss how this relates to the symptoms she is experiencing, her family history, and treatment options, including ovulation induction and referral to a reproductive endocrinologist. The key element for coding the evaluation and management (E/M) level of this visit is

* (A) medical and family history
  (B) physical examination
  (C) complexity of medical decision making
* (D) face-to-face time
  (E) coordination of care

The patient described presented for a counseling visit that involved mostly education about her diagnosis and the options she faced. The term counseling refers to discussion with the patient or family of the following:

- Diagnostic results
- Prognosis
- Treatment options
- Instructions
- Risk factor reduction
- Patient and family education

In the setting where counseling, with or without coordination of care, involves more than 50% of the face-to-face time with the physician, coding for the E/M level is based on time. In order to use time to determine the level of service, the following must be documented in the medical record:

- Extent of counseling
- Amount of time spent counseling
- Total time for the visit

The time spent coordinating care with other members of the health care team, in this case with the reproductive endocrinologist, is not included in the face-to-face time spent with the patient. This type of non-face-to-face time was taken into account when calculating the total work involved in a typical encounter and is included in the service. The difficulty in tracking and documenting such non-face-to-face time led to a decision to use solely face-to-face time as the basis for the E/M levels in the outpatient setting. In the hospital or nursing facility, the time factor is based on the total time in the patient care unit.

Physical examination and history taking were completed during a previous encounter and do not enter into coding decisions for this visit. Likewise, although the complexity of medical decision making in this case may be considered moderate or extensive, this is reflected in the time spent explaining the diagnosis and treatment options and is thus compensated appropriately using a time-based E/M level. The same holds true for the nature of the presenting problem.

American College of Obstetricians and Gynecologists. CPT coding in obstetrics and gynecology—2004. Washington, DC: ACOG; 2003.

American College of Obstetricians and Gynecologists. Frequently asked questions in obstetric and gynecologic coding. 2nd ed. Washington, DC: ACOG; 2005.

American Medical Association. Current procedural terminology—2005. Chicago (IL): AMA; 2004.

# 40

## Evaluation of hematuria

A 50-year-old asymptomatic woman is found to have five red blood cells per high-power field on a routine urinalysis. The test also noted the presence of proteinuria but was otherwise unremarkable. Urine culture was negative. A 24-hour urine protein collection showed 400 mg of protein. The most likely cause of her hematuria and proteinuria is

　　　　(A) bladder cancer
　　*　(B) glomerulonephritis
　　　　(C) hemolysis
　　　　(D) renal lithiasis
　　　　(E) interstitial cystitis

The value of routine urinalysis as a screening test for bladder cancer or asymptomatic bacteriuria is questioned and the test is not recommended by the U.S. Preventive Services Task Force. Such screening for infection is reasonable in high-risk groups such as pregnant women. Microscopic hematuria is defined as 3–5 erythrocytes per high-power field, and is relatively common, with a prevalence of 2–5%. Dipstick testing is not sufficiently specific and is too sensitive to be used as the basis for initiating evaluation. The risk of serious urologic disease in asymptomatic patients with microscopic hematuria is low, approximately 2%.

In women, urinary tract infection should be ruled out early by culture. The urinalysis should be repeated a few days later before any workup is initiated. If persistent hematuria is found, whether routinely or secondary to symptoms, the initial step is to look for findings suggestive of glomerular disease. Proteinuria or casts should prompt measurement of serum creatinine, blood urea nitrogen (BUN), creatinine clearance, and complete blood count. More than 300 mg of protein in 24 hours suggests the kidney is the source of the hematuria. Figures 40-1 and 40-2 show the initial evaluation and urologic evaluation of asymptomatic microscopic hematuria for low- and high-risk patients, respectively. Low-risk patients are younger than 40 years and have negative histories for smoking, chemical exposure, irritative voiding symptoms, and gross hematuria.

In a study with renal biopsy of patients in whom no other source of hematuria was identified, 16% had a glomerular source. Immunoglobulin (Ig) A nephropathy was the most common source of hematuria.

The remainder of the evaluation should address an assessment of the collecting tract. Possible diagnoses include benign and malignant tumors of the bladder, ureters, or kidney; renal lithiasis; polycystic kidney disease; trauma; vascular malformations; and interstitial cystitis. Other causes can include strenuous exercise and thin basement membrane disease. In the presence of proteinuria, the other options are less likely. Although hematuria can be detected with hemolysis, intact red cells are not seen. Cancers account for approximately 5% and are more common in women older than 65 years, smokers, phenacetin users, and individuals with occupational exposure to chemicals in the leather, dye, and rubber industries.

Evaluation should include assessment of the lower and upper urinary tracts. Cystourethroscopy permits direct visualization and biopsy of strictures, stones, diverticulae, trabeculation, inflammation, and tumors. Using an intravenous pyelogram is the traditional method of imaging the entire renal system, but ultrasonography is safer, less expensive, and appropriate for use during pregnancy. It is being replaced in some centers with a computerized tomography urogram without contrast, which is more sensitive for the presence of stones. Cytology of voided urine is less sensitive but more specific than cystoscopy for the detection of bladder cancer.

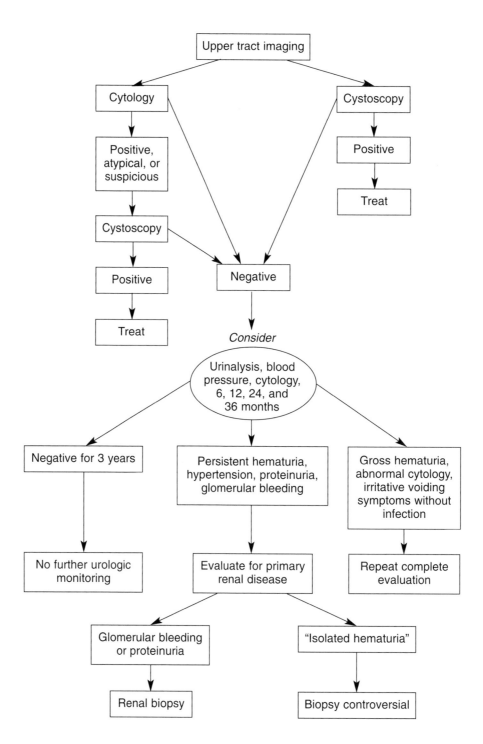

**FIG. 40-1.** Suggested follow-up regimen for low-risk patients with asymptomatic microscopic hematuria and an initial negative urologic evaluation. (Modified from Grossfeld GD, Wolf JS Jr, Litwin MS, Hricak H, Shuler CL, Agerter DC, et al. Evaluation of asymptomatic microscopic hematuria in adults: the American Urological Association best practice policy—part II: patient evaluation, cytology, voided markers, imaging, cystoscopy, nephrology evaluation, and follow-up. Urology 2001; 57:609.)

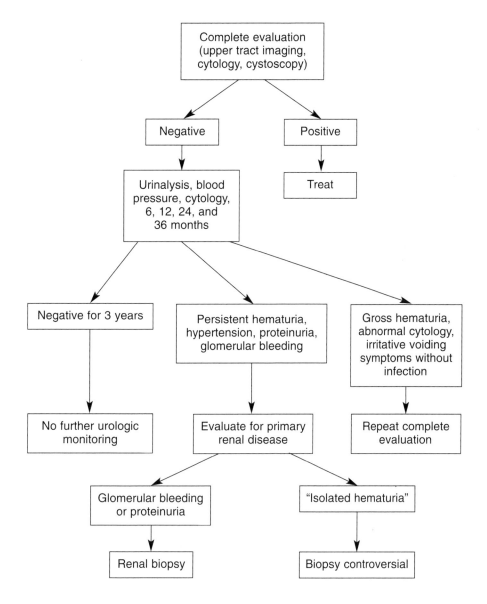

**FIG. 40-2.** Suggested follow-up regimen for high-risk patients with asymptomatic microscopic hematuria and an initial negative urologic evaluation. (Modified from Grossfeld GD, Wolf JS Jr, Litwin MS, Hricak H, Shuler CL, Agerter DC, et al. Evaluation of asymptomatic microscopic hematuria in adults: the American Urological Association best practice policy—part II: patient evaluation, cytology, voided markers, imaging, cystoscopy, nephrology evaluation, and follow-up. Urology 2001;57:609.)

Cohen RA, Brown RS. Clinical practice. Microscopic hematuria. N Engl J Med 2003;348:2330–8.

Grossfeld GD, Litwin MS, Wolf JS, Hricak H, Shuler CL, Agerter DC, et al. Evaluation of asymptomatic microscopic hematuria in adults: the American Urological Association best practice policy—part I: definition, detection, prevalence, and etiology. Urology 2001; 57:599–603.

Grossfeld GD, Litwin MS, Wolf JS Jr, Hricak H, Shuler CL, Agerter DC, et al. Evaluation of asymptomatic microscopic hematuria in adults:

the American Urological Association best practice policy—part II: patient evaluation, cytology, voided markers, imaging, cystoscopy, nephrology evaluation, and follow-up. Urology 2001;57:604–10.

Grossfeld GD, Wolf JS Jr, Litwin MS, Hricak H, Shuler CL, Agerter DC, et al. Asymptomatic microscopic hematuria in adults: summary of the AUA best practice policy recommendations. Am Fam Physician 2001;63:1145–54.

Sutton JM. Evaluation of hematuria in adults. JAMA 1990;263: 2475–80.

# 41

## Mortality data in adolescents

A distraught mother tells you of her concerns about her 16-year-old daughter's increasingly reckless behavior and attitude. She has come home intoxicated on several occasions, frequently seems sullen, withdrawn, and depressed, and her grades in school have dropped. A week ago, she was involved in a minor automobile accident. She has been associating with gang members and her most recent boyfriend has abused her. The mother believes the girl is sexually active and also using illegal substances. She is afraid "something might happen" to her daughter. You agree that her daughter's pattern of behavior is of concern and counsel her that a girl of her age has the greatest risk of mortality from

* (A) motor vehicle accident
(B) homicide
(C) suicide
(D) drug overdose

Adolescence is a time of growth and burgeoning autonomy as teenagers transition from childhood to adulthood. Adolescents tend to be a healthy subgroup of the population and death is infrequent. However, immaturity and a sense of invulnerability can drive many adolescents to partake in risky and potentially fatal behaviors. Up to 70% of all deaths in adolescents and young adults can be attributed to one of four causes:

1. Motor vehicle accident

2. Homicide

3. Suicide

4. Other accidental death

Death from a motor vehicle accident has traditionally been the most common cause of mortality among adolescents, both male and female. Even though the mortality rate has been decreasing over the past 20 years, motor vehicle accidents continue to be the leading cause of death among adolescents and young adults regardless of race, ethnicity, and sex. Thrill-seeking behaviors and lack of foresight frequently lead adolescents to drive in an unsafe and dangerous manner.

Greater awareness of seat belt use and the dangers of driving under the influence have contributed to the decline in mortality from accidents. Unfortunately, motor vehicle accidents still account for 32–43% of all deaths in adolescent girls and young women. Alcohol and illegal substances are a frequent companion to such behaviors and compound the problem. Up to 30% of all adolescents admit to riding in an automobile with an intoxicated driver, and 12% admit to driving while intoxicated.

Homicide and suicide are increasingly common among adolescent girls and account for 8–11% of mortality in all females aged 15–24 years. Although broad characterizations across racial categories are problematic, statistics show that African-American adolescent girls show a greater percentage of homicide deaths than suicide; however, the reverse is true for white and Hispanic girls. The percentage of adolescent girls that have considered suicide is significantly higher among whites and Hispanics than African Americans, as are the numbers who are successful in their attempts. Hispanic adolescents in particular are more apt to consider and attempt suicide than any other racial and ethnic grouping. Among white adolescent girls, suicide is responsible for a greater number of deaths than homicide. Although substance abuse is common among teenagers of all ages and ethnicity, actual death from drug overdose remains uncommon (Fig. 41-1; see color plate). For the adolescent described, counseling by a professional counselor is advisable.

Centers for Disease Control and Prevention, National Centers for Injury Prevention and Control. Web-based Injury Statistics Query and Reporting System (WISQARS). Available at: http://www.cdc.gov/ncipc/wisqars/. Retrieved June 4, 2005.

Federal Interagency Forum on Child and Family Statistics. America's children: key national indicators of well-being, 2005. Federal Interagency Forum on Child and Family Statistics. Washington, DC: U.S. Government Printing Office; 2005.

Grunbaum JA, Kann L, Kinchen S, Ross J, Hawkins J, Lowry R, et al. Youth risk behavior surveillance—United States, 2003 [published errata appear in MMWR Morb Mortal Wkly Rep 2004;53:536; MMWR Morb Mortal Wkly Rep 2005;54:608]. MMWR Surveill Summ 2004; 53(2):1–96.

# 42

## Graves' disease in nonpregnant women

A 32-year-old woman, gravida 1, para 1, returns for follow-up of her Graves' disease 1 year after giving birth. The condition was diagnosed at 14 weeks of gestation when she presented with palpitations, heat intolerance, and a small, symmetric goiter. Her laboratory test results at that time showed a thyroid-stimulating hormone (TSH) level of 0.01 µU/mL, free thyroxine ($T_4$) level of 4.7 ng/mL, and the presence of thyrotropin receptor antibodies. She is being treated with low-dose propylthiouracil (PTU) with normalization of her $T_4$ and TSH. She is on no other medication. She recently finished breastfeeding and is ready to conceive another child. She wishes to stop the PTU. Her examination is unremarkable with a normal-sized, nontender thyroid. The best management for this patient is to stop PTU and to

*   (A) follow serial laboratory test results
    (B) start methimazole (Tapazole)
    (C) treat with radioactive iodine
    (D) add a β-blocker
    (E) refer for thyroidectomy

Graves' disease is the most common cause of hyperthyroidism. Onset typically occurs between ages 30 and 40 years, and risk is highest for women, patients with a family history of Graves' disease, and individuals with other autoimmune disorders. The disease is an autoimmune process in which antibodies formed act on the TSH receptor and stimulate the thyroid gland without a negative feedback system. Graves' disease presents with common symptoms of hyperthyroidism and a diffusely enlarged thyroid gland that is usually soft and symmetric (Box 42-1). Patients with Graves' disease often have features related to the immune system that are not seen in other forms of thyrotoxicosis, such as ophthalmopathy, orbitopathy, or dermopathy. Most patients have a very low or undetectable TSH or serum thyrotropin and high serum concentrations of $T_4$ and triiodothyronine ($T_3$). Approximately 90% of patients with Graves' disease will have thyrotropin receptor antibodies present although the diagnosis frequently is made without this test when the classic manifestations are present.

When hyperthyroidism occurs in pregnancy, Graves' disease is the cause in 85–90% of patients. Medical therapy is the preferred treatment in pregnancy with PTU being the drug of choice in the United States. Studies have shown that methimazole has been associated with aplasia cutis. Radioiodine is contraindicated in pregnancy, and surgery requires pretreatment with antithyroid drugs to render the patient euthyroid.

In pregnancy, antithyroid drugs cross the placenta. Pregnancy itself usually does have an ameliorating effect on Graves' disease with the dose of antithyroid drugs required often decreasing as pregnancy progresses. Complications of uncontrolled hyperthyroidism include miscarriage, placental abruption, low birth weight, preeclampsia, and preterm delivery. In addition, congestive heart failure and thyroid storm may occur. Patients initially need counseling and education about the risks of hyperthyroidism and the effects on maternal and fetal well-being. Obstetricians may follow and treat hyperthyroidism in pregnancy, but questions of treatment following pregnancy often remain.

In most parts of the world and in pregnancy, antithyroid drugs are the treatment of choice for Graves' disease. The decision to use antithyroid drugs as primary treatment must be weighed against the risks and benefits of the more definitive therapy with radioiodine or surgery. The preference of the patient is paramount in the decision process.

This patient has completed 1 year of antithyroid therapy and now desires conception. It would be safe and acceptable to discontinue PTU and to monitor thyroid function for possible recurrence (Fig. 42-1). The risk of recurrence after being euthyroid on antithyroid medications is 30–50%. Exact markers for recurrence cannot be predicted but many retrospective studies show that patients with severe degrees of hyperthyroidism, including large goiters and high levels of antithyrotropin-receptor antibodies, have a lower likelihood of remission. Patients with milder disease and smaller goiters are felt to have higher remission rates. If a patient discontinues therapy, lifelong follow-up is required in case of recurrence and because spontaneous hypothyroidism can develop in some patients even decades later.

In patients who elect to have radioactive iodine therapy, recommendations are to wait for 6 months after treatment to allow thyroid function to normalize before conception.

Antithyroid drugs are usually stopped for approximately 1 week prior to radioiodine treatment. The patient is then followed every 4–6 weeks until the patient is euthyroid and clinically stable. Most patients actually become hypothyroid within 3 months requiring full thyroid replacement, but up to 20% will require a second dose of radioiodine.

Beta-blockers play an important role in the management of Graves' disease, but not in the euthyroid state or as prevention. They are used in the acute setting to alleviate and provide relief from symptoms such as palpitations, anxiety, tremor, and heat intolerance. Surgery usually is reserved for patients who are intolerant to antithyroid drugs, have large goiters, or have suspicion of malignancy.

---

**BOX 42-1**

**The Six Basic Signs and Symptoms of Graves' Disease**

General
  Weight loss
  Heat intolerance
  Thyroid enlargement
  Increased gastrointestinal motility
  Weakness
  Insomnia
Cardiorespiratory
  Tachycardia
  Atrial fibrillation
  Shortness of breath
  Systolic murmur
Ocular
  Burning
  Irritation
  Proptosis
  Decreased blinking

Dermatologic
  Pruritus
  Warm and moist skin
  Alopecia
  Sweating
  Separation of nail from nail bed
Central nervous system
  Anxiety
  Agitation
  Restlessness
  Emotional lability
  Memory loss
  Hyperreflexia
Reproductive
  Oligomenorrhea
  Amenorrhea
  Gynecomastia
  Decreased libido

Streetman DD, Khanderia U. Diagnosis and treatment of Graves disease. Ann Pharmacother 2003;37:1101.

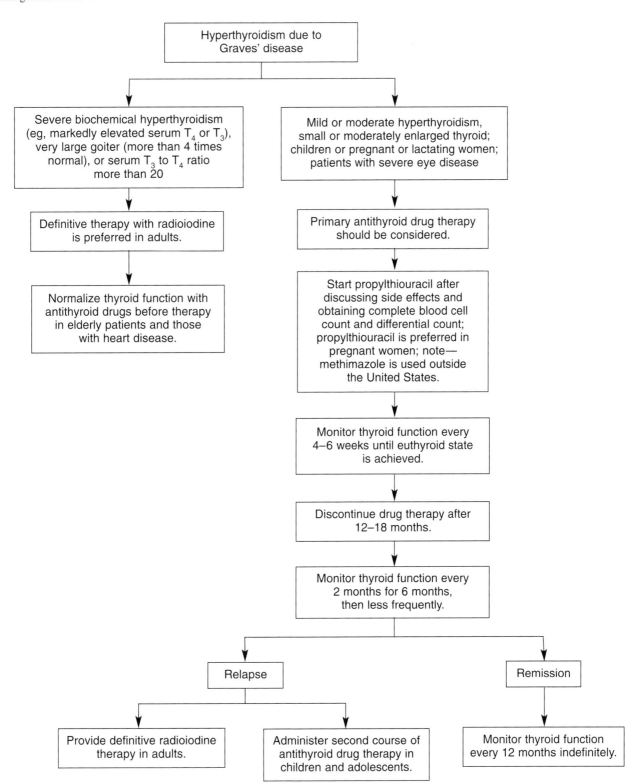

**FIG. 42-1.** Algorithm for the use of antithyroid drugs among patients with Graves' disease. (Streetman DD, Khanderia U. Diagnosis and treatment of Graves disease. Ann Pharmacother 2003;37:1101.)

American Association of Clinical Endocrinologists medical guidelines for clinical practice for the evaluation and treatment of hyperthyroidism and hypothyroidism. American Association of Clinical Endocrinologists. Endocr Pract 2002;8:457–69.

Cooper DS. Antithyroid drugs. N Engl J Med 2005;352:905–17.

Cooper DS. Hyperthyroidism. Lancet 2003;362:459–68.

Lazarus JH. Thyroid disorders associated with pregnancy: etiology, diagnosis, and management. Treat Endocrinol 2005;4:31–41.

Streetman DD, Khanderia U. Diagnosis and treatment of Graves disease. Ann Pharmacother 2003;37:1100–9.

# 43

## Long-term health risks of polycystic ovary syndrome

A 35-year-old nulligravid woman comes to your office and requests routine care. She has a lifelong history of oligomenorrhea with menses every 2–6 months. She has been overweight since adolescence and currently weighs 102.1 kg (225 lb) and is 1.6 m (63 in.) tall. Her examination is normal with the exception of mild acne and facial hair and a waist circumference of 1.04 m (41 in.). The fasting glucose and lipid profile (high-density lipoprotein cholesterol [HDL-C]; low-density lipoprotein cholesterol [LDL-C]; triglycerides [TRG]) most consistent with her diagnosis are

|       | Glucose Level* | HDL-C* | LDL-C* | TRG* |
|-------|----------------|--------|--------|------|
| * (A) | 105            | 35     | 136    | 250  |
| (B)   | 66             | 61     | 100    | 83   |
| (C)   | 200            | 68     | 110    | 120  |
| (D)   | 100            | 50     | 86     | 140  |

*In milligrams per deciliter.

Polycystic ovary syndrome (PCOS) is one of the most common female hormonal disorders and affects an estimated 5–10% of women. However, PCOS is a diagnosis of exclusion after other conditions known to cause irregular menses and hyperandrogenism have been ruled out. An international consensus group has suggested that two of the following are necessary to establish the diagnosis:

- Oligoovulation or anovulation
- Elevated levels of circulating androgens
- Clinical manifestations of androgen excess
- Polycystic ovaries diagnosed with ultrasonography

Women with PCOS usually present with reproductive issues (irregular menses or infertility) or symptoms of androgen excess (acne or hirsutism). Such women are at substantial risk of metabolic and subsequent cardiovascular disease similar to patients with metabolic syndrome (syndrome X). Both PCOS and metabolic syndrome are characterized by hyperinsulinism, glucose intolerance, obesity with an increased waist–hip ratio, and lipid abnormalities, all known risk factors for cardiovascular disease. Both insulin resistance and elevated androgens contribute to the atherogenic lipid profiles and glucose intolerance. Patients with PCOS are at increased risk for an elevated fasting blood glucose or abnormal 2-hour glucose tolerance test, hypertriglyceridemia, elevated very-low-density lipoprotein cholesterol (VLDL-C) and LDL-C levels, and decreased levels of HDL-C. Most PCOS patients have normal fasting glucose concentrations; approximately 30% have impaired glucose tolerance. Fasting glucose measurements are poor predictors of type 2 diabetes mellitus.

The patient described is likely to have fasting glucose and lipid levels that correspond to option A. She has mildly elevated fasting glucose level, low HDL-C, high LDL-C, and high triglycerides.

Ehrmann DA. Polycystic ovary syndrome. N Engl J Med 2005;352: 1223–36.

Legro RS, Kunselman AR, Dodson WC, Dunaif A. Prevalence and predictors of risk for type 2 diabetes mellitus and impaired glucose tolerance in polycystic ovary syndrome: a prospective, controlled study in 254 affected women. J Clin Endocrinol Metab 1999;84:165–9.

Revised 2003 consensus on diagnostic criteria and long-term health risks related to polycystic ovary syndrome (PCOS). The Rotterdam ESHRE/ARSRM-Sponsored PCOS Consensus Workshop Group. Hum Reprod 2004;19:41–7.

# 44

## Differential diagnosis of pigmented vulvar lesion

A 47-year-old woman, gravida 2, para 2, presents for a periodic health examination. She has made regular visits; her last visit was 18 months ago. She has a negative history for sexually transmitted diseases and no prior abnormal cytology. She has been in a monogamous sexual relationship for the past 5 years and had a tubal ligation as her contraceptive method. Physical examination reveals an area of pigmentation on her vulva (Fig. 44-1; see color plate). The patient is unaware of this lesion and has not previously been told of its presence by her partner or health care provider. A punch biopsy of the lesion is shown (Fig. 44-2; see color plate). The most appropriate next step is colposcopy with

*    (A) wide local excision
      (B) unilateral radical vulvectomy
      (C) topical steroid therapy
      (D) follow-up every 3–4 months
      (E) no further intervention

The differential diagnosis of pigmented lesions of the vulva is extensive and includes both benign and malignant lesions and human papillomavirus (HPV)-associated infectious lesions, such as warts, vulvar intraepithelial neoplasia, and squamous carcinoma (Box 44-1).

Approximately 10–12% of women have some pigmented lesion on their vulva. Of all vulvar pigmented lesions, benign lentigines are the most common, and are present in up to 7% of all patients. These are small macules, which reveal increased basal layer pigmentation histologically. Vulvar melanosis is a term that describes larger, benign, irregularly bordered melanotic macules that resemble melanoma.

Although only 0.1% of moles occur on the vulva, 2.8% of all melanomas occur there. In addition, 8–11% of all vulvar malignancies are melanomas. Vulvar melanomas are typically diagnosed at a later stage than melanomas at other sites. It is unclear if this is due to the tumor location or if there is a true difference in behavior of melanomas of the vulvar skin. It is therefore important to carefully examine any pigmented lesion of the vulva and to sample any suspicious areas.

In the management of melanoma, tumor depth and width are important in determining prognosis. It is known that melanomas with a depth less than 1.5 mm have an excellent prognosis. In patients with clean surgical margins of 2 cm, local recurrence is rare. Thus, excision with a reasonably wide margin may be curative in early lesions.

The HPV-related lesions of the vulva have a tendency to be multifocal as well as to extend microscopically beyond the boundaries visible to the naked eye. Therefore, an important component to the workup of a patient with a pigmented vulvar lesion is colposcopy to determine visible margins and to allow for adequate excision.

Vulvar intraepithelial neoplasia (VIN) lesions can be white (hypopigmented), red (hypervascular), or brown (hyperpigmented). Although the most common symptom of VIN is pruritus, 50% of patients have no symptoms. The punch biopsy in this patient reveals VIN III. Given the high progression rate as well as the frequent association with an invasive focus, excision is warranted with an aggressive attempt to achieve negative surgical margins. Radical excision would be warranted if an invasive focus was found on biopsy. Given that this sample reveals full thickness VIN but no invasive focus, such extensive excision would not be necessary for this patient. There is no place for topical steroid therapy in the treatment of preinvasive lesions of the vulva. This option for therapy would be more appropriate for a diagnosis of dermatitis, lichen sclerosis, or other inflammatory conditions of the vulva.

---

**BOX 44-1**

**Differential Diagnosis of Pigmented Lesions of the Vulva**

Benign lesions
- Nevi
- Lentigines
- Melanosis
- Postinflammatory hyperpigmentation
- Seborrheic keratosis
- Human papillomavirus-associated lesions
  —Warts
  —Vulvar intraepithelial neoplasia (VIN)

Malignant lesions
- Squamous carcinoma
- Melanoma

After the diagnosis and adequate excision have been confirmed, close follow-up with colposcopy every 3–4 months is recommended in the management of patients with a history of VIN. In this case, however, treatment is warranted for the lesion as well as to rule out any associated invasive focus. Thus, doing nothing at this point or waiting for 3–4 months to follow up would risk progression of her disease.

Joura EA. Epidemiology, diagnosis and treatment of vulvar intraepithelial neoplasia. Curr Opin Obstet Gynecol 2002;14:39–43.

Medeiros F, Nascimento AF, Crum CP. Early vulvar squamous neoplasia: advances in classification, diagnosis, and differential diagnosis. Adv Anat Pathol 2005;12:20–6.

Rock B. Pigmented lesions of the vulva. Dermatol Clin 1992;10: 361–70.

van Seters M, van Beurden M, de Craen AJ. Is the assumed natural history of vulvar intraepithelial neoplasia III based on enough evidence? A systematic review of 3322 published patients. Gynecol Oncol 2005;97:645–51.

Trimble EL. Melanomas of the vulva and vagina. Oncology 1996; 10:1017–23; discussion 1024.

# 45

## Indications for influenza vaccination

A healthy, 22-year-old woman, gravida 1, comes to the office for her first obstetric visit in early December. She is at 6 weeks of gestation. She has never received an influenza vaccine. Your best recommendation to reduce her risk of symptomatic influenza is

    (A) vaccinate immediately with attenuated vaccine

\*   (B) vaccinate immediately with inactivated influenza vaccine

    (C) wait until the second trimester, then vaccinate with attenuated vaccine

    (D) wait until the second trimester, then vaccinate with inactivated vaccine

    (E) treat with amantadine if she develops influenza during pregnancy

Influenza is associated with an increased risk of morbidity and mortality in pregnant women, especially in the second and third trimesters. Influenza A may cause viral pneumonia. In the 1918 influenza pandemic, 50% of 1,350 pregnant women studied developed pneumonia with a 27% overall mortality rate. Similarly, in the 1957 influenza pandemic, pregnant women also had increased mortality; in England and New York City, approximately 10% of fatalities occurred in pregnant women. Influenza is also associated with increased hospitalizations in children younger than 2 years.

Inactivated influenza vaccines have been licensed since 1945. In healthy adults, the efficacy rates for preventing influenza are 70–90%. The World Health Organization, in conjunction with national centers around the world, such as the Centers for Disease Control and Prevention (CDC), perform surveillance of influenza activity. Every year, the U.S. Food and Drug Administration (FDA) assembles an advisory group to make recommendations on the composition of the next season's vaccine. The vaccine produced yearly is targeted against the strains felt most likely to be involved in the next season's influenza outbreak.

In the northern hemisphere, the peak influenza season is December to March, and in the southern hemisphere it is May to September. Therefore, in the northern hemisphere, the best time to vaccinate is early October through mid-November. For the pregnant patient, vaccine should be given when she comes to the office in any trimester from October through May, the end of the influenza season. The recommendation to vaccinate in the first trimester was added by the CDC in 2004. Reports show the safety of inactivated vaccine in the first trimester. The CDC has concluded that the benefits of the vaccine outweigh any theoretical risks of thimerosal preservative in multidose vials. The vaccine is most effective in patients younger than 65 years. If the vaccine strains match the circulating strains of influenza A and B, illness will be prevented in 70–90% of adults. Inactivated vaccine is less effective in the elderly, but still decreases hospitalizations by 70% and death by 85%. The vaccine also is indicated in breast-feeding women, to decrease exposure of her infant to influenza, and to minimize the risk of decreased milk supply in an acutely infected woman with fever, exhaustion, and other influenza symptoms.

In 2003, the FDA approved for use an attenuated live intranasal vaccine (Flumist). The vaccine contains two influenza A and one influenza B live attenuated strains. Healthy, nonpregnant individuals, aged 5–49 years, without high-risk conditions, and who are not contacts of severely immunocompromised individuals may receive either the live attenuated or the inactivated vaccine. Children younger than 5 years should be vaccinated as well as caregivers of children younger than 5 years. Antiviral drugs should not be used for 48 hours before the patient receives Flumist and also should not be administered for 2 weeks after the vaccine is given. Because live, attenuated vaccines can theoretically revert to a wild type virus, the vaccines should not be used in pregnant women. No live influenza vaccine safety data are currently available for pregnant women.

Patients who do not receive influenza vaccine and are exposed to influenza may receive medication for prophylaxis against or treatment of influenza. The M2 ion channel inhibitors prevent viral uncoding early in the replication cycle of influenza A. Amantadine and rimantadine are the two M2 blockers currently available. They can be used for chemoprophylaxis against influenza A. Amantadine and rimantadine administered within hours of the onset of symptoms also reduce the duration of influenza A illness. However, the drug class adamantanes are embryotoxic and teratogenic in rodents, so they should be used only in pregnant women when the potential for complications from influenza outweighs the risk from the antiviral drug. A high level of resistance to amantadine and rimantadine was observed among the circulating influenza A viruses in 2005–2006. Neither drug was recommended for use in the 2005–2006 influenza season. Resistance to circulating strains may need to be evaluated in future influenza seasons.

Neuraminidase inhibitors, such as zanamivir (Relenza) and oseltamivir, prevent the release of influenza virus from infected cells, thus preventing both influenza viruses A and B from infecting other cells. Oseltamivir is approved for prophylaxis as well as treatment. Zanamivir is approved by the Food and Drug Administration only for treatment of influenza. Neuraminidase inhibitors are associated with skeletal abnormalities after high-dose in utero rat exposure. Safety and efficacy in human pregnancy have not been studied with any of these antiviral agents. The American College of Obstetricians and Gynecologists recommends that these four antiviral drugs not be used as a substitute for vaccination in pregnancy. They should be used in pregnancy only if the potential benefits outweigh the unknown risks of these medications.

Antiviral drugs for prophylaxis and treatment of influenza. Med Lett Drugs Ther 2004;46:85–7.

High levels of adamantane resistance among influenza A (H3N2) viruses and interim guidelines for use of antiviral agents—United States. 2005–06 influenza season. Centers for Disease Control and Prevention. MMWR Morb Mortal Wkly Rep 2006;55:44–6.

Ie S, Rubio ER, Alper B, Szerlip HM. Respiratory complications of pregnancy. Obstet Gynecol Surv 2001;57:39–46.

Influenza vaccination and treatment during pregnancy. ACOG Committee Opinion No. 305. American College of Obstetricians and Gynecologists. Obstet Gynecol 2004;104:1125–6.

Poehling KA, Edwards KM. Prevention, diagnosis, and treatment of influenza: current and future options. Curr Opin Pediatr 2001;13:60–4.

Prevention and control of influenza: recommendations of the Advisory Committee on Immunization Practices (ACIP). Centers for Disease Control and Prevention. MMWR Recomm Rep 2005;54(RR-8):1–40.

# 46

## Fetal cardiovascular malformations and inheritance patterns

A healthy 30-year-old woman, gravida 3, para 2, is seen for her first prenatal visit. She emigrated from South America 2 years ago. Her first pregnancy resulted in a full-term, 2,629-g (5.8-lb) infant that was sick at birth and died when 2 weeks old. She only remembers being told that the baby had a heart condition. Her second child, the product of a term pregnancy, is healthy. She notes that her sister experienced similar problems, with heart "problems" diagnosed in two of her four children. You recommend a fetal echocardiogram. The cardiac anomaly most compatible with this medical history is

*   (A) hypoplastic left heart
    (B) truncus arteriosus
    (C) tetralogy of Fallot
    (D) transposition of the great vessels
    (E) Ebstein's anomaly

Congenital heart anomalies are the most common birth defects with an estimated prevalence of 8–10 infants with birth defects in every 1,000 live births. Cardiovascular malformations represent a leading cause of infant mortality and may occur in isolation, in the setting of chromosomal abnormalities, or as part of complex anomaly syndromes; 75% of cardiovascular malformations occur in isolation and are believed to be sporadic. For parents, the risk of recurrence is an important issue to be addressed.

Hypoplastic left heart syndrome (HLHS) is believed to be a type of a left ventricular outflow tract obstruction. Components of the complex malformation syndrome include hypoplastic left ventricle, hypoplasia of the aorta, aortic stenosis and bicuspid aortic valve, and coarctation of the aorta. Analysis of the recurrence risk has documented patterns that suggest polygenic influence with a recurrence risk of 1–2%. Other studies have documented recurrence rates compatible with an autosomal dominant pattern suggesting a single gene defect.

The Baltimore–Washington Infant Study, 1981–1989, a study of the distribution of familial, social, medical, and occupational factors among 4,390 infants with cardiovascular malformations and 3,572 control infants, found the rate of affected first-degree relatives highest at 8% in infants with HLHS. In a smaller study of probands with HLHS (N = 38), cardiovascular malformations were confirmed in 19.3% of 379 first-degree relatives when assessed by clinical examination and echocardiography. The type of malformation was predominantly (72%) left-sided obstructive lesions. This is in contrast to the rate of 2% of cardiovascular malformations identified in first-degree relatives of probands with d-transposition of the great vessels. A study of four families clearly documented a recurrent risk consistent with autosomal dominant

inheritance with greater than 50% of first-degree relatives affected by a component of the obstruction. Therefore, the cardiac anomaly suspected in this family is HLHS. In families with a known history of left ventricular obstruction, counseling and evaluation should be considered because of the higher risk of recurrence.

Truncus arteriosus, also known as common aortic pulmonary trunk, is suspected when a single large ventricular outflow tract is identified with ultrasonography. This cardiovascular malformation is rare, with an incidence of 3 per 100,000 live births. The risk is increased in the fetuses of pregnancies affected by pregestational diabetes mellitus. It may occur as part of the DiGeorge sequence, and identification prenatally should prompt karyotype analysis, including evaluation for 22q11 microdeletions. Recurrence risk is estimated at 1% with one affected sibling and 3% with two affected siblings. Familial clustering is rare.

Tetralogy of Fallot, one of the more common cardiovascular malformations with an incidence of 2 out of 10,000 live births, accounts for 5–10% of the malformations. Anatomically, this anomaly consists of ventricular septal defect, right ventricular outflow tract obstruction, aorta overriding interventricular septum, and right ventricular hypertrophy. Recurrence risk is 2.5% with one affected fetus and increases to 8% with two affected siblings. Tetralogy of Fallot may be associated with velocardiofacial syndrome, DiGeorge syndrome, CHARGE (coloboma, heart anomaly, choanal atresia, retardation, genital and ear anomalies), and VATER (anomalies of the vertebral, anal, tracheal, esophageal, and renal and radius systems) associations. Long-term outcome is generally good with 90% 30-year survival in infants that survive a complete repair (operative repair is associated with a risk of 1–3% postoperative mortality).

Transposition of the great vessels is an anomaly in which the pulmonary artery arises from the left ventricle and the aorta originates from the right ventricle, resulting in two separate circulations. Its incidence is 2 in 10,000 live births and the anomaly accounts for 10% of all congenital heart defects in infants. Almost all cases are isolated malformations with a normal karyotype. Risk of recurrence is 1.5% with one affected sibling and 5% with two affected siblings.

Ebstein's anomaly is rare; it occurs in 1 in 20,000 live births and accounts for 0.3–0.6% of all cardiovascular malformations. Tricuspid valvular dysplasia occurs as a result of displacement of the septal and posterior leaflets and adherence to the ventricular wall. Diagnosed in utero, the anomaly has a poor prognosis with a high risk of fetal death in utero and neonatally. Ebstein's anomaly has been linked to lithium exposure in pregnancy. Recent controlled studies suggest that the magnitude of risk is much smaller than previously thought, and in some case–control studies of Ebstein's anomaly, lithium exposure was not identified.

Bianchi DW, Crombleholme TM, D'Alton ME. Fetology diagnosis and management of the fetal patient. New York: McGraw-Hill; 2000. p. 377–81, 389–402, 425–35.

Cohen LS, Friedman JM, Jefferson JW, Johnson EM, Weiner ML. A reevaluation of risk of in utero exposure to lithium [published erratum appears in JAMA 1994;271:1485]. JAMA 1994;271:146–50.

Loffredo CA, Chokkalingam A, Sill AM, Boughman JA, Clark EB, Scheel J, et al. Prevalence of congenital cardiovascular malformations among relatives of infants with hypoplastic left heart, coarctation of the aorta, and d-transposition of the great arteries. Am J Med Genet A 2004;124:225–30.

McBride KL, Pignatelli R, Lewin M, Ho T, Fernbach S, Menesses A, et al. Inheritance analysis of congenital left ventricular outflow tract obstruction malformations: segregation, multiplex relative risk, and heritability. Am J Med Genet A 2005;134:180–6.

Wessels MW, Berger RM, Frohn-Mulder IM, Roos-Hesselink JW, Hoogeboom JJ, Mancini GS, et al. Autosomal dominant inheritance of left ventricular outflow tract obstruction. Am J Med Genet A 2005; 134:171–9.

# 47

## Date rape

Following a normal gynecologic examination, a 17-year-old adolescent asks you for information about date rape. She tells you she is concerned because date rape happened to a friend last year. You inform her that the greatest risk factor for date rape is

* (A) age
  (B) college attendance
  (C) use of prescription antianxiety medications
  (D) history of previous sexual assault

Approximately 15–40% of adolescents have used some form of violence against their dating partners, including forms of violence that could result in serious injury. The most common victims of dating violence include adolescent females and young adult women aged 16–24 years. The perpetrator is often a known acquaintance, boyfriend, or date. High-risk groups of adolescents may include minorities, postpartum females, individuals of low educational or socioeconomic status, and those with a history of past violent behaviors. Firearm use and use or abuse of recreational drugs or alcohol also may enhance the likelihood of abuse or violence in relationships.

Student surveys regarding dating aggression, both perpetration and victimization, reveal that men and women reported similar amounts of overall aggression, but differed on the types of violence used and experienced. Young adult women reported greater sexual assault and attempted rape. Other factors associated with risk for date rape include an early sexual debut and a history of previous sexual abuse (Box 47-1). Factors protective against dating violence include the following:

- Consistent refusal of unwanted sex
- Consistent use of safe sex practices
- Social competency skills
- Group activities
- Refusal of mind-altering substances
- Avoiding unprotected drinks

Most research on dating violence has been conducted on white college women. However, more reports of research on minority populations and other risk groups, such as school dropouts and postpartum women, are emerging. Sexual victimization may result in high rates of sexually transmitted diseases, poor contraceptive use, and unwanted pregnancy.

---

**BOX 47-1**

**Risk Factors for Date Rape Associated With Physical and Sexual Aggression**

Associated risk factors
- Early age at first dating
- Date-specific behaviors
- Early sexual debut
- Substance or alcohol use
- History of sexual assault
- Acceptance of dating violence
- Previous violent dating relationship
- Previous violent behavior

Possibly associated risk factors
- School dropouts
- Postpartum states
- Availability of firearms

Data from Rickert VI, Vaughan RD, Wiemann CM. Adolescent dating violence and date rape. Curr Opin Obstet Gynecol 2002;14:495–500.

---

Some forms of sexual assault or dating violence may include drug-facilitated assaults. Such substances may be used to facilitate assault on males or females. Drugs administered before assault may cause sedation or amnesia that can result in the victim being unable to resist and being unaware of any sexual events. Drugs most commonly used include flunitrazepam (Rohypnol) and gamma-aminobutyric acid (GABA).

Violence and dating relationships can have both immediate and long-term consequences, including risk for future physical or sexual assault, sexually transmitted diseases, unwanted pregnancy, childhood sexual assault, and development of eating disorders. Whether or not risk factors are present, prevalence is still highest in adolescent girls and young adult women aged 16–24 years.

Lewis SF, Femouw W. Dating violence: a critical review of the literature. Clin Psychol Rev 2001;21:105–27.

Rickert VI, Vaughan RD, Wiemann CM. Adolescent dating violence and date rape. Curr Opin Obstet Gynecol 2002;14:495–500.

Slaughter L. Involvement of drugs in sexual assault. J Reprod Med 2000;45:425–30.

Wingood GM, DiClemente RJ, McCree DH, Harrington KF, Davies SL. Dating violence and the sexual health of black adolescent females. Pediatrics 2001;107:E72.

# 48

# Benefits of glycemic control in microvascular disease

Type 2 diabetes mellitus was diagnosed in a 60-year-old woman 5 years ago. She is concerned because her mother, who has diabetes mellitus, developed renal failure and retinopathy. The patient has been treated with oral hypoglycemic agents with moderately good results, but she has questions about the benefits of future therapy. In addition to better glucose control, you tell her that the major advantage of targeted intensive therapy to attain normal glycemic levels in patients with type 2 diabetes mellitus is

      (A)  fewer urinary tract infections

\*    (B)  fewer microvascular complications

      (C)  increased fructosamine levels

      (D)  fewer myocardial infarctions

      (E)  less peripheral vascular disease

More than 7% of individuals in the United States are known to have diabetes mellitus. However, because of the associated microvascular and macrovascular disease, diabetes mellitus accounts for almost 14% of the health care expenditures in this country, at least one half of which is related to complications such as myocardial infarctions, strokes, end-stage renal disease, retinopathy, and foot ulcers. In 2002, direct medical and indirect expenditures attributable to diabetes mellitus were estimated to be $132 billion.

The United Kingdom Prospective Diabetes Study confirmed that intensive therapy in type 2 diabetes mellitus decreased microvascular complications. Investigators followed 4,000 patients with newly diagnosed type 2 diabetes mellitus for 10 years. The study was designed to compare the efficacy of different treatment regimens (diet, sulfonylureas, metformin, and insulin) on glycemic control and the complications of diabetes mellitus. The risk for any diabetes mellitus-related endpoint was 12% lower in the intensive-therapy group and 10% lower for any diabetes-related death. It was estimated that 19.6 patients would have to be treated to prevent any single endpoint in one patient in 10 years. Most of the risk reduction in the intensive therapy group was due to a 25% risk reduction in microvascular disease (ie, retinopathy, nephropathy, or neuropathy). No reduction in infections or macrovascular disease (eg, myocardial infarction or peripheral vascular disease) was observed.

Intensive therapy in patients with type 2 diabetes mellitus results in an increased chance of hypoglycemia. Patients in the intensive therapy group had more hypoglycemic episodes largely due to the hypoglycemic nature of insulin, as well as oral hypoglycemic drugs that stimulate release of insulin from pancreatic β-cells (eg, the sulfonylureas).

A possible side effect associated with these glucose control improvements is weight gain. Weight gain was greater in patients who received insulin (4.0 kg) than in those who received sulfonylureas, such as chlorpropamide (2.6 kg) or glibenclamide (1.7 kg). A subsequent cost-effectiveness analysis found that intensive therapy significantly increased treatment costs. However, these costs were largely offset by a reduction in the cost of complications and an increased time free of complications. The Diabetes Control and Complications Trial Study for type 1 diabetes mellitus similarly demonstrated that improved glycemic control in diabetic patients reduced the incidence of diabetic microvascular complications.

Fructosamine is a glycated serum protein that reflects mean glucose over the prior 1–3 weeks. Lower levels generally correlate with better glucose control.

Abraira C, Colwell J, Nuttall F, Sawin CT, Henderson W, Comstock JP, et al. Cardiovascular events and correlates in the Veterans Affairs Diabetes Feasibility Trial. Veterans Affairs Cooperative Study on Glycemic Control and Complications in Type II Diabetes. Arch Intern Med 1997;157:181–8.

The effect of intensive treatment of diabetes on the development and progression of long-term complications in insulin-dependent diabetes mellitus. Diabetes Control and Complications Trial Research Group. N Engl J Med 1993;329:977–86.

Gray A, Raikou M, McGuire A, Fenn P, Stevens R, Cull C, et al. Cost effectiveness of an intensive blood glucose control policy in patients with type 2 diabetes: economic analysis alongside randomised controlled trial (UKPDS 41). United Kingdom Prospective Diabetes Study Group. BMJ 2000;320:1373–8.

Intensive blood-glucose control with sulphonylureas or insulin compared with conventional treatment and risk of complications in patients with type 2 diabetes (UKPDS 33). UK Prospective Diabetes Study (UKPDS) Group [published erratum appears in Lancet 1990;354:602]. Lancet 1998;352:837–53.

Vijan S, Hofer TP, Hayward RA. Estimated benefits of glycemic control in microvascular complications in type 2 diabetes. Ann Intern Med 1997;127:788–95.

# 49

## Tamoxifen use and adverse effects

Estrogen receptor-positive stage II breast cancer was diagnosed 2 years ago in a 66-year-old woman. She recently had benign endometrial polyps resected hysteroscopically. She is about to complete her second year of tamoxifen citrate (Nolvadex) therapy and asks what can be done to prevent recurrence of endometrial disease. In addition to discontinuing tamoxifen, the most appropriate therapy is

(A) progesterone
\* (B) aromatase inhibitor
(C) raloxifene hydrochloride (Evista)
(D) endometrial ablation
(E) hysterectomy with bilateral salpingo-oophorectomy (BSO)

Because the selective estrogen receptor modulator, tamoxifen, has been shown to reduce recurrence of estrogen receptor-positive breast cancer, it is widely used as adjuvant therapy. Unfortunately, use of tamoxifen in women with a uterus increases the risk of endometrial polyps and neoplasia. Given that this patient has already developed endometrial polyps during tamoxifen therapy, polyps might well recur if she continues this medication following resection.

In 2004, based on clinical trials of the aromatase inhibitors, anastrozole (Arimidex), letrozole (Femara), and exemestane (Aromasin), the American Society of Clinical Oncology (ASCO) issued a report indicating that appropriate adjuvant treatment of postmenopausal women with hormone receptor-positive breast tumors should include aromatase inhibitors. The ASCO recommendations indicated that aromatase inhibitors were appropriate for women who cannot tolerate tamoxifen, as in the patient described, and that appropriate candidates should consider aromatase inhibitor therapy as initial adjuvant therapy or following tamoxifen therapy.

Although both tamoxifen and aromatase inhibitors can cause vasomotor symptoms, their side effect profiles vary. Unlike tamoxifen, aromatase inhibitors do not cause endometrial or thromboembolic disease. Aromatase inhibitors, in contrast to tamoxifen, lower background estrogen levels, leading to loss of bone mineral density and a potential risk of fractures. Accordingly, attention to adequate calcium and vitamin D intake, monitoring of bone density, and, in selected patients, treatment with bisphosphonates are appropriate in women who receive long-term aromatase inhibitor therapy.

Although progesterone might prevent future endometrial polyps with ongoing tamoxifen use, its use is not recommended in this setting. In contrast with the findings from the Trial of Combination Estrogen–Progestin Therapy, data from the Women's Health Initiative clinical trial of estrogen-only therapy in menopausal women after hysterectomy found no increased risk of breast cancer, suggesting that it is the progestin component of combination hormone therapy that increases breast cancer risk. Thus, prescribing oral progestin therapy may not be appropriate in this patient. Interestingly, use of the progestin-releasing intrauterine device prevents endometrial polyp recurrence in women who take tamoxifen.

Raloxifene may reduce recurrence risk in women treated for hormone receptor-positive breast cancer. In addition, raloxifene does not cause endometrial disease. However, because there are few data to support the use of raloxifene as adjuvant therapy, such use does not currently represent standard therapy following initial treatment for receptor-positive breast cancer. Both raloxifene and tamoxifen have been shown to be effective for breast cancer prophylaxis in high-risk women.

Endometrial ablation does not remove all endometrial tissue. Accordingly, if the patient were to continue tamoxifen therapy following ablation, polyps might recur. Given that discontinuation of tamoxifen and initiation of aromatase inhibitor therapy have the potential to prevent recurrence of both endometrial disease and breast cancer in this patient, appropriate therapeutic goals can be achieved without subjecting her to hysterectomy and BSO.

Anderson GL, Limacher M, Assaf AR, Bassford T, Beresford SA, Black H, et al. Effects of conjugated equine estrogen in postmenopausal women with hysterectomy: the Women's Health Initiative randomized controlled trial. Women's Health Initiative Steering Committee. JAMA 2004;291:1701–12.

Breast cancer. American College of Obstetricians and Gynecologists. Obstet Gynecol 2004;104 suppl:11S–6S.

Gardner FJ, Konje JC, Abrams KR, Brown LJ, Khanna S, Al-Azzawi F, et al. Endometrial protection from tamoxifen-stimulated changes by a levonorgestrel-releasing intrauterine system: a randomised controlled trial. Lancet 2000;356:1711–7.

Winer EP, Hudis C, Burstein HJ, Wolff AC, Pritchard KI, Ingle JN, et al. American Society of Clinical Oncology technology assessment on the use of aromatase inhibitors as adjuvant therapy for postmenopausal women with hormone receptor-positive breast cancer: status report 2004. J Clin Oncol 2005;23:619–29.

# 50

## Association of anal and urinary incontinence

A menopausal woman is being evaluated for urge urinary incontinence. She recently was involved in an automobile accident in which she experienced possible nerve damage. She answers affirmatively to a questionnaire that asks if she has experienced any fecal incontinence. The best test to evaluate this problem is

* * (A) anal manometry
  * (B) barium enema
  * (C) colonoscopy
  * (D) endoanal ultrasonography
  * (E) rectal examination

Fecal incontinence is estimated to affect 2–25% of women in their lifetime. Fecal incontinence is estimated to also be present in 20% of women with urinary incontinence. Patients with urinary incontinence have an elevated risk of fecal incontinence. The risk factors that are associated with one may be found with the other. A survey of women with organ prolapse or urinary incontinence found that urinary incontinence, abnormal anal sphincter tone, and irritable bowel syndrome were associated with fecal incontinence. It is important to look for this symptom because it worsens the quality of life of the patient significantly more than urinary incontinence alone. Studies that have examined specific subtypes of incontinence found a relationship between urinary and fecal urgency, which suggests a common visceral motility disorder.

The best test to evaluate the neurologic function of the continence mechanism is manometry. Anal manometry involves measurement of resting and squeeze pressures and assessment of rectal sensation, compliance, rectoanal inhibitory reflex, and rectoanal contractile response to filling. It can be used to assess urgency fecal incontinence that might be caused by irritable bowel syndrome.

Barium enema and colonoscopy are used to evaluate the bowel for anatomic lesions and sources of bleeding and pain, but are not generally useful for evaluation of incontinence. These tests would be helpful if the symptoms were due to a change in stools (eg, onset of diarrhea).

Endoanal ultrasonography is a useful test for evaluation of the sphincter muscle. It can reveal defects in the integrity of the internal and external anal sphincter (eg, due to unrepaired fourth-degree lacerations). Defects of this kind often cause passive incontinence rather than urgency. Physical examination is neither sensitive nor specific enough to be relied on to make a diagnosis, but the sense of decreased rectal tone may be appreciated by the examiner.

Fialkow MF, Melville JL, Lentz GM, Miller EA, Miller J, Fenner DE. The functional and psychosocial impact of fecal incontinence on women with urinary incontinence. Am J Obstet Gynecol 2003;189: 127–9.

Jackson SL, Weber AM, Hull TL, Mitchinson AR, Walters MD. Fecal incontinence in women with urinary incontinence and pelvic organ prolapse. Obstet Gynecol 1997;89:423–7.

Manning J, Eyers AA, Korda A, Benness C, Solomon MJ. Is there an association between fecal incontinence and lower urinary dysfunction? Dis Colon Rectum 2001;44:790–8.

Nelson R, Norton N, Cautley E, Furner S. Community-based prevalence of anal incontinence. JAMA 1995;274:559–61.

Soligo M, Salvatore S, Milani R, Lalia M, Malberti S, Digesu GA, et al. Double incontinence in urogynecologic practice: a new insight. Am J Obstet Gynecol 2003;189:438–43.

# 51

## Cardiovascular disease during menopause

A 48-year-old woman, gravida 2, para 2, visits your office for her periodic examination. Her menses have become further apart and lighter and her last menstrual period occurred 6 months ago. She is without complaints except for hot flushes, which do not interfere with activities or sleep. Family history is positive for colon cancer in her father at age 59 years, but there is no history of premature heart disease. The patient has no medical history for illnesses or surgery except for a postpartum bilateral tubal ligation. A complete review of systems is negative for disease. Physical examination shows a blood pressure of 124/83 mm Hg, weight 68 kg (150 lb), and height 1.6 m (63 in.). Her body mass index (weight in kilograms divided by height in meters squared [kg/m²]) is 26.6. Her fasting profile reveals a low-density lipoprotein (LDL) cholesterol level of 139 mg/dL, a high-density lipoprotein (HDL) cholesterol level of 45 mg/dL, triglyceride level of 189 mg/dL, and blood glucose level of 98 mg/dL. To reduce her risk of heart disease, you advise her that the most important step consistent with current guidelines is to start

       (A) low-dose hormone therapy
       (B) a statin cholesterol-lowering agent
       (C) a low-dose aspirin daily
   *   (D) an exercise program and begin an American Heart Association prudent diet
       (E) vitamin E

Cardiovascular disease is the number one killer of menopausal women. Risk factors for heart disease have been well delineated along with therapeutic interventions to reduce morbidity and mortality. Although many interventions have been recommended over the years to reduce risk of heart disease, many have been shown not to be effective. Low-dose aspirin has been recommended to prevent myocardial infarction. Most of the data on aspirin for the prevention of cardiovascular events come from studies in men. However, in the largest study published to date, almost 40,000 women older than 45 years without a history of coronary artery disease, cerebrovascular disease, or cancer were randomized to receive placebo or aspirin, 100 mg daily, and were monitored for a mean of 10 years. No differences were observed between the groups in regard to risk of myocardial infarction or any major cardiovascular event. Gastrointestinal bleeding that required transfusion was more common in the aspirin group. Subgroup analyses showed that aspirin did significantly reduce the risk of major cardiovascular events, ischemic stroke, and myocardial infarction among women aged 65 years or older. In younger women not at high risk for heart disease, risks may outweigh benefits.

Antioxidant vitamins also have been recommended as a preventive measure in reducing risk of heart disease without definitive proof. In a large study involving patients with vascular disease randomized to vitamin E, 400 international units, vs placebo, no significant differences were observed in the incidence of cancer or deaths related to cancer and cardiovascular outcomes including death. A significantly increased risk in heart failure and related complications was seen in the vitamin E group. This study supports the results of a recent meta-analysis that found no benefit and a slightly higher rate of death in patients who took high-dose vitamin E. Similarly, the largest randomized, placebo-controlled trial of hormone therapy, the Women's Health Initiative, did not show a reduction in coronary heart disease (CHD).

The Third Report of the Expert Panel on Detection, Evaluation, and Treatment of High Blood Cholesterol in Adults (Adult Treatment Panel III or ATP III) presents the updated recommendations for cholesterol testing and management from the National Cholesterol Education Program. Although ATP III advises attention to intensive treatment of patients with CHD, its major new feature is a focus on primary prevention. The new recommendations emphasize lowering LDL cholesterol levels in the whole population and keeping cholesterol levels low with initial adoption of a diet low in saturated fat and cholesterol, maintenance of a healthy weight, and regular physical activity.

In a meta-analysis of dietary trials and pharmacotherapy, lowering serum cholesterol by means of a change in diet was shown to lower the risk of CHD without the adverse side effects associated with drugs such as statins. In addition, physical activity was shown to favorably modify several risk factors for heart disease, including lowering LDL cholesterol and triglyceride levels, raising HDL cholesterol levels, improving insulin sensitivity, and lowering blood pressure. The ATP III reports document the case for the efficacy and safety of primary prevention through lifestyle changes. In the case described, where there is no personal or family history of CHD or other high-risk factors, diet and exercise constitute the first line of prevention. Because LDL cholesterol is the most atherogenic lipoprotein, levels of increasing risk have been classified (Table 51-1). In patients with an elevated LDL cholesterol level higher than 130 mg/dL and multiple risk factors for heart disease, primary prevention with statin therapy has been efficacious and cost-effective.

**TABLE 51-1.** Adult Treatment Panel III (ATP III) Classification of Total Cholesterol and Low-Density Lipoprotein (LDL) Cholesterol

| Cholesterol (mg/dL) | Classification |
| --- | --- |
| Total cholesterol | |
| Less than 200 | Desirable |
| 200–239 | Borderline high |
| 240 or higher | High |
| LDL cholesterol | |
| Less than 100 | Optimal |
| 100–129 | Near optimal/above optimal |
| 130–159 | Borderline high |
| 160–189 | High |
| 190 or higher | Very high |

National Cholesterol Education Program. Adult Treatment Panel III Report. Bethesda (MD): NHLBI; 2001. p. II-5. Available at: http://www.nhlbi.nih.gov/guidelines/cholesterol/atp3_rpt.pdf. Retrieved June 15, 2005.

Lonn E, Bosch J, Yusuf S, Sheridan P, Pogue J, Arnold JM, et al. Effects of long-term vitamin E supplementation on cardiovascular events and cancer: a randomized controlled trial. The HOPE and HOPE-TOO Trial Investigators. JAMA 2005;293:1338–47.

Miller ER 3rd, Pastor-Barriuso R, Dalal D, Riemersma RA, Appel LJ, Guallar E. Meta-analysis: high-dosage vitamin E supplementation may increase all-cause mortality. Ann Intern Med 2005;142:37–46.

Ridker PM, Cook NR, Lee IM, Gordon D, Gaziano JM, Manson JE, et al. A randomized trial of low-dose aspirin in the primary prevention of cardiovascular disease in women. N Engl J Med 2005;352:1293–304.

Rossouw JE, Anderson GL, Prentice RL, LaCroix AZ, Kooperberg C, Stefanick ML, et al. Risks and benefits of estrogen plus progestin in healthy postmenopausal women: principal results from the Women's Health Initiative randomized controlled trial. Writing Group for the Women's Health Initiative Investigators. JAMA 2002;288:321–33.

# 52

## Evaluation of rhinosinusitis

A 27-year-old woman presents with an 11-day history of an upper respiratory tract infection, headache, postnasal drip, unilateral facial pain, and nasal discharge. She states that some of her symptoms have resolved but she continues to have nasal discharge. The complaint mentioned by the patient that is most consistent with acute bacterial rhinosinusitis is

*    (A) symptoms for greater than 10 days
      (B) headache
      (C) unilateral facial pain
      (D) persistent nasal discharge
      (E) postnasal drip

Acute rhinosinusitis is one of the most common conditions for which patients seek care. Most episodes of sinusitis are viral in nature. Despite this, most patients assume that they have an infection of bacterial origin. Compounding this is the fact that physicians incorrectly diagnose acute bacterial rhinosinusitis 50% of the time. It is estimated that acute bacterial rhinosinusitis is responsible for only one in every eight infections and that progression of a viral infection to a bacterial infection occurs in only 0.5–2% of cases.

Recognition of the factors associated with acute bacterial rhinosinusitis is crucial in order to determine when antibiotic therapy is necessary. Symptoms of rhinosinusitis are common, and vague complaints can easily be confused with unrelated conditions. Postnasal drip and nasal discharge are common in both viral and bacterial rhinosinusitis. Discharge is usually clear or yellow. Greenish tint is frequently normal but may be suggestive of bacterial infection. Headache and facial pain are commonly reported symptoms but are nonspecific complaints that may or may not be representative of acute bacterial rhinosinusitis. Migraines, tension headaches, temporomandibular joint pain, eye disease, and dental conditions also may cause anterior or unilateral facial pain and discomfort of a similar nature.

Cluster headaches in particular often feature acute episodes of rhinorrhea. Symptoms that initially improve but then worsen may be indicative of a progressive or bacterial infection. Acute viral rhinosinusitis usually resolves without intervention within 7–10 days, and two thirds of bacterial rhinosinusitis cases will resolve without medication. However, recent consensus guidelines propose that any infection lasting for more than 10–14 days is consistent with acute bacterial rhinosinusitis. Infections of less than 10 days' duration are most likely viral in nature and do not require antibiotic coverage in the absence of severe or complicating factors. After 10–14 days of symptoms, it can be assumed that bacterial infection is present and antibiotics may be started.

Incaudo GA. Diagnosis and treatment of allergic rhinitis and sinusitis during pregnancy and lactation. Clin Rev Allergy Immunol 2004; 27:159–77.

Meltzer EO, Hamilos DL, Hadley JA, Lanza DC, Marple BF, Nicklas RA, et al. Rhinosinusitis: establishing definitions for clinical research and patient care. Otolaryngol Head Neck Surg 2004;131 suppl:S1–S62.

Scheid DC, Hamm RM. Acute bacterial rhinosinusitis in adults: part I. Evaluation [published erratum appears in Am Fam Physician 2006;73:33]. Am Fam Physician 2004;70:1685–92.

Scheid DC, Hamm RM. Acute bacterial rhinosinusitis in adults: part II. Treatment [published erratum appears in Am Fam Physician 2006;73:33]. Am Fam Physician 2004;70:1697–704.

# 53

## Cervical cytology screening

A 25-year-old woman has had three consecutive normal annual cervical cytologic screening results. According to American College of Obstetricians and Gynecologists (ACOG) guidelines, when liquid-based cervical cytology screening is used, the appropriate interval for her next screening is

　　　(A) 6 months
＊　　(B) 1 year
　　　(C) 2 years
　　　(D) 3 years
　　　(E) 5 years

Cervical cancer mortality has decreased by one half in the past 30 years mostly as a result of cervical screening. Screening identifies the precursor lesion, cervical intraepithelial neoplasia, allowing for treatment before the development of invasive disease.

The conventional Pap test has been performed for more than 50 years by sampling the cervix with a brush or spatula and smearing the exfoliated material onto a glass slide. Following fixation and staining, the cells are examined microscopically by a cytopathologist. In 1996, the U.S. Food and Drug Administration (FDA) approved the use of a liquid-based preparation of the exfoliated sample. The sample is placed in a liquid fixative and processed in the laboratory before staining and microscopic examination. This process allows for removal of contaminating material such as blood and mucus. Two commercially available tests use the liquid-based collection method:

- ThinPrep. Filters the collected specimen and deposits the filtered cells onto a slide for staining

- SurePath. Uses enrichment of the sample to extract the cells

The sensitivity of the traditional Pap test for detection of cervical cancer and its precursors is estimated to be lower than the 60–85% previously reported. Studies used to establish the accuracy of newer screening technologies indicate that the sensitivity of the traditional Pap test may be as low as 50%. The newer liquid-based technique detects more low- and high-grade intraepithelial lesions than does the traditional slide-based Pap test, which should result in an increased sensitivity. The magnitude of increase in sensitivity of the thin-layer technology over the traditional Pap test is uncertain. The specificity of the thin-layer techniques has not been well studied. Specificity is important in cervical cytology screening, because false-positive test results will lead to unnecessary procedures and subsequent costs.

The U.S. Preventive Services Task Force reviewed the data regarding new technologies in cervical cancer screening. The task force concluded that insufficient evidence exists to recommend the routine use of new technologies in cervical cancer screening. It has not been demonstrated that screening using the liquid-based technologies reduces cervical cancer incidence or mortality when compared to screening by the traditional Pap test.

Recommendations for screening intervals have changed in recent years; ACOG currently recommends that women younger than 30 years undergo annual screening. Women older than 30 years may have cervical cytology screening every 2–3 years if they have three consecutive negative test results. Although ACOG does not support altering the interval of screening based on test performed, the American Cancer Society recommends cervical cytology every 2 years for women younger than 30 years if thin-layer technology is used. Limited data exist to support a screening interval of more than 1 year. The overall magnitude of increase in sensitivity between conventional and liquid-based screening is small.

This patient had received three consecutive negative cervical cytology test results. Provided that the test result remains negative, the screening interval could be extended to every 2–3 years after age 30 years. Intervals greater than 3 years are not recommended regardless of history. Women infected with human immunodeficiency virus should be screened at 6-month intervals for the first year after diagnosis and then annually thereafter if the test results are negative.

Cervical cytology screening. ACOG Practice Bulletin No. 45. American College of Obstetricians and Gynecologists. Obstet Gynecol 2003; 102:417–27.

Screening for cervical cancer: recommendations and rationale. US Preventive Services Task Force, Agency for Healthcare Research and Quality. Rockville (MD): AHRQ; 2003.

Smith RA, Cokkinides V, Eyre HJ. American Cancer Society guidelines for the early detection of cancer 2005. CA Cancer J Clin 2005;55: 31–44; quiz 55–6.

# 54

## Treatment of vulvar lichen planus

A 58-year-old woman presents with progressively worsening vulvar burning, pruritus, and dyspareunia for 1 year. Genital examination reveals erosions and erythema of the vestibule (Fig. 54-1; see color plate) and oral lesions are also noted (Fig. 54-2; see color plate). The best topical treatment for the genital lesions is

    (A) clobetasol propionate (Cormax, Temovate)
    (B) testosterone
    (C) estrogen
    (D) betamethasone valerate
\*   (E) hydrocortisone acetate

Lichen planus is one of the three "lichen" disorders of the vulva, the others being lichen simplex chronicus and lichen sclerosus. Lichen planus is characterized by chronic and debilitating symptoms in the vulva and vagina. These symptoms include itching, irritation, burning, and dyspareunia. Examination of the vulva and vagina reveals an inflamed erythematous epithelium or frank erosions. A white reticulate pattern, Wickham striae, may be seen surrounding the inflamed or erosive areas (Fig. 54-1). Advanced cases can lead to vaginal stenosis and intravaginal adhesions.

The oral lesions of lichen planus are virtually pathognomonic of the disorder. These oral lesions appear as erythema at the gingival-dentate junction (Fig. 54-2). The oral lesions of lichen planus also may appear as lacy white plaques. When oral and vulvar lesions are present, the disease is termed the vulvovaginal gingival syndrome. Skin lesions may be present, appearing as "violaceous papules" on the flexor surfaces or striae.

The diagnosis of lichen planus is based mostly on clinical findings as described previously. Biopsy of genital lesions may reveal hyperkeratosis, thinning of the epidermis, and mononuclear cell infiltrates. Histology is not always confirmatory, particularly in the presence of erosions.

Two studies have confirmed the usefulness of 25-mg vaginal hydrocortisone suppositories in the treatment of lichen planus. Symptomatic relief of vulvar burning, pruritus, and dyspareunia is achieved with hydrocortisone acetate. Vaginal stenosis does not appear to improve with the hydrocortisone suppositories. Therapy usually is initiated as twice daily dosing, tapering down to maintenance doses when symptoms are controlled. Long-term maintenance therapy often is required to prevent relapse.

Two small series have demonstrated efficacy in treating erosive lichen planus with tacrolimus. Tacrolimus is a topical ointment that acts as an immunosuppressant. Currently approved by the U.S. Food and Drug Administration (FDA) for atopic dermatitis, this therapy may emerge as a viable alternative for those patients with erosive lichen planus refractory to hydrocortisone. Concerns about the drug's side effects may limit its use.

Estrogen and testosterone have not been shown to be effective in the treatment of lichen planus. Topical estrogen is indicated for treatment of symptomatic vulvovaginal atrophy. Topical testosterone was once used to treat lichen sclerosus, but has been mostly abandoned because it has been shown to be less effective than high-potency topical steroids, such as clobetasol propionate.

Betamethasone valerate and clobetasol are more potent topical steroids than hydrocortisone. They have not been proven effective for lichen planus. Although theoretically any topical steroid would be effective in treating the disorder, chronic use of high-potency topical steroids may lead to dermal atrophy. Thus, use of the steroid preparation with the lowest potency for a chronic condition such as lichen planus is recommended. High-potency topical steroids are indicated for lichen sclerosis.

Anderson M, Kutzner S, Kaufman RH. Treatment of vulvovaginal lichen planus with vaginal hydrocortisone suppositories. Obstet Gynecol 2002;100:359–62.

Foster DC. Vulvar disease. Obstet Gynecol 2002;100:145–63.

Lewis FM. Vulval lichen planus. Br J Dermatol 1998;138:569–75.

Lotery HE, Galask RP. Erosive lichen planus of the vulva and vagina. Obstet Gynecol 2003;101:1121–5.

# 55

## Office infertility workup

A 28-year-old nulligravid woman and her husband consult you for evaluation of primary infertility. They have been attempting pregnancy for 13 months using unprotected sexual intercourse concentrated midcycle. Her cycles are regular, every 30–32 days. She notes fairly severe dysmenorrhea for which she has taken birth control pills in the past and currently takes nonsteroidal antiinflammatory drugs (NSAIDs) around the clock during her menses. She has no history of abdominal surgery, abnormal Pap test results, or major medical problems. She has a history of chlamydia that was treated with outpatient antibiotics while she was in college. Her husband is a healthy 32-year-old male with no history of sexually transmitted diseases. He has never fathered a child. Physical examination reveals the woman's cervix is normal without evidence of inflammation. Bimanual examination reveals a small anteverted uterus that is mobile and nontender. There are no adnexal masses and rectovaginal examination is normal. The most appropriate test to perform in this patient to establish fallopian tube patency is a diagnostic

      (A)  sonohysterogram
\*    (B)  hysterosalpingogram (HSG)
      (C)  hysteroscopy
      (D)  laparoscopy

Infertility is defined as the inability to conceive after 1 year of unprotected sexual intercourse. Historical data have shown that in a given cycle there is approximately a 20% chance of conception in a normal couple. This puts the likelihood of conception after 12 months at approximately 93%. Factors found in association with infertility can be classified into four groups, each of which are important in approximately 25% or more of infertility cases:

1. Male factor (ie, azospermia or oligospermia)

2. Ovulatory dysfunction

3. Anatomic causes (ie, tubal blockage, abnormal cervical mucus, or obstruction)

4. Unexplained infertility

In most cases, the actual causal relationship between the finding of a given abnormality on diagnostic testing and infertility is uncertain. Data indicate an established correlation with impaired fertility and abnormal semen analysis, tubal blockage on hysterosalpingography or laparoscopy, and laboratory assessment revealing impaired ovulation. Causes of tubal blockage include a history of peritonitis (ie, appendicitis or pelvic inflammatory disease, endometriosis, or previous pelvic surgery). The patient described has a history of chlamydia, a known contributor to pelvic adhesions. She also notes a history of dysmenorrhea, which could be consistent with endometriosis. Her cycles are regular, which suggests she ovulates most of the time. Therefore, assessment of her pelvic anatomy to look specifically at tubal patency would be warranted as the initial workup.

Tubal abnormalities can be diagnosed accurately by both HSG and laparoscopy. Laparoscopy with chromopertubation is in most cases considered the criterion standard for evaluation of tubal anatomy because it not only reveals the same proximal tubal obstruction that HSG shows but also more effectively reveals partial tubal obstruction, peritoneal adhesions, and evidence of endometriosis.

Endometriosis occurs with a higher frequency in infertile women than in fertile women. Surgical treatment of endometriosis in severe cases can positively affect fertility. However, effectiveness of treatment of mild to moderate cases is controversial. Given that laparoscopy is significantly more expensive and carries a higher inherent risk, many specialists argue for HSG, the less expensive, safer study, which, in many abnormal cases, can obviate the need for laparoscopy. In addition, assisted reproductive technologies have become quite advanced with excellent success rates in patients who have tubal obstruction. Practitioners have moved away from the more invasive surgical approach (ie, laparoscopy with ablation of endometriosis or adhesions) toward in vitro fertilization (IVF) techniques, which have proved to be highly successful. For example, women who have an HSG that reveals tubal blockage may proceed to IVF without the need for an additional invasive procedure. Women with a normal HSG who may be candidates for donor insemination or ovulation induction may consider several cycles of such treatment before moving on to the more invasive test. Before an invasive approach is tried, an HSG should be done to evaluate her pelvic anatomy, including uterine cavity and fallopian tube architecture and patency.

Recently, sonohysterography has been considered an alternative to HSG in the evaluation of pelvic structures. It is inexpensive compared to both HSG and laparoscopy and does not involve the higher levels of radiation entailed in the fluoroscopy in HSG. This method is excellent for evaluation of the uterine cavity and can reveal hydrosalpinges. However, the accuracy of sonohysterography in the diagnosis of partial or even complete tubal blockage in the absence of dilation does not seem to be as good as that of HSG. Part of the limitations of the technique may be due to the echogenicity of the bowel, which typically drape the tubes and can make evaluation of the narrow lumen of the tubes difficult and unclear.

Hysteroscopy frequently is used in the evaluation and sometimes treatment of the infertile patient. It is an effective measure in evaluation of the uterine cavity when there is a high index of suspicion for endometrial pathologic conditions. The effectiveness of surgical treatment of endometrial conditions as part of the management of infertility is not clear. Hysteroscopy does not reveal tubal pathology and would thus be an inadequate diagnostic tool in this patient.

Laparoscopy often is considered the criterion standard for evaluation of the fallopian tubes. However, laparoscopy is much more invasive and expensive than HSG and is reasonable only when it would favorably affect fertility. Given this patient's normal examination and relatively mild symptoms of dysmenorrhea, the risk–benefit ratio would not justify this level of invasion. The use of an HSG as a first step in the patient's workup would be much more prudent.

Surgical evaluation and treatment of infertility involves fine, microsurgical technique, which minimizes adhesion formation and promotes tubal patency and health. Laparotomy is known to result in significantly more adhesion formation than laparoscopy and thus has no place in the diagnostic workup of the infertile patient.

Balasch J. Investigation of the infertile couple: investigation of the infertile couple in the era of assisted reproductive technology: a time for reappraisal. Hum Reprod 2000;15:2251–7.

Hull MG, Glazener CM, Kelly NJ, Conway DI, Foster PA, Hinton RA, et al. Population study of causes, treatment, and outcome of infertility. Br Med J (Clin Res Ed) 1985;291:1693–7.

Marcoux S, Maheux R, Berube S. Laparoscopic surgery in infertile women with minimal or mild endometriosis. Canadian Collaborative Group on Endometriosis. N Engl J Med 1997;337:217–22.

Radic V, Canic T, Valetic J, Duic Z. Advantages and disadvantages of hysterosonosalpingography in the assessment of the reproductive status of uterine cavity and fallopian tubes. Eur J Radiol 2005;53:268–73.

# 56

## Relationship between prevalence and positive predictive value

A recent trial of a new screening test for a sexually transmitted disease (STD) reports a positive predictive value of 47.5%. The prevalence of the disease in the study population is 10%. Because you practice in a population that is at lower risk, with a disease prevalence of 5%, you know that, compared with the published report, the positive predictive value for the STD in your clinic will be

\*     (A) lower
       (B) the same
       (C) slightly higher
       (D) twice as high

It is increasingly difficult for physicians to maintain and improve their knowledge base as medicine becomes more and more sophisticated and specialized. Understanding how to interpret new information within the context of the individual physician's patient population is a fundamental skill that all physicians should possess.

The positive predictive value (PPV) in the clinic described will be lower than that in the published report. The PPV is the proportion of patients with a positive test result who actually have the disease. The PPV is calculated by the formula, $a / a + b$, where $a$ = true positive and $b$ = false positive. The prevalence is the proportion of patients in the population who actually have the disease. The prevalence is calculated using the formula, $e / e + f$,

where $e$ represents the total number of individuals with the disease and $f$ represents the total number of individuals without the disease (Tables 56-1 and 56-2).

Prevalence is positively related to PPV (ie, the higher the prevalence, the higher the PPV), but it is not a one-to-one relationship. For example, for a screening test with a sensitivity of 90% ($a / a + c$) and specificity of 11% ($d / b + d$), used in a population of 1,000 with a prevalence of 10%, the PPV is 47.4% (Table 56-3).

Using the same screening test in a population with a lower prevalence yields a lower PPV. For example, with a prevalence of 5%, the PPV is 30.2% (Table 56-4). If, on the other hand, the population prevalence is higher, the PPV increases. For example, with a prevalence of 20%, the PPV is 67.2% (Table 56-5).

**TABLE 56-1.** Definition of Terms for Interpreting Clinical Value of Information

| Term | Definition | Formula |
| --- | --- | --- |
| Sensitivity | Proportion of individuals with condition who test positive | $a / a + c$ |
| Specificity | Proportion of individuals without condition who test negative | $d / b + d$ |
| Positive predictive value | Proportion of individuals with positive test who have condition | $a / a + b$ |
| Negative predictive value | Proportion of individuals with negative test who do not have the condition | $d / c + d$ |
| Prevalence | Proportion of individuals who have the condition | $e / e + f$ |

Modified from U.S. Preventive Services Task Force. Guide to clinical preventive services: report of the U.S. Preventive Services Task Force. 2nd ed. Baltimore (MD): Williams & Wilkins; 1996. table 2, p. xliii.

**TABLE 56-2.** Explanation of Formulas for Calculating Prevalence

|  | Disease Present | Disease Absent | Total |
|---|---|---|---|
| **Positive test result** | a | b | a + b |
| **Negative test result** | c | d | c + d |
| **Total** | e | f | e + f |

where a = true positive; b = false positive; c = false negative; d = true negative; e = total number with disease; f = total number without disease.

Modified from U.S. Preventive Services Task Force. Guide to clinical preventive services: report of the U.S. Preventive Services Task Force. 2nd ed. Baltimore (MD): Williams & Wilkins; 1996. table 2, p. xliii.

**TABLE 56-3.** Positive Predictive Value (PPV) and Prevalence of 10% for a Sexually Transmitted Disease (STD)

|  | STD Present | STD Absent | Total |
|---|---|---|---|
| **Positive test result** | 90 | 100 | 190 |
| **Negative test result** | 10 | 800 | 810 |
| **Total** | 100 | 900 | 1,000 |

PPV = a / a + b = 90/190 = 47.4%

**TABLE 56-4.** Positive Predictive Value (PPV) and Prevalence of 5% for a Sexually Transmitted Disease (STD)

|  | STD Present | STD Absent | Total |
|---|---|---|---|
| **Positive test result** | 45 | 104 | 149 |
| **Negative test result** | 5 | 846 | 851 |
| **Total** | 50 | 950 | 1,000 |

PPV = a / a + b = 45/149 = 30.2%

**TABLE 56-5.** Positive Predictive Value (PPV) and Prevalence of 20% for a Sexually Transmitted Disease (STD)

|  | STD Present | STD Absent | Total |
|---|---|---|---|
| **Positive test result** | 180 | 88 | 268 |
| **Negative test result** | 20 | 712 | 732 |
| **Total** | 200 | 800 | 1,000 |

PPV = a / a + b = 180/268 = 67.2%

Agency for Healthcare Research and Quality. Guide to clinical preventive services, 2005: recommendations of the U.S. Preventive Services Task Force. Rockville (MD): AHRQ; 2005. AHRQ Publication No. 05-0570. Available at: http://www.ahrq.gov/clinic/pocketgd. Retrieved September 27, 2006.

Armitage P, Berry G, Mathews JNS. Statistical methods in medical research. 4th ed. Oxford: Blackwell Science; 2002:692–8.

Grimes DA, Schulz KF. Clinical research in obstetrics and gynecology: a Baedeker for busy clinicians. Obstet Gynecol Surv 2002;57:S36–S53.

Sackett DL, Straus SE, Richardson WS, Rosenberg W, Haynes RB. Evidence-based medicine: how to practice and teach EBM. 2nd ed. Edinburgh: Churchill Livingstone; 2000. p. 67–93, 249.

# 57

## Pyelonephritis in pregnancy

A 25-year-old primigravid woman comes to your office at 24 weeks of gestation with fever, shaking chills, and right-sided flank pain. She also has pain with urination and increased urinary frequency. Her temperature is 38°C (100.4°F) and her lungs are clear. She has right costovertebral angle tenderness. Results of a urine culture show 10,000 colony-forming units per mL (cfu/mL) for *Escherichia coli*, sensitive to all antibiotics tested. She is admitted to the hospital for 3 days and is treated with intravenous ceftriaxone for 3 days. She completes a 7-day course of an oral cephalosporin as an outpatient. Follow-up care relative to her urinary system should include

*     (A) nitrofurantoin suppression
        (B) no further antibiotics
        (C) ciprofloxacin (Cipro) suppression
        (D) urine cultures when symptomatic

Acute pyelonephritis is one of the most common reasons for antepartum hospitalization, occurring in 1–2% of all pregnancies. It also may occur postpartum. The diagnosis is made with analysis of clinical signs and symptoms and laboratory data. The presenting symptoms are fever, shaking chills, nausea, vomiting, flank pain, dysuria, or increased frequency of urination. Examination may reveal costovertebral angle tenderness. The Infectious Diseases Society of America consensus definition of pyelonephritis accepts a clean-catch urine showing 10,000 cfu/mL or greater as laboratory evidence to corroborate a clinically established diagnosis. This is different from the 100,000 cfu/mL value for the diagnosis of asymptomatic bacteriuria. Antimicrobial sensitivities should be performed on the infecting urine organism. The most common etiologic bacteria are *Escherichia coli*, *Klebsiella, Enterobacter* species, and *Proteus* species. Gram-positive organisms, which are found more often in the third trimester, include *Enterococcus faecalis* and group B streptococci.

Maternal complications of pyelonephritis in pregnancy involve multiple organ systems and include anemia due to endotoxin hemolysis with elevated lactate dehydrogenase. Transient renal dysfunction, respiratory insufficiency including adult respiratory distress syndrome, and septicemia also may occur. Pregnancy complications include increased uterine contractions, with or without cervical change. Earlier studies noted increased spontaneous abortions, preterm labor and delivery, and low-birth-weight neonates. However, more recent studies show that aggressive therapy may reduce these complications.

Because of the severe complications that may accompany acute pyelonephritis in pregnancy, most experts advise inpatient hospitalization and parenteral antibiotic therapy. Antibiotics should cover the usual pathogenic bacteria, be safe in pregnancy, achieve high concentrations in the renal parenchyma, and concentrate in the urine. Inpatient treatment is started empirically with cephalosporins, ureidopenicillins, or amino and carboxypenicillin derivatives with or without clavulanic acid. Aminoglycosides may be used, but are associated with potential fetal ototoxicity, enhanced clearance resulting in subtherapeutic levels near term, and they may exacerbate renal insufficiency; so they are used as second-line medications. Ampicillin is not used because of antimicrobial resistance for many urinary tract pathogens, and ampicillin also may cause an increase in resistant organisms with long-term use. After the patient's symptoms have eased somewhat and she is afebrile for 48 hours, she may be sent home to complete a course of antibiotics, which is effective against the isolated uropathogen. The optimal duration of this treatment is not known. Many practitioners use 7–10 days of antimicrobials.

Antibiotic suppression for the duration of pregnancy and for 4–6 weeks postpartum is recommended to decrease the risk of recurrent pyelonephritis. Nitrofurantoin has been shown in multiple studies to be safe and effective for suppression throughout pregnancy and postpartum. Ciprofloxacin, a quinoline, is contraindicated in pregnancy secondary to potential fetal abnormalities. A urine culture for "test of cure" and then frequent urine cultures are recommended for screening for recurrent bacteriuria.

Pyelonephritis may occur in any trimester of pregnancy, with the majority occurring in the second and third trimester, but up to 20% of cases occur in the first trimester. With increasing stasis in the ureters, due to the enlarging uterus, patients are thought to be at increased risk of recurrence as the pregnancy advances. Urinary tract manipulation at the time of delivery also may increase the risk of postpartum pyelonephritis. The diagnosis and treatment of pyelonephritis remains a clinical challenge due to the complexities of the pathogenic bacteria, the changes in the genitourinary system during pregnancy, and the maternal response to the infection.

Hill JB, Sheffield JS, McIntire DD, Wendel GD. Acute pyelonephritis in pregnancy. Obstet Gynecol 2005;105:18–23.

Millar LK, DeBuque L, Wing DA. Uterine contraction frequency during treatment of pyelonephritis in pregnancy and subsequent risk of preterm birth. J Perinat Med 2003;31:41–6.

Wing DA. Pyelonephritis in pregnancy, treatment options for optimal outcomes. Drugs 2001;61:2087–96.

# 58

## Calcium and vitamin D supplements in postmenopausal women

A 45-year-old woman with a 40-pack-per-year history of tobacco use and pernicious anemia (vitamin $B_{12}$ deficiency) is interested in osteoporosis prevention. Your initial discussion centers on smoking cessation and confirmation of the efficacy of her vitamin $B_{12}$ therapy. You counsel her that the most important first-line pharmacologic strategy for osteoporosis prevention is

      (A) sodium fluoride
*    (B) vitamin D and calcium
      (C) bisphosphonates
      (D) calcitriol (vitamin $D_3$)
      (E) parathyroid hormone

Prevention and treatment of osteoporosis consist of nondrug and drug or hormonal therapy. Nondrug therapy of osteoporosis consists of three components:

1. Diet
2. Exercise
3. Cessation of smoking

In addition, affected patients should avoid, if possible, drugs that increase bone loss (eg, corticosteroids) and maximize therapy for other risk factors, such as pernicious anemia.

Postmenopausal women should take adequate supplemental elemental calcium, in divided doses, at mealtime. Total calcium intake, inclusive of dietary calcium, should approximate 1,500 mg/d. Women also should ingest a total of 800 international units of vitamin D daily. Higher doses are required for women who have malabsorption or rapid metabolism of vitamin D due to concomitant anticonvulsant drug therapy.

Although recent evidence suggests that vitamin and calcium supplementation may be of limited benefit, such dietary supplementation should still be recommended. In addition to its beneficial effects on the skeleton, calcium supplementation may affect serum lipids favorably. Furthermore, calcium intake has been shown to be inversely associated with cardiovascular disease in postmenopausal women.

Dietary calcium intake may be estimated by multiplying the number of dairy servings consumed per day by 300 mg. One serving is 240 mL (8 oz) of milk or yogurt, 480 mL (16 oz) of cottage cheese, or 28.4 g (1 oz) of hard cheese. Hence, it can be difficult to consume enough extra calcium by means of diet alone. Calcium supplements or increased intake of dairy products should be recommended if dietary calcium intake is below recommended levels. Calcium supplements may be preferable to dietary modification in patients with inadequate calcium intake because of the high prevalence of lactose intolerance. Calcium citrate may be the best first-line calcium supplement because it is well absorbed when not taken with a meal, and some data suggest it is better absorbed than calcium carbonate even when taken with a meal.

After the nonpharmacologic means and calcium and vitamin D supplementation have been implemented, pharmacotherapy may be used. This may include a bisphosphonate, a selective estrogen-receptor modulator, estrogen, and nasal calcitonin. Hormone therapy was once considered the primary therapy for postmenopausal women with osteoporosis. Estrogen has the additional advantages of controlling menopausal symptoms. However, data from the Women's Health Initiative (WHI) revealed that estrogen–progestin therapy does not reduce the risk of coronary heart disease, and increases the risk of breast cancer, stroke, and venous thromboembolic events. For patients who do not choose to take hormone therapy or those for whom HT is contraindicated, other antiresorptive agents are now the drugs of choice.

Given the availability of other therapies, fluoride is not recommended for the treatment of patients with osteoporosis. Calcitriol is a second-tier choice for the treatment of women with osteoporosis after all other modalities have been used. Parathyroid hormone is a third-line agent that increases trabecular bone, not cortical bone.

NIH Consensus Conference. Optimal calcium intake. NIH Consensus Development Panel on Optimal Calcium Intake. JAMA 1994;272: 1942–8.

Rosen CJ. Clinical practice. Postmenopausal osteoporosis. N Engl J Med 2005;353:595–603.

Tucker KL, Hannan MT, Qiao N, Jacques PF, Selhub J, Cupples LA, et al. Low plasma vitamin $B_{12}$ is associated with lower BMD: the Framingham Osteoporosis Study. J Bone Miner Res 2005;20:152–8.

# 59

## Salpingitis treatment

A 15-year-old adolescent presents with new onset of vaginal discharge and lower abdominal pain. She has a temperature of 37.8°C (100°F). Mucopurulent cervical discharge is noted on vaginal speculum examination. Cervical motion and adnexal tenderness are noted on bimanual examination. The patient, who lives at home with her parents, indicates she would prefer to avoid hospitalization. The most appropriate initial antibiotic regimen is

(A) intravenous cefotetan disodium (Cefotan) plus doxycycline
(B) intravenous doxycycline plus gentamicin
\* (C) intramuscular ceftriaxone plus oral doxycycline and oral metronidazole
(D) oral levofloxacin (Levaquin) plus oral metronidazole

Pelvic inflammatory disease (PID) represents a common infectious disorder of the upper genital tract in women, and includes endometritis, salpingitis, tuboovarian abscess, and pelvic peritonitis. Although the sexually transmitted pathogens, *Chlamydia trachomatis* and *Neisseria gonorrhoeae*, are responsible for many cases of PID, other organisms commonly encountered in the vagina, including anaerobes, enteric Gram-negative rods, and streptococci also are associated with this diagnosis. Regardless of culture results, appropriate regimens for treating PID must cover these pathogens. Clinicians who treat patients with PID should be aware of the sexually transmitted diseases treatment guidelines issued and periodically updated by the Centers for Disease Control and Prevention (CDC).

Because rapid treatment initiation of PID lowers subsequent risk of tubal infertility and ectopic pregnancy, treatment should start promptly. Treatment regimens for PID should include 14 days of antibiotic therapy. Although some clinicians continue to recommend that all women with diagnosed PID be hospitalized to allow inpatient monitoring and intravenous antibiotics, the decision whether or not to hospitalize patients with PID should be individualized. No data suggest that hospitalization improves outcomes for adolescents with diagnosed PID. Likewise, no data suggest parenteral antibiotic regimens are more effective in the treatment of PID than are oral

regimens. Hospitalization is appropriate for women with diagnosed PID who meet any of the following criteria:

- Surgical emergencies (eg, appendicitis) cannot be excluded
- Pregnancy
- Patient does not respond to oral antibiotics, or is not able to follow or tolerate an outpatient oral antibiotic regimen
- Severe illness, nausea and vomiting, or high fever is present
- A tuboovarian abscess is suspected or diagnosed

The symptoms and signs observed in this 15-year-old adolescent support a clinical diagnosis of PID. Given her desire to be treated as an outpatient, ambulatory management is reasonable if the clinician determines that the patient is likely to adhere to the recommended antibiotic regimen. If she has a good relationship with her parents, who are willing and able to facilitate their daughter's treatment, this would increase confidence that ambulatory management will be successful.

Intravenous cefotetan plus doxycycline represents a parenteral regimen recommended by the CDC guidelines. However, given the considerations reviewed previously, an antibiotic regimen that does not require frequent parenteral administration is more appropriate for this adolescent (Box 59-1). Intravenous doxycycline plus gentamicin does not represent a regimen recommended by the CDC. Intramuscular ceftriaxone or cefoxitin with probenecid or

---

**BOX 59-1**

**Outpatient Regimen to Combat Pelvic Inflammatory Disease**

Ceftriaxone, 250 mg intramuscularly in a single dose

*or*

Cefoxitin, 2 g intramuscularly in a single dose and probenecid, 1 g orally administered concurrently in a single dose

*or*

Other parenteral third-generation cephalosporin (eg, ceftizoxime or cefotaxime)

*plus*

Doxycycline, 100 mg orally twice a day for 14 days

*with or without*

Metronidazole, 500 mg orally twice a day for 14 days

Pelvic inflammatory disease. Sexually transmitted diseases treatment guidelines, 2006. Centers for Disease Control and Prevention [published erratum appears in MMWR Recomm Rep 2006;55(36):997]. MMWR Recomm Rep 2006;55(RR-11):1–94.

other parenteral third-generation cephalosporin plus oral doxycycline and oral metronidazole represents an appropriate ambulatory antibiotic regimen. Ceftriaxone covers *N gonorrhoeae*, the doxycycline covers *C trachomatis*, and anaerobic coverage is accomplished with metronidazole. Although the levofloxacin-based regimen is one of the oral antibiotic regimens included in the CDC guidelines, quinolone antibiotics are not appropriate for patients younger than 18 years because studies in immature animals have demonstrated cartilage erosions in weight-bearing joints.

Ness RB, Soper DE, Holley RL, Peipert J, Randall H, Sweet RL, et al. Effectiveness of inpatient and outpatient treatment strategies for women with pelvic inflammatory disease: results from the Pelvic Inflammatory Disease Evaluation and Clinical Health (PEACH) Randomized Trial. Am J Obstet Gynecol 2002;186:929–37.

Pelvic inflammatory disease. Sexually transmitted diseases treatment guidelines, 2006. Centers for Disease Control and Prevention [published erratum appears in MMWR Recomm Rep 2006;55(36):997]. MMWR Recomm Rep 2006;55(RR-11):1–94.

# 60

## Patient advocacy

A pregnant patient with Crohn's disease and recurrent perineal fistulae is a member of a health maintenance organization (HMO) plan. She wishes to have a primary cesarean delivery to avoid damage to a previous fistulae repair. Her insurance company refuses to precertify the surgery despite multiple discussions with your office staff. In these circumstances, the physician should

(A) submit the bill using a false diagnostic code
* (B) call the medical director of the health plan
(C) refuse to perform the surgery
(D) bill the patient outside the insurance plan
(E) obtain a second opinion

Physicians have a responsibility to advocate for their patients in the interest of beneficence and justice. They should have the interests of the patient at heart and try to help them regardless of compensation. They also are morally obligated to be truthful and not to engage in behavior that is deceitful. This includes the necessity for accurate coding of the services that they provide.

When a physician or insurer purposefully processes claims incorrectly to enhance reimbursement, it should be considered dishonest behavior. Such actions may be subject to civil and criminal penalties.

Claims may be denied for several reasons. A common reason for the denial of claims is coding errors on the part of physicians, who are responsible for educating themselves and their staff about how to link *Current Procedural Terminology* (CPT) codes and *International Classification of Diseases,* Ninth Revision, *Clinical Modification* (ICD-9-CM) diagnostic codes and the proper use of modifiers. Other common problems are inappropriate bundling of procedures by the payer and denying procedures done on the same day as an evaluation and management (E/M) visit. In this case scenario, the issue is more complex and involves medical decision making about the appropriate way to manage the patient. Physicians should keep in mind that patients also have a responsibility for the plans they select and the level of coverage they are entitled to according to their contracts.

The American College of Obstetricians and Gynecologists (ACOG) has recommended seven steps for appealing denied claims:

1. Negotiate, using accepted coding standards; done in a polite and direct manner, this is more likely to succeed than confrontation.

2. Have office staff contact the claims department of the insurer to discuss reasons for denial, and document this.

3. If this fails, directly contact the HMO's medical director.

4. Involve the state medical society, especially if patterns of abuse emerge.

5. Contact ACOG for assistance.

6. Send copies of the correspondence to your state insurance commissioner.

7. Involve the patient, who may be able to encourage policy revision if repeated complaints about coverage are received.

To transfer care of the patient to another physician only delays care. Refusal to care for the patient likewise does not fulfill the obligation toward the patient and is tantamount to abandonment.

American College of Obstetricians and Gynecologists. Coding responsibility. ACOG Committee Opinion 249. Washington, DC: ACOG; 2001.

American College of Obstetricians and Gynecologists. Inappropriate reimbursement practices by third-party payers. ACOG Committee Opinion 250. Washington, DC: ACOG; 2001.

# 61

## Skin cancer screening

A 39-year-old black woman presents with a raised lesion on her left shoulder. Biopsy reveals a small basal cell skin cancer. She states that she worked as a lifeguard for 6 years when she was in her twenties. She has an 18-year history of smoking and states that she has occasionally had warts on her hands in the past. Her mother had a basal cell carcinoma removed at age 63 years. Given her medical history, the risk factor that puts the patient at greatest risk for basal cell skin cancer is

      (A) female sex
      (B) history of smoking
      (C) history of warts on her hands
      (D) family member with basal cell carcinoma
\*    (E) history of prolonged sun exposure

Skin cancer remains the most common of all cancer types. In the United States, more than 1.3 million new cases are detected annually, and one in six individuals will develop skin cancer at some point in their lifetime. The incidence of skin cancer is growing at a rate faster than any other cancer today, and it has been estimated that this rate will continue to grow by 5% each year. In most instances, these cancers are benign basal cell carcinomas. Some cancer types, such as squamous cell carcinoma and melanoma, can carry significant mortality. Multiple risk factors exist for developing skin cancer (Table 61-1).

In reviewing this patient's history, it is important to note that women tend to have fewer skin cancers than men. Smoking has been associated with squamous cell carcinoma; however, no such relationship exists with basal cell cancers or melanoma. Genital human papillomavirus (HPV) infection has been well established as a precursor to vulvar and cervical cancer, but, to date, no connection has been proven between HPV infection and skin cancer at other sites. Certain melanoma types exhibit hereditary occurrence patterns, but nonmelanoma tumors are not familial in occurrence.

This patient's single most important risk factor for skin cancer is the same as it is for most of the population: prolonged exposure to ultraviolet radiation from the sun. All skin cancers are much more common among fair-skinned individuals than among dark-skinned individuals. It is much less likely for individuals of color to develop skin cancer, but it is important to remember that all individuals with significant sun exposure are at risk for development of skin cancer regardless of their skin color.

Recent studies have shown that blacks with diagnosed melanoma have lower survival rates and tend to present with more advanced disease than lighter skinned individuals. It is thought that a low level of awareness of skin cancer risk may exist in the African-American community and that both physician and patient may overlook dark-colored lesions on dark skin. It is vitally important, there-

**TABLE 61-1.** Risk Factors for Skin Cancer

| Risk Factor | Nonmelanoma Skin Cancer | Melanoma |
|---|---|---|
| Age | Increases with age | Peaks in early adulthood |
| Family history | No risk | Familial risk |
| Sex | Significant male preponderance | Slight male preponderance |
| Geography | Increased near equator | Increased near equator |
| Human papillomavirus | Genital (+), extragenital (−) | No risk |
| Occupation | Outdoor workers | Indoor workers |
| Prior skin cancer | Increased risk | Increased risk |
| Race | More common in whites | More common in whites |
| Smoking | Basal (−), squamous (+) | No risk |
| Skin type | Fair complexion, red or blond hair | Fair complexion, red or blond hair |
| Sun exposure | Cumulative exposure is the greatest risk factor | Intense exposure, blistering sunburn increases risk |

Modified from Jerant AF, Johnson JT, Sheridan CD, Caffrey TJ. Early detection and treatment of skin cancer. Am Fam Physician 2000;62:357–68, 375–6, 381–2.

fore, that the physician counsel all patients on the risk of skin cancer, encourage liberal use of sunscreens, and perform screening skin examinations on all individuals at risk regardless of their skin color.

Bellows CF, Belafsky P, Fortgang IS, Beech DJ. Melanoma in African-Americans: trends in biological behavior and clinical characteristics over two decades. J Surg Oncol 2001;78:10–6.

De Hertog SA, Wensveen CA, Bastiaens MT, Kielich CJ, Berkhout MJ, Westendorp RG, et al. Relation between smoking and skin cancer. Leiden Skin Cancer Study. J Clin Oncol 2001;19:231–8.

Jerant AF, Johnson JT, Sheridan CD, Caffrey TJ. Early detection and treatment of skin cancer. Am Fam Physician 2000;62:357–68, 375–6, 381–2.

Pfister H. Chapter 8: human papillomavirus and skin cancer. J Natl Cancer Inst Monogr 2003;31:52–6.

U.S. Preventive Services Task Force. Counseling for skin cancer: recommendations and rationale. Washington, DC: Office of Disease Prevention and Health Promotion; 2001.

U.S. Preventive Services Task Force. Screening for skin cancer: recommendations and rationale. Washington, DC: Office of Disease Prevention and Health Promotion; 2001.

# 62

## Nonsteroidal antiinflammatory drug use in the elderly

A 70-year-old obese woman comes to the office for a periodic examination. She is hypertensive and has coronary artery disease, which was diagnosed 6 months ago. She has been treated medically and is doing well. She was treated in the past with naproxen sodium for low back and knee pain, but now asks about the risks of using this pain reliever. At therapeutic doses, the most common and concerning side effect of naproxen sodium is

    (A) liver function abnormalities
    (B) acute renal failure
\*   (C) gastrointestinal complications
    (D) myocardial infarction
    (E) clotting problems

Pain-related complaints account for up to 80% of visits to physicians. Older patients more often report chronic pain in major joints, back, legs, and feet. In evaluating patients, a detailed history and characteristics of the pain should be noted along with precipitating events, history of treatments including hospitalizations, and stressful life events. Functional status including activities of everyday life should be assessed to estimate impairment and tolerance of pain. A broad understanding of nonsteroidal antiinflammatory drugs (NSAIDs) is then needed to counsel aging patients and prescribe these medications safely. These drugs are classified into two groups:

1. Conventional NSAIDs or nonselective NSAIDs

2. Newer selective NSAIDs known as cyclooxygenase (COX)-2 inhibitors

Nonselective NSAIDs inhibit two forms of cyclooxygenase: COX-1 and COX-2. Whereas COX-1 generates prostaglandins believed to be involved in gastrointestinal (GI) mucosal protection, vascular homeostasis, and platelet aggregation, COX-2 is induced at sites of inflammation and generates prostaglandins that mediate inflammation and pain. Inhibition of COX-1 is believed to be primarily responsible for the NSAID-induced gastrointestinal adverse events.

The choice of NSAID is frequently dictated by convenience, cost, and risk. No particular NSAID is consistently more effective for pain relief than another. Responses to individual drugs vary greatly from patient to patient. Therefore a few trials of different classes of NSAIDs may be necessary to optimize the individual patient's therapy (Appendix E).

Adverse GI side effects are the most common and concerning risk for NSAIDs. Frequently, patients who take NSAIDs are unaware of or unconcerned about GI complications. In reality, 10–20% of patients have dyspepsia while taking an NSAID and 2–4% of patients develop clinically significant gastric or duodenal ulcers if treated for at least a year. In patients hospitalized with NSAID-induced upper GI bleeding, the mortality rate is approximately 5–10%. Dyspepsia may be a warning sign for GI complications; however, many patients have no symptoms before a serious complication. It is therefore important to identify factors that increase the risk of complications and to determine methods for reducing the risk (Box 62-1). The occurrence of NSAID-induced GI side effects is time dependent. Studies have shown, how-

BOX 62-1

**Risk Factors for Nonsteroidal Antiinflammatory Drug–Associated Gastroduodenal Ulcers**

Established risk factors
- Advanced age (linear increase in risk)
- History of ulcer
- Concomitant administration of corticosteroids
- Higher doses of nonsteroidal antiinflammatory drugs, including the use of more than one nonsteroidal antiinflammatory drug
- Concomitant administration of anticoagulants
- Serious systemic disorder

Possible risk factors
- Concomitant infection with *Helicobacter pylori*
- Cigarette smoking
- Consumption of alcohol

Wolfe MM, Lichtenstein DR, Singh G. Gastrointestinal toxicity of nonsteroidal antiinflammatory drugs. N Engl J Med 1999;340:1889. Copyright ©1999 Massachusetts Medical Society. All rights reserved.

ever, that significant deleterious effects can be seen as soon as 7 days after initiation of treatment with indomethacin and within 2–3 months with other nonselective NSAIDs.

When risk factors are recognized, several strategies can be used to reduce GI complications. A co-prescription with a gastroprotective agent (misoprostol) is recommended in individuals older than 60 years and those with a history of peptic ulcer or GI bleeding. Although misoprostol is effective in preventing NSAID-induced ulcers, it has a number of adverse effects, including diarrhea and abdominal pain. A second strategy is to use COX-2 inhibitors, which have been shown to have an improved GI profile compared to nonselective NSAIDs.

One of the COX-2 inhibitors, rofecoxib (Vioxx), has been associated with a fivefold higher risk of myocardial infarction compared to naproxen. The adverse effects are dose-related and seem to manifest themselves in the early months of use. Rofecoxib is currently off the market. Although cardiovascular concerns may not extend to another COX-2 inhibitor, celecoxib, confirmation about its safety and that of the newer COX-2 inhibitors is needed. Nonselective NSAIDs have not been associated with myocardial infarction.

Renal effects of NSAIDs are rare (1.1 case of renal failure per 10,000 person-years) but significant. Users of NSAIDs have a threefold greater risk for developing acute renal failure than nonusers. The risks are greater with long-term therapy and a higher daily dose. Therefore, using the lowest effective dose is prudent to try to decrease renal and GI complications in the elderly. Additional risk factors that increase adverse renal effects with use of NSAIDs are hypertension, diabetes, heart failure, and use of cardiovascular drugs.

Hepatic and hematologic effects are uncommon. Small elevation of one or more liver test findings may occur in patients taking NSAIDs, and notable elevations (3–4 times normal) of transaminases have been reported in 1% of patients. Patients usually are asymptomatic, and discontinuation or dose reduction results in normalization of transaminases. The hematologic effects reported are aplastic anemia, agranulocytosis, and thrombocytosis.

Bombardier C, Laine L, Reicin A, Shapiro D, Burgos-Vargas R, Davis B, et al. Comparison of upper gastrointestinal toxicity of rofecoxib and naproxen in patients with rheumatoid arthritis. VIGOR Study Group. N Engl J Med 2000;343:1520–8.

Maxwell SR, Webb DJ. COX-2 selective inhibitors—important lessons learned. Lancet 2005;365:449–51.

Rahme E, Barkun AN, Adam V, Bardou M. Treatment costs to prevent or treat upper gastrointestinal adverse events associated with NSAIDs. Drug Saf 2004;27:1019–42.

Richy F, Bruyere O, Ethgen O, Rabenda V, Bouvenot G, Audran M, et al. Time dependent risk of gastrointestinal complications induced by non-steroidal anti-inflammatory drug use: a consensus statement using a meta-analytic approach. Ann Rheum Dis 2004;63:759–66.

Wolfe MM, Lichtenstein DR, Singh G. Gastrointestinal toxicity of nonsteroidal antiinflammatory drugs. N Engl J Med 1999;340:1888–99.

# 63

## Indications for varicella vaccination

A 20-year-old primigravid woman comes to your office for her first prenatal visit. She has no history of chickenpox. Varicella immunoglobulin (Ig) G serology shows her to be varicella susceptible. She is Rh-negative, and her husband is Rh-positive. She plans to breastfeed. The earliest safe time to administer her first dose of varicella vaccine is

       (A) in the third trimester
\*   (B) immediately after delivery
       (C) 6 weeks postpartum
       (D) after she weans the baby
       (E) after the baby has been immunized at 1 year

Varicella (chickenpox) is caused by varicella-zoster virus, a member of the herpesvirus family. It is contagious; 95% of household contacts who are susceptible contract the virus. Varicella usually causes mild disease in children, which lasts 4–5 days with vesicles erupting and then crusting over. Complications can arise in approximately 1% of children younger than 15 years. These complications include secondary bacterial infection of the lesions, hepatitis, arthritis, encephalitis, pneumonia, hemorrhagic complications, and Reye's syndrome. The mortality rate in children in the United States is 2 per 100,000. Infants less than 1 year of age may have more severe infection, because their immune system is not yet well developed.

In temperate climates, only 2% of infections are in patients 20 years old and older. In the subtropics and tropics, 20–50% of infections occur in adolescents and adults. Adults are more likely to develop encephalitis or pneumonia, and to succumb to the infection. Pregnant women are at increased risk of pneumonia and death from chickenpox infection. Approximately 5% of U.S. women are seronegative for varicella.

Varicella is also a teratogen; 0.4–2% of fetuses of nonimmune women exposed at less than 20 weeks of gestation develop the congenital varicella syndrome. Exposure to active varicella infection between 5 days before birth and 2 days after birth may result in severe varicella infection in the newborn. Varicella immune globulin used in pregnancy may reduce severity of symptoms when there is a risk of maternal infection. Acyclovir also may be used to attenuate the peripartum neonatal infection.

As with all herpes viruses, after initial infection there is latent virus in nerve roots. Latent virus may reactivate with a painful vesicular rash in a dermatome distribution (shingles). Approximately 15% of previously infected individuals will develop shingles. The incidence of shingles is approximately 74 per 100,000 in children younger than 10 years, 300 per 100,000 in adults aged 35–44 years, and 1,200 per 100,000 in individuals older than 75

years. The shingles vesicles must come in direct contact with a susceptible individual for infection with varicella to occur.

A live, attenuated varicella vaccine was first developed in Japan in 1974. The vaccine has been improved, and was introduced in the United States in 1995. Currently, it is recommended to vaccinate healthy infants at age 12–18 months. Catch-up vaccination in older children and vaccination of susceptible adolescents and adults is also recommended. The best seroconversion occurs with two doses in adults. Only one dose is required in children. Varicella vaccine in adolescents and adults produces detectable levels of varicella antibodies in 97–100% of patients 1–6 years after vaccination. Clinically, there is an 80% reduction in the expected number of varicella patients, and patients with chickenpox usually have fewer lesions.

Varicella vaccine is contraindicated in patients with cellular immunodeficiencies such as human immunodeficiency virus (HIV). It may be given to patients with humoral immunodeficiencies such as agammaglobulinemia. The Centers for Disease Control and Prevention (CDC) have published detailed recommendations for vaccination of individuals with immunocompromised conditions. Adverse reactions to the varicella vaccine include injection site reactions and mild varicellalike rash. Severe adverse reactions to varicella vaccine are unlikely; one trial found a rate of 2.9 per 100,000. Vaccination has not been shown to transmit varicella zoster virus between immunocompetent individuals. It has also been shown to be safe in children who reside in households with cancer patients without putting the cancer patient at risk.

Herpes zoster incidence is decreased in patients who receive varicella vaccine. A study with a new booster varicella vaccine (with a distinct formulation from that used for varicella vaccination in susceptible patients) showed herpes zoster incidence decreases in older adults given this booster vaccination.

Some clinicians recommend varicella IgG screening before conception with vaccination before pregnancy for susceptible women. Routine prenatal screening with the intent to vaccinate susceptible women postpartum may be cost-effective. Postpartum vaccination is safe in breast-feeding women. Varicella vaccine virus is not found in breast milk. Blood or blood products administered within 6 weeks of live virus vaccines may inhibit their effectiveness. However, an exception to this is Rh D immune globulin. The volume administered is so small; interference with immunization has not been documented. Women should avoid pregnancy for 1 month after vaccination.

Live attenuated vaccines should not be administered to pregnant women. There is a theoretical risk of reversion to a wild type and exposure of the fetus to a potential teratogen. Inadvertent varicella vaccine exposure in pregnancy is being followed with a registry. After the first 362 reported pregnancies with vaccination exposure within 3 months of pregnancy or during pregnancy, no congenital varicella syndrome cases have been diagnosed. However,

these are preliminary data, and vaccination should be avoided in pregnancy. A pregnancy test before vaccination of reproductive-aged females is not currently recommended by the CDC. Confusion between varicella zoster immune globulin (VZIG) and live attenuated varicella vaccine has been responsible for some of the inadvertent administration of varicella vaccine in pregnant women exposed to the virus.

Bohlke K, Galil K, Jackson LA, Schmid DS, Starkovich P, Loparev VN, et al. Postpartum varicella vaccination: is the vaccine virus excreted in breast milk? Obstet Gynecol 2003;102:970–7.

Faix RG. Immunization during pregnancy. Clin Obstet Gynecol 2002;45:42–58.

Koren G, Money D, Boucher M, Aoki F, Petric M, Innocencion G, et al. Serum concentrations, efficacy, and safety of a new, intravenously administered varicella zoster immune globulin in pregnant women. J Clin Pharmacol 2002;42:267–74.

Shields KE, Galil K, Seward J, Sharrar RG, Cordero JF, Slater E. Varicella vaccine exposure during pregnancy: data from the first 5 years of the pregnancy registry. Obstet Gynecol 2001;98:14–9.

Skull SA, Wang EL. Varicella vaccination—a critical review of the evidence. Arch Dis Child 2001;85:83–90.

# 64

## Family history of mental retardation

A 32-year-old woman comes to the office for preconception counseling. She has one child, a 5-year-old girl with moderate mental retardation. An abnormal biochemical screen for Down syndrome occurred during that pregnancy, and an amniocentesis was performed with findings of a normal karyotype. She reports that she drank 1–2 glasses of wine per day before she knew she was pregnant. She smoked approximately one half of a pack of cigarettes per day but was able to decrease to 2–3 cigarettes per day. The pregnancy ended in preterm labor at approximately 34 weeks with delivery of a 2,000-g neonate. The infant required ventilator support for a few days, but after 2 weeks of hospitalization the infant was able to go home. The patient is concerned about the chance of giving birth to another infant with mental retardation and seeks advice on what steps can be taken to determine or prevent this risk. You recommend

      (A) assessment of cervical length in pregnancy
      (B) complete abstinence from alcohol and cigarette use
\*   (C) maternal DNA analysis
      (D) cervical fetal fibronectin measurement after 20 weeks of gestation
      (E) serial level II ultrasonography

Mental retardation is estimated to affect 1–3% of the general population, depending on the diagnostic criteria used. With known etiologies, the timing of the insult is prenatal in approximately 50–70% of cases. The known etiologies that occur prenatally are generally genetic and include fragile X syndrome (1–2% of individuals with mental retardation), Down syndrome, mutations in the gene encoding *MECP2*, and subtelomeric rearrangements.

Other prenatal causes are structural central nervous system abnormalities and, less commonly, growth restriction, congenital infection, toxin, and radiation exposure.

Fragile X syndrome is the most common inherited form of mental retardation and is estimated to affect 1 in 1,500 males and 1 in 2,500 females. Fragile X demonstrates an atypical pattern of expression. Although its inheritance is X-linked, it is neither recessive nor dominant; 20% of males who inherit the gene are not affected, 50% of females who are heterozygous will exhibit some mild cognitive behavioral abnormality, and 30% are clearly mentally retarded.

Fragile X is a site on the long arm of the X chromosome (Xq27.3), and the molecular basis is related to the fragile X mental retardation-1 gene. Mutations in this gene are related to an expansion of triplet cytosine-guanine-guanine. Expansions in the range of 50–200 copies are labeled as premutations. Premutations, previously thought to be asymptomatic, have recently been linked to mild cognitive and behavioral deficits, increased risk of intention tremor and gait ataxia with aging, and possibly premature ovarian failure (or early menopause). The carrier rate of premutations is estimated at 1 in 295 females and 1 in 810 males. When transmitted by the mother to the child, premutations can expand to the full mutation. Premutations with at least 90–100 cytosine-guanine-guanine repeats are likely to expand to full mutations. The full mutation is accompanied by greater than 200 copies of the cytosine-guanine-guanine triplet. If this degree of expansion is accompanied by methylation and inactivation of the fragile X mental retardation-1 gene, then mental retardation is likely. Phenotypic findings associated with fragile X in males include autistic behavior, macroorchidism, narrow face and large jaw, and speech and language problems. These findings are more difficult to detect in females.

Standard karyotype does not reliably demonstrate fragile X. To assess the number of cytosine-guanine-guanine repeats and the methylation of the fragile X mental retardation-1 gene—the two characteristics that correlate the best with mental retardation—DNA-based molecular testing is needed. Information regarding whether the mother carries the fragile X gene and expansion of the cytosine-guanine-guanine triplet would allow her to make an informed decision about future pregnancy as well as prenatal testing.

Results from studies on the effect of smoking during pregnancy and cognitive outcome are contradictory. The findings of some studies demonstrate differences with delayed cognitive development in offspring of mothers who smoked during pregnancy. In contrast, other studies show no differences in cognitive development. A study of 578 same-sex sibling pairs, where the mother smoked during one pregnancy but not during the other pregnancy, did document deficits in spelling and reading but not in arithmetic. This may be the most convincing evidence of the effect of smoking on cognitive function, because the

environmental, maternal, and familial circumstances were similar for both siblings. However, none of the reports labeled these children as mentally retarded.

Although there is no definition of a safe alcohol intake in pregnancy, the degree of exposure related by this patient is an unlikely source of the child's mental retardation. It is strongly recommended that pregnant women abstain completely from alcohol intake. Fetal alcohol syndrome and fetal alcohol effects have been reported with chronic alcohol use and binge drinking (5 or more drinks on one occasion). The prevalence of fetal alcohol syndrome has been estimated to be 3–5 out of 1,000 live births but as high as 2–4 per 100 among heavy drinkers (binge drinking and minimum of 1–3 drinks per day). The syndrome consists of prenatal and postnatal growth restriction, cranial facial dysmorphology, and neurodevelopmental abnormalities, including mental retardation. Most children with fetal alcohol syndrome are mildly to moderately retarded with average IQ scores of 65–70. In children exposed in pregnancy to 14.2 g (0.5 oz) of alcohol daily, less severe fetal alcohol effects have been observed, but deficits in cognitive function are reported.

Prematurity is generally not a major cause of mental retardation, with the exception that extremely premature infants are much more at risk of mental retardation than term infants. Cervical length and cervicovaginal evaluation for fetal fibronectin may be helpful in assessing the risk of recurrent preterm birth but not mental retardation.

Level II prenatal ultrasonography is useful in the detection of fetal central nervous system abnormalities. However, because the previous child did not demonstrate any such abnormality, the risk would not be assumed to be elevated.

Chiriboga CA. Fetal alcohol and drug effects. Neurologist 2003;9: 267–79.

Croen LA, Grether JK, Selvin S. The epidemiology of mental retardation of unknown cause. Pediatrics 2001;107:E86–E90.

Genetics and molecular diagnostic testing. ACOG Technology Assessment No. 1. American College of Obstetricians and Gynecologists. Obstet Gynecol 2002;100:193–211.

Hagerman PJ, Hagerman RJ. The fragile-X premutation: a maturing perspective [published erratum appears in Am J Hum Genet 2004;75:352]. Am J Hum Genet 2004;74:805–16.

Lassen K, Oei TP. Effects of maternal cigarette smoking during pregnancy on long-term physical and cognitive parameters of child development. Addict Behav 1998;23:635–53.

Screening for fragile X syndrome. ACOG Committee Opinion No. 338. American College of Obstetricians and Gynecologists. Obstet Gynecol 2006;107:1483–5.

Shapiro LR. The Fragile X syndrome. A peculiar pattern of inheritance. N Engl J Med 1991;325:1736–8.

# 65

## Appendectomy in the third trimester of pregnancy

A 16-year-old adolescent, gravida 1, with an intrauterine pregnancy at 35 weeks of gestation, arrives in labor and delivery with abdominal pain and uterine contractions. She reports good fetal movement, one episode of chills, increasing nausea, anorexia, and occasional uterine contractions. Her blood pressure is 110/70 mm Hg, temperature 38°C (100.4°F); pulse and respirations are within normal limits. The abdominal examination is soft with tenderness in the right lower quadrant with rebound. No masses are palpated. Fetal heart rate is 150 beats per minute with moderate variability. She has uterine contractions, which are palpated as mild to moderate every 4 minutes. Pelvic examination reveals the cervix to be long and closed. She has a white blood cell count of 14,800/mm$^3$ with an increased number of bands and a normal urinalysis. The most appropriate diagnostic test is

        (A) computed tomography (CT) scan of the abdomen and pelvis
*    (B) ultrasonography of the abdomen and pelvis
        (C) amniocentesis
        (D) abdominal X-ray series

Appendicitis is the most common nongynecologic surgical emergency in pregnancy. It occurs in approximately 1 in 1,440 pregnancies. Failure to diagnose appropriately and proceed with prompt surgical excision may result in appendicular rupture with peritonitis or abscess formation and a secondary poor outcome for fetus and mother.

Historically, the appendix was considered to be displaced as pregnancy progressed. However, more recent imaging studies and surgical findings have demonstrated the appendix often is accessible in the right lower quadrant.

The diagnosis of appendicitis in the pregnant patient is made more complex compared to diagnosis in the nonpregnant patient because pregnancy adds additional dimensions to the differential diagnosis. The classic symptoms of gastrointestinal distress and elevated white blood cell count remain a common part of the presenting scenario. Acute infectious diseases in pregnancy also may be accompanied by premature labor. The differential diagnosis includes infectious etiologies of the upper genital structures and chorioamnionitis as well as pathologic processes of the gastrointestinal tract (inflammatory bowel disease) and pyelonephritis. Adnexal torsion also may result in a similar clinical presentation.

A high index of suspicion may prompt further evaluation by either traditional or spiral CT scan. In the nonpregnant patient, obtaining a CT scan has resulted in accurate diagnoses of appendicitis in most patients, but it is not the best choice for the patient described.

Ultrasonography would be the best diagnostic test for this patient. Table 65-1 shows a comparison of sensitivity and specificity of ultrasonography and CT scan in the diagnosis of appendicitis. Although ultrasonography is

**TABLE 65-1.** Sensitivity and Specificity of Ultrasonography and Computed Tomography Scan in the Diagnosis of Appendicitis

| Test | Sensitivity (%) | Specificity (%) |
|---|---|---|
| Ultrasonography | 0.86 (0.83–0.88) | 0.81 (0.78–0.84) |
| Computed tomography scan | 0.94 (0.91–0.95) | 0.95 (0.93–0.96) |

Data from Terasawa T, Blackmore CC, Bent S, Kohlwes RJ. Systematic review: computed tomography and ultrasonography to detect acute appendicitis in adults and adolescents. Ann Intern Med 2004;141:537–46.

less sensitive and specific than a CT scan, it does not expose the patient to radiation as does the CT scan.

Other laboratory or diagnostic tests may be ordered to exclude disease processes in the differential diagnosis. Plain X-rays of the abdomen may assist visualization of disorders such as bowel obstruction or ileus, but add little to the diagnosis of acute appendicitis. Amniocentesis may be considered if there is a high suspicion of chorioamnionitis and may assist in the management of the differential diagnosis in a patient with this clinical scenario.

A recent large series of 9,753 appendectomies included 94 women who were pregnant, with 24.5% in the third trimester of pregnancy. Perforation of the appendix occurred in 26.1% of cases of those women who were in the third trimester. In a patient with acute appendicitis, early surgical intervention is recommended.

Ames Castro M, Shipp TD, Castro EE, Ouzounian J, Rao P. The use of helical computed tomography in pregnancy for the diagnosis of acute appendicitis. Am J Obstet Gynecol 2001;184:954–7.

Popkin CA, Lopez PP, Cohn SM, Brown M, Lynn M. The incision of choice for pregnant women with appendicitis is through McBurney's point. Am J Surg 2002;183:20–2.

Ueberrueck T, Koch A, Meyer L, Hinkel M, Gastinger I. Ninety-four appendectomies for suspected acute appendicitis during pregnancy. World J Surg 2004;28:508–11.

# 66

## Cardioprotective effects of hormone therapy

A 49-year-old woman, gravida 2, para 2, presents with increasingly severe hot flushes and night sweats. Her menses have become progressively lighter and farther apart. Her last menstrual period was 4 months ago. She has tried over-the-counter herbal preparations with no relief. She has been reluctant to start hormone therapy (HT) since reading newspaper reports regarding a large study being stopped early because of health problems. You inform her that the estrogen–progestin arm of the Women's Health Initiative concluded that the condition associated with the highest risk was

    (A) stroke
    (B) coronary heart disease
    (C) breast cancer
    (D) colon cancer
\*    (E) venous thromboembolic event

The Women's Health Initiative (WHI) was the largest randomized placebo-controlled trial of HT in menopausal women. More than 27,000 menopausal women aged 50–79 years were randomized to placebo vs conjugated equine estrogen, 0.625 mg, plus medroxyprogesterone acetate, 2.5 mg (estrogen and progesterone) daily if they had a uterus (N = 16,608) or placebo vs conjugated equine estrogen, 0.625 mg alone (E), if they had undergone a hysterectomy (N = 10,739). The primary purpose of the study was to assess the effects of HT on risk of coronary artery disease (CAD). Observational data had accumulated suggesting a significant reduction in CAD in HT users. Because some studies had suggested a possible association of use with breast cancer, the primary adverse outcome was the incidence of breast cancer. Although the study was planned for 9 years, the estrogen and progesterone arm was discontinued in May 2002 after an average follow-up of 5.2 years. Preliminary data analysis had shown no decrease in CAD but a trend toward increased incidence of CAD (Table 66-1) and breast cancer. Other adverse events in the estrogen and progesterone arm included an increase in stroke and venous thromboembolism. No differences in rates of

death were noted. Significant reductions were seen in colon cancer and hip fracture. The greatest absolute increase in risk was for venous thromboembolism (Table 66-1).

The estrogen vs placebo arm of the study was discontinued in February 2004 after an average follow-up of 6.8 years. Although no increase in breast cancer or CAD was seen, there was an increased risk of stroke in this arm of the study (Table 66-2).

Caution must be used when trying to apply the results of WHI to a 49-year-old woman with symptoms of severe estrogen deficiency, as in the patient described. The average age of women in the WHI was 63.2 years, but the average age of initiating HT in clinical practice is much younger. Guidelines established by the American College of Obstetricians and Gynecologists recommend the use of HT in symptomatic women using the lowest effective dose for the shortest possible duration. When a woman discontinues HT, risk assessment and screening should follow the same criteria as for a woman who is in the early stages of menopause. It also should take into account bone mineral density measurements based on age and other risk factors for osteoporosis.

**TABLE 66-1.** Relative and Absolute Increased Risks and Benefits of Use of Conjugated Equine Estrogen 0.625 mg Plus Medroxyprogesterone Acetate 2.5 mg in the Women's Health Initiative: Data From Various WHI Studies

| Event | Overall Hazard Ratio | Unadjusted 95% Confidence Interval | Adjusted 95% Confidence Interval | Absolute Increased Risk per 10,000 Women Per Year | Absolute Increased Benefit per 10,000 Women per Year |
|---|---|---|---|---|---|
| Coronary heart disease* | 1.24 | 1.00–1.54 | 0.97–1.60 | 6 | |
| Breast cancer[†] | 1.24 | 1.01–1.54 | 0.97–1.59 | 8 | |
| Stroke[‡] | 1.31 | 1.02–1.68 | 0.93–1.84 | 7 | |
| Venous thromboembolism[§] | 2.06 | 1.58–2.82 | 1.26–3.55 | 18 | |
| Colorectal cancer[‖] | 0.63 | 0.43–0.92 | 0.32–1.24 | | 6 |
| Hip fractures[¶] | 0.67 | 0.47–0.96 | 0.41–1.10 | | 5 |
| Total fractures[¶] | 0.76 | 0.69–0.83 | – | | 47 |
| Diabetes mellitus[#] | 0.79 | 0.67–0.93 | – | | 15 |

*Manson JE, Hsia J, Johnson KC, Rossouw JE, Assaf AR, Lasser NL, et al. Estrogen plus progestin and the risk of coronary heart disease. N Engl J Med 2003;349:523–34.

[†]Chlebowski RT, Hendrix SL, Langer RD, Stefanick ML, Gass M, Lane D, et al. Influence of estrogen plus progestin on breast cancer and mammography in healthy postmenopausal women: the Women's Health Initiative Randomized Trial. JAMA 2003:289:3243–53.

[‡]Wassertheil-Smoller S, Hendrix SL, Limacher M, Heiss G, Kooperberg C, Baird A, et al. Effect of estrogen plus progestin on stroke in postmenopausal women: the Women's Health Initiative: a randomized trial. JAMA 2003;289:2673–84.

[§]Cushman M, Kuller LH, Prentice R, Rodabough RJ, Psaty BM, Stafford RS, et al. Estrogen plus progestin and risk of venous thrombosis. JAMA 2004;292:1573–80.

[‖]Chlebowski RT, Wactawski-Wende J, Ritenbaugh C, Hubbell FA, Ascensao J, Rodabough RJ, et al. Estrogen plus progestin and colorectal cancer in postmenopausal women. N Engl J Med 2004:350:991–1004.

[¶]Cauley JA, Robbins J, Chen Z, Cummings SR, Jackson RD, LaCroix AZ, et al. Effects of estrogen plus progestin on risk of fracture and bone mineral density: the Women's Health Initiative randomized trial. JAMA 2003;290:1729–38.

[#]Margolis KL, Bonds DE, Rodabough RJ, Tinker L, Phillips LS, Allen C, et al. Effect of oestrogen plus progestin on the incidence of diabetes in postmenopausal women: results from the Women's Health Initiative Hormone Trial. Diabetologia 2004;47:1175–87.

**TABLE 66-2.** Relative and Absolute Risks and Benefits of Use of Conjugated Equine Estrogen, 0.625 mg, Alone in the Women's Health Initiative Trial

| Event | Overall Hazard Ratio | Unadjusted 95% Confidence Interval | Adjusted 95% Confidence Interval | Absolute Increased Risk per 10,000 Women Per Year | Absolute Increased Benefit per 10,000 Women per Year |
|---|---|---|---|---|---|
| Coronary heart disease | 0.91 | 0.75–1.12 | 0.72–1.15 | | −5 |
| Breast cancer | 0.77 | 0.59–1.01 | 0.57–1.06 | | −7 |
| Stroke | 1.39 | 1.10–1.77 | 0.97–1.99 | +12 | |
| Venous thromboembolism | 1.33 | 0.99–1.79 | 0.86–2.08 | +7 | |
| Pulmonary embolism | 1.34 | 0.87–2.06 | 0.70–2.55 | +3 | |
| Colorectal cancer | 1.08 | 0.75–1.55 | 0.63–1.86 | +1 | |
| Hip fractures | 0.61 | 0.41–0.91 | 0.33–1.11 | | −6 |
| Total fractures | 0.70 | 0.63–0.79 | 0.59–0.83 | | −56 |

Data from Women's Health Initiative Steering Committee. Effects of conjugated equine estrogen in postmenopausal women with hysterectomy. JAMA 2004;291:1701–12.

Anderson GL, Limacher M, Assaf AR, Bassford T, Beresford SA, Black H, et al. Effects of conjugated equine estrogen in postmenopausal women with hysterectomy: the Women's Health Initiative randomized controlled trial. Women's Health Initiative Steering Committee. JAMA 2004;291:1701–12.

Hormone therapy [special issue]. American College of Obstetricians and Gynecologists. Obstet Gynecol 2004;104(suppl).

Rossouw JE, Anderson GL, Prentice RL, LaCroix AZ, Kooperberg C, Stefanick ML, et al. Risks and benefits of estrogen plus progestin in healthy postmenopausal women: principal results from the Women's Health Initiative randomized controlled trial. Women's Health Initiative Steering Committee. JAMA 2002;288:321–33.

# 67

## Male contribution to infertility

A 27-year-old nulligravid woman reports a 1-year history of unprotected sexual intercourse with her husband without conception. Her menses are regular and monthly. She has experienced no changes in menstrual flow or premenstrual symptoms. She denies pelvic pain and dyspareunia. She has no history of sexually transmitted diseases. Her medical history is uncomplicated and her immunizations are current. She used oral contraceptives for 3 years before her marriage. The most appropriate next step in her workup is

     (A) hysterosalpingography
     (B) diagnostic laparoscopy
\*   (C) semen analysis
     (D) home urinary luteinizing hormone (LH) test
     (E) postcoital test

Infertility is the absence of pregnancy despite 1 year of unprotected intercourse. Currently, 15% of all couples are affected by the condition, and it has been shown that the rate of infertility is continuing to increase each year. Infertility can be related to female factors, male factors, or combined factors and has many different causes. In 15% of infertile couples, however, no identifiable reason for infertility can be ascertained. When a woman presents with complaints of infertility, it is important to elicit a history that takes into account both the woman and her male partner. The goal of the initial workup for the woman is to assess for normal ovulation, identify factors that may limit tubal patency, evaluate timing of intercourse and sexual habits, and recognize medical conditions that may be associated with subfertility. In most cases, this can be accomplished easily at the initial evaluation.

Hysterosalpingography (HSG) may be indicated if sufficient suspicion for tubal occlusion exists. A history of pelvic inflammatory disease, endometriosis, and abdominal surgery may indicate the need for HSG. Laparoscopy has traditionally played a part in the workup for infertility. However, recent advances in assisted reproductive technologies (ART) may limit its usefulness in many situations. Some physicians will now choose to bypass laparoscopy and proceed with ART on the basis of its proven success in achieving pregnancy. The invasiveness of laparoscopy and the potential for complications may outweigh the benefit. Home urinary LH tests are helpful in assessing for the presence of ovulation and as an aid to the timing of sexual intercourse in cases of unexplained infertility where the workup for both partners has not revealed a cause. Postcoital testing, formerly thought to be useful in diagnosing cervical factors associated with infertility, has now been shown to be of limited value.

Review of this woman's history reveals that she possesses no real risk factors for infertility. Her menses are regular, so it can be assumed that she is ovulating monthly. She gives no history consistent with tubal occlusion and she has no ongoing medical concerns. The most appropriate next step in the workup is analysis of her husband's semen. Male factor infertility accounts for up to one third of all cases of infertility and should be assessed early in the workup of this case. Semen analysis is inexpensive, noninvasive, and easily obtained. When identified early, male subfertility may allow the physician to forego or postpone many aspects of the female workup that are both expensive and invasive. Moreover, treatment of male infertility may allow the couple to proceed with natural conception, sparing the cost of ART as well as the potential risk for multiple gestations.

Isaksson R, Tiitinen A. Present concept of unexplained infertility. Gynecol Endocrinol 2004;18:278–90.

Kolettis PN. Evaluation of the subfertile man [published erratum appears in Am Fam Physician 2003;68:1266]. Am Fam Physician 2003;67:2165–72.

Speroff L, Glass RH, Kase NG. Clinical gynecologic endocrinology and infertility. 6th ed. Philadelphia (PA): Lippincott Williams & Wilkins, 1999. p. 1015–42.

Strandell A. Surgery in contemporary infertility. Curr Womens Health Rep 2003;3:367–74.

# 68

## Follow-up after hepatitis B vaccine for proof of immunity

A 42-year-old woman comes to the office for her periodic health examination. She completed her series of hepatitis B vaccinations 6 months ago and asks about the need for follow-up testing. The appropriate testing would be

* (A) hepatitis B surface antibody titer
  (B) hepatitis B surface antigen titer
  (C) hepatitis B core antibody titer
  (D) hepatitis B e antigen titer
  (E) none needed

The hepatitis B vaccination is a series of three intramuscular injections with the second and third doses administered at 1 and 6 months, respectively, after the first injection. The vaccines licensed for use in the United States are made by recombinant DNA techniques. The recommended site of injection is the deltoid muscle in adults; administration in the buttock decreases the immunogenicity of the vaccine. Vaccination is recommended by the Centers for Disease Control and Prevention (CDC) for all infants regardless of maternal serologic status.

For adults, CDC recommends vaccination of high-risk groups (Box 68-1). The vaccine is 80–90% effective in preventing hepatitis B infection, and the effectiveness approaches 100% if a protective antibody response develops after vaccination. Determining the schedule and need for follow-up testing after vaccination is important to ensure protection from hepatitis B infection in high-risk groups.

Postvaccination testing for serologic response uses the assay for the hepatitis B surface antibody. Testing for vaccine response is not necessary after routine vaccination of infants, children, or adolescents. The testing for immunity is recommended for those individuals at high risk for exposure. These groups include infants born to hepatitis B surface antigen–positive mothers, dialysis patients, and human immunodeficiency virus (HIV)-infected individuals. Additionally, health care workers should have postvaccination testing due to the occupational risk from exposure to injury from sharp instruments.

The management of postexposure prophylaxis depends on the individual's antibody response to vaccination. For individuals exposed to hepatitis B who lack the appropriate antibody response, administration of hepatitis B immune globulin may be necessary. Postvaccination testing for immune response should be performed 1–6 months after completion of the vaccination series. For patients who do not develop hepatitis B surface antibodies after vaccination, revaccination is recommended. Additionally, these individuals should be tested for mark-

ers of past or present infection with hepatitis B. The antibody response after one revaccination dose is 15–25% and after three doses is 30–50%.

The immunologic memory from hepatitis B immunization appears to last at least 15 years. Recent data from long-term follow-up of children immunized as infants indicated that immunity wanes after 15 years and booster vaccination augmented the vaccine response in most indi-

---

**BOX 68-1**

**High-Risk Groups Recommended for Hepatitis B Virus (HBV) Vaccination**

- Individuals with occupational risk
- Clients and staff of institutions for the developmentally disabled
- Hemodialysis patients
- Recipients of clotting factor concentrates
- Household contacts and sex partners of HBV carriers
- Adoptees from countries where HBV infection is endemic
- International travelers
- Intravenous drug users
- Sexually active homosexual and bisexual men
- Sexually active heterosexual men and women in the following groups:
  —Other recently acquired sexually transmitted diseases
  —Commercial sex workers
  —Individuals who have a history of sexual activity with more than one partner in the previous 6 months
- Inmates of long-term correctional facilities

Modified from Hepatitis B virus: a comprehensive strategy for eliminating transmission in the United States through universal childhood vaccination. Recommendations of the Immunization Practices Advisory Committee (ACIP). MMWR Recomm Rep 1991;40(RR-13):1–19.

viduals. However, neither the CDC nor the European Consensus Group on Hepatitis B Immunity recommends booster vaccinations in immunocompetent individuals.

A positive test result for hepatitis B surface antigen titer indicates current active infection. A positive assay result for hepatitis B core antibody signals prior infection with hepatitis B. Presence of hepatitis B e antigen identifies an individual with hepatitis B (chronic or acute) who is highly infectious.

Are booster immunizations needed for lifelong hepatitis B immunity? European Consensus Group on Hepatitis B Immunity. Lancet 2000; 355:561–5.

Hepatitis B virus: a comprehensive strategy for eliminating transmission in the United States through universal childhood vaccination. Recommendations of the Immunization Practices Advisory Committee (ACIP). MMWR Recomm Rep 1991;40(RR-13):1–25.

Lu CY, Chiang BL, Chi WK, Chang MH, Ni YH, Hsu HM, et al. Waning immunity to plasma-derived hepatitis B vaccine and the need for boosters 15 years after neonatal vaccination. Hepatology 2004; 40:1415–20.

# 69

## Cancer screening in postmenopausal women

A healthy 50-year-old woman comes to the office for her periodic medical examination. Her last three liquid-based cytology results have been normal. She recently quit smoking after a 25-packs-per-year history. Her mother and sister have breast cancer. In addition to mammography, the best screening test for this patient is

      (A) *BRCA1* and *BRCA2* gene mutation screening
      (B) chest X-ray
\*   (C) colonoscopy
      (D) cervical cytologic screening
      (E) ultrasonography of the ovaries

Evidence for different tests can be examined according to the National Cancer Institute's Physician Data Query Program. Breast cancer screening for women aged 40–64 years should consist of annual mammography and clinical breast examination. Although there is good evidence for mammography screening in this age group, studies are less certain for women older than 70 years and younger than 40 years. According to American Cancer Society (ACS) recommendations, women may choose whether or not to also perform breast self-examination.

The decision whether or not to undergo genetic testing for familial types of breast cancer has serious implications for asymptomatic patients. It is more common to test family members who have breast cancer before considering testing those who have not developed the disease.

Spiral computed tomography (CT) scanning has been increasingly used in an effort to identify early lung cancer. The ACS has historically maintained that individuals at high risk for lung cancer (smokers) may choose screening on an individual basis, but ACS recommends that CT scanning not be performed in asymptomatic individuals. The U.S. Preventive Services Task Force (USPSTF) makes no recommendation for or against CT scanning. Chest X-ray as a screening modality for lung cancer is not

recommended. The ongoing collaborative National Lung Cancer Screening Trial should provide more information in the future.

The USPSTF found fair to good evidence that several screening methods are effective in reducing mortality from colorectal cancer in patients older than 50 years. Fecal occult blood testing (FOBT) has decreased mortality by 20%. Testing should be done after abstaining from foods and medications that can affect results and on three separate occasions. There is evidence that sigmoidoscopy alone or in combination with FOBT every 5 years reduces mortality, particularly when screening results in removal of dysplastic polyps. Colonoscopy has the potential to detect neoplasia in the proximal colon that may be missed on sigmoidoscopy, but this must be balanced against the increased risk of complications. It should be performed every 10 years unless polyps are detected. The USPSTF did not find direct evidence that colonoscopy decreases mortality, but it may be extrapolated from sigmoidoscopy studies and case–control studies. Double-contrast barium enema is less sensitive than colonoscopy with no direct evidence that it reduces mortality rates.

Newer recommendations on the frequency of cervical cytologic screening advise screening every 2–3 years for patients older than 30 years with three consecutive normal results and no abnormal results. Cytologic screening has significantly decreased mortality from cervical cancer.

According to the American College of Obstetricians and Gynecologists (ACOG), recommended screening for ovarian cancer in asymptomatic women should consist of annual pelvic examination. However, insufficient data exist to prove the efficacy of annual pelvic examination, ultrasonography, and serum CA 125 antigen as screening tests. The latter two tests have been done serially in high-risk women, but no data support this management strategy. Proteomic serum profiling was reported to discriminate patients with ovarian cancer from normal controls and from those with benign disease. Unfortunately, the results have not been reproducible.

Franco EL, Duarte-Franco E, Rohan TE. Evidence-based policy recommendations on cancer screening and prevention. Cancer Detect Prev 2002;26:350–61.

Mulshine JL, Sullivan DC. Clinical practice. Lung cancer screening. N Engl J Med 2005;352:2714–20.

Petricoin EF, Ardekani AM, Hitt BA, Levine PJ, Fusaro VA, Steinberg SM, et al. Use of proteomic patterns in serum to identify ovarian cancer. Lancet 2002;359:572–7.

Ransohoff DF. Lessons from controversy: ovarian cancer screening and serum proteomics. J Natl Cancer Inst 2005;97:315–9.

Screening for Colorectal Cancer; Screening for Breast Cancer; Lung Cancer Screening. US Preventive Services Task Force. Available at: http://www.preventiveservices.ahrq.gov. Retrieved October 5, 2005.

Schoenfeld P, Cash B, Flood A, Dobhan R, Eastone J, Coyle W, et al. Colonoscopic screening of average-risk women for colorectal neoplasia. CONCeRN Study Investigators. N Engl J Med 2005;352:2061–8.

Smith RA, Cokkinides V, Eyre HJ. American Cancer Society guidelines for the early detection of cancer, 2004. American Cancer Society. CA Cancer J Clin 2004;54:41–52.

# 70

## Management of postpartum depression

A 32-year-old woman, gravida 1, para 1, comes to your office for her 6-week postpartum visit accompanied by her mother and infant. She states that her infant son is doing well, but she is tired of nursing frequently and has little appetite. When you ask her if her husband is helping, you learn that they had been considering separation long before the baby was born. She tells you that she is devastated and exhausted from inability to sleep, even when she has the opportunity to sleep between feedings. At this point, the baby starts crying and the patient's mother tries to soothe him without success. Your patient makes no attempt to reach for the baby. The best next step in the care of this patient is

(A) hemoglobin and thyroid function tests
* (B) detailed clinical assessment of emotional status
(C) outpatient treatment with an antidepressant
(D) outpatient psychotherapy
(E) hospitalization in a psychiatric unit

Postpartum depression occurs in 10–15% of parturients. Impediments to diagnosis include the following:

- First-time mothers believe that what they experience is normal

- Societal pressures to be a "good mother" make acknowledgment of depression a shameful prospect.

- Exhaustion and low energy can be confused with thyroid dysfunction or anemia.

Symptoms of postpartum depression are the same as for major depression with the addition of decreased maternal functioning. An effective tool to screen for postpartum depression is the Edinburgh Postnatal Depression Scale (Box 70-1). The depression scale is a 10-item self-rated instrument that can be administered easily at the postpartum visit. A score of more than 12 is 100% sensitive and 95.5% specific in detecting postpartum depression. A positive score should prompt the clinician to pursue a thorough evaluation for depression. Treatment is indicated when postpartum depression is diagnosed. It should be noted that interpersonal psychotherapy has been shown to be as effective as pharmacotherapy for treatment of clinical depression. Research demonstrates that the ideal treatment for depression is a course of both antidepressants and psychotherapy.

Women at increased risk for postpartum depression are those with marital or partner dissatisfaction, poor social support, history of previous mood disorder, or family history of depression. Because up to 90% of women who

**BOX 70-1**

## Edinburgh Postnatal Depression Scale

Instructions for users:
1. The mother is asked to underline the response that comes closest to how she has been feeling in the previous 7 days.
2. All 10 items must be completed.
3. Care should be taken to avoid the possibility of the mother discussing her answers with others.
4. The mother should complete the scale herself, unless she has limited English or has difficulty reading.
5. The instrument may be used at 6–8 weeks to screen postnatal women. The child health clinic, postnatal check-up, or a home visit may provide suitable opportunities for its completion.

Name: _____

Address: _____

Baby's age: _____

As you recently had a baby, we would like to know how you are feeling. Please UNDERLINE the answer that comes closest to how you have felt IN THE PAST 7 DAYS, not just how you feel today.

Here is an example, already completed.

    I have felt happy
        Yes, all the time
        <u>Yes, most of the time</u>
        No, not very often
        No, not at all

This would mean: "I have felt happy most of the time" during the past week. Please complete the other questions in the same way.

In the past 7 days:

1. I have been able to laugh and see the funny side of things
    As much as I always could
    Not quite as much now
    Definitely not so much now
    Not at all

2. I have looked forward with enjoyment to things
    As much as I ever did
    Rather less than I used to
    Definitely less than I used to
    Hardly at all

*3. I have blamed myself unnecessarily when things went wrong
    Yes, most of the time
    Yes, some of the time
    Not very often
    No, never

4. I have been anxious or worried for no good reason
    No, not at all
    Hardly ever
    Yes, sometimes
    Yes, very often

*5. I have felt scared or panicky for no very good reason
    Yes, quite a lot
    Yes, sometimes
    No, not much
    No, not at all

*6. Things have been getting on top of me
    Yes, most of the time I haven't been able to cope at all
    Yes, sometimes I haven't been coping as well as usual
    No, most of the time I have coped quite well
    No, I have been coping as well as ever

*7. I have been so unhappy that I have had difficulty sleeping
    Yes, most of the time
    Yes, sometimes
    Not very often
    No, not at all

*8. I have felt sad or miserable
    Yes, most of the time
    Yes, quite often
    Not very often
    No, not at all

*9. I have been so unhappy that I have been crying
    Yes, most of the time
    Yes, quite often
    Only occasionally
    No, not ever

*10. The thought of harming myself has occurred to me
    Yes, quite often
    Sometimes
    Hardly ever
    Never

Response categories are scored 0, 1, 2, and 3 according to increased severity of the symptom.

*Items marked with an asterisk are reverse scored (ie, 3, 2, 1, and 0). The total score is calculated by adding together the scores for each of the 10 items.

© 1987 The Royal College of Psychiatrists. The Edinburgh Postnatal Depression Scale may be photocopied by individual researchers or clinicians for their own use without seeking permission from the publishers. The scale must be copied in full and all copies must acknowledge the following source: Cox JL, Holden JM, Sagovsky R. (1987) Detection of postnatal depression. Development of the 10-item Edinburgh Postnatal Depression Scale. British Journal of Psychiatry, 150, 782–786. Written permission must be obtained from the Royal College of Psychiatrists for copying and distribution to others or for republication (in print, online, or by any other medium). Translations of the scale, and guidance as to its use, may be found in Cox JL, Holden J. (2003) Perinatal Mental Health: A Guide to the Edinburgh Postnatal Depression Scale. London: Gaskell.

have had previous postpartum depression have a recurrence and up to 70% of women with bipolar disorder relapse after delivery, it is essential to do prenatal screening. Prophylactic postpartum treatment with antidepressants is indicated for new mothers with previous postpartum depression and with lithium for those with bipolar disorder. Because lithium is secreted at high levels in breast milk and may cause toxicity in the nursing infant, breastfeeding is contraindicated.

Postpartum psychosis, a rare disorder, occurs in 0.2% of childbearing women. The clinical picture is most often manic in nature, with symptoms that include inability to sleep for several nights, agitation, expansive or irritable mood, avoidance of the infant, and delusions or hallucinations about the infant. Patients who are not showing interest in their baby should be asked if they have thoughts about the baby being "possessed" or if they hear voices telling them to do anything to the baby. Suicide and infanticide are real risks. The presence of such ideation or plans represents a medical emergency that requires referral to a psychiatrist, psychiatric hospitalization, and treatment with neuroleptics or mood stabilizers. This patient's lack of responsiveness to her baby's crying is a concern that requires immediate further assessment of her emotional status.

Although "postpartum blues" are common and occur in 50–85% of all women postpartum, they are transitory and relatively mild. Blues symptoms include affective instability, rapidly fluctuating mood, tearfulness, irritability, and anxiety but do not affect maternal functioning. Symptoms usually peak 4–5 days postpartum and remit spontaneously by day 10. Typically, no specific treatment beyond support and reassurance is needed.

Thyroid dysfunction and anemia should be ruled out to decrease misdiagnosis of depression. Hypothyroidism is seen in 5% of postpartum women and causes symptoms of low mood, lack of motivation, weight gain, anxiety, and fatigue. Sometimes this is preceded by hyperthyroidism with symptoms of rapid weight loss, agitation, and panic. Hemoglobin and thyroid function tests are always indicated when patients present with symptoms of fatigue; however, in this case, further assessment of the patient's emotional status is more critical.

When mothers are depressed, they often are either less interactive with their babies or inappropriately intrusive, each of which can affect the child's developing sense of self and psychologic well-being. Children of mothers with postpartum depression are more likely to exhibit behavioral problems (eg, sleeping and eating difficulties, temper tantrums, hyperactivity, delay in cognitive development, emotional and social dysregulation, and early onset of depressive illness). Obstetrician–gynecologists are in a pivotal position to affect the social, emotional, and cognitive development of children by becoming skilled in the detection and treatment of mood disorders in postpartum women.

Bowes WA, Katz VL. Postpartum care. In: Gabbe SG. Niebyl JR, Simpson JL, editors. Obstetrics: normal and problem pregnancies. 4th ed. Philadelphia (PA): Churchill Livingstone; 2002. p. 701–26.

Brockington I. Postpartum psychiatric disorders [Review]. Lancet 2004;363:1077–8.

Clay EC, Seehusen DA. A review of postpartum depression for the primary care physician. [Review.] South Med J 2004;97:157–61; quiz 162.

Cox JL, Holden JM, Sagovsky R. Detection of postnatal depression. Development of the 10-item Edinburgh Postnatal Depression Scale. Br J Psychiatry 1987;150:782–6.

Gjerdingen D. The effectiveness of various postpartum depression treatments and the impact of antidepressant drugs on nursing infants. J Am Board Fam Pract 2003;16:372–82.

# 71

## Risk of failed vaginal birth after cesarean delivery

A 33-year-old woman, gravida 3, para 2, is seen at 32 weeks of gestation. The patient has a history of a primary low transverse cesarean delivery performed for arrest of labor as primigravida. She has a Bishop score of less than 4. Her second child was a 3,800-g infant by spontaneous vaginal delivery. The finding associated with the highest likelihood of a successful vaginal birth after a cesarean delivery (VBAC) is

      (A) epidural anesthesia
\*   (B) previous successful VBAC
      (C) induced labor
      (D) Bishop score less than 4
      (E) maternal age younger than 35 years

A previous successful VBAC is probably the best predictor of future VBAC success. A prior vaginal delivery and, particularly, a prior VBAC are associated with a higher rate of successful trial of labor compared with patients with no prior vaginal delivery. Various studies have reported 90% or more of such women deliver vaginally with a trial of labor. One study showed that compared to women without a history of previous VBAC, women with a previous VBAC were seven times more likely to have a successful VBAC. The higher rate of successful trials of labor was explained by lower rates of cesarean delivery for both fetal distress and labor dystocia. Identifying which women will be successful can help to decrease perinatal morbidity and mortality. Women who have had a previous successful VBAC, those who had a previous cesarean delivery for a nonrecurring indication, and those whose fetuses weighed less than 4,000 g at delivery are more likely to have successful VBAC attempts. Among women with one previous cesarean delivery and one previous vaginal delivery, mothers whose most recent delivery was vaginal had a higher rate of successful VBAC and shorter duration of labor than mothers whose most recent delivery was cesarean.

A Bishop score of 4 or more at the beginning of labor is a strong indicator for successful VBAC. Not unlike labor outside a VBAC setting, a favorable cervix increases the success rate for vaginal delivery sixfold. An important point for any scoring system is that it should be applied at the time of admission, not at the last prenatal visit. Application before the onset of labor would not be valid. Cervical dilation and effacement often change dramatically between the last prenatal examination and the time of admission.

The vaginal delivery rate is significantly higher in patients with spontaneous labor compared with induced labor. Care should be taken in the choice of induction agent. The use of prostaglandins for induction of labor in women with a previous cesarean delivery should be discouraged. Induction agents to consider in VBAC include oxytocin and mechanical methods. The safety of oxytocin for augmentation of contractions during a trial of labor after a previous low-transverse cesarean delivery has been examined in several studies. On average, 80% of women with spontaneous onset of labor delivered vaginally vs 68% who received oxytocin.

Most women who have undergone cesarean delivery because of dystocia also can have a successful VBAC, but the percent may be lower (50–80%) than for women with nonrecurring indications (75–86%). The success rate is higher if surgery was performed in the latent phase of labor and lower if performed after full dilation. If the prior cesarean delivery for dystocia was performed before complete cervical dilation (5–9 cm), 67–73% of VBAC attempts are successful compared with only 13% if the prior cesarean delivery was performed after complete cervical dilation.

Patients aged 35 years or older compared with younger patients are more prone to have a failed trial of labor after a prior cesarean delivery. After adjusting for confounding variables, maternal age of 35 years or older was associated with a lower rate of successful vaginal delivery in patients without prior vaginal delivery.

A VBAC is not a contraindication to epidural anesthesia, and adequate pain relief may encourage more women to choose a trial of labor. Success rates for VBAC are similar in women who do and do not receive epidural analgesia, as well as in those women who receive other types of pain relief. Epidural analgesia rarely masks the signs and symptoms of uterine rupture.

Bujold E, Hammoud AO, Hendler I, Berman S, Blackwell SC, Duperron L, et al. Trial of labor in patients with a previous cesarean section: does maternal age influence the outcome? Am J Obstet Gynecol 2004;190:1113–8.

Gyamfi C, Juhasz G, Gyamfi P, Stone JL. Increased success of trial of labor after previous vaginal birth after cesarean. Obstet Gynecol 2004;104:715–9.

Hendler I, Bujold E. Effect of prior vaginal delivery or prior vaginal birth after cesarean delivery on obstetric outcomes in women undergoing trial of labor. Obstet Gynecol 2004;104:273–7.

Induction of labor for vaginal birth after cesarean delivery. ACOG Committee Opinion No. 271. American College of Obstetricians and Gynecologists. Obstet Gynecol 2002;99:678–80.

Lydon-Rochelle M, Holt VL, Easterling TR, Martin DP. Risk of uterine rupture during labor among women with a prior cesarean delivery. N Engl J Med 2001;345:3–8

Macones GA, Hausman N, Edelstein R, Stamilio DM, Marder SJ. Predicting outcomes of trials of labor in women attempting vaginal birth after cesarean delivery: a comparison of multivariate methods with neural networks. Am J Obstet Gynecol 2001;184:409–13.

Mankuta DD, Leshno MM, Menasche MM, Brezis MM. Vaginal birth after cesarean section: trial of labor or repeat cesarean section? A decision analysis. Am J Obstet Gynecol 2003;189:714–9.

Sims EJ, Newman RB, Hulsey TC. Vaginal birth after cesarean: to induce or not to induce. Am J Obstet Gynecol 2001;184:1122–4.

Vaginal birth after previous cesarean delivery. ACOG Practice Bulletin No. 54. American College of Obstetricians and Gynecologists. Obstet Gynecol 2004;104:203–12.

# 72

## Use of antiviral treatment

A 65-year-old woman with asthma comes to your office for her periodic health maintenance examination in early November. She visited a friend in a nursing home yesterday. Today she was called by her friend and told there is an outbreak of influenza B at the nursing home. They spent several hours together, in the common areas of the nursing home, where there were residents who did not feel well. She is scheduled to receive her influenza vaccination today. She asks if there is anything else she can do to avoid becoming infected with influenza B. Your best advice is to begin taking

* (A) oseltamivir phosphate (Tamiflu)
   (B) acyclovir
   (C) amantadine
   (D) rimantadine
   (E) zanamivir (Relenza)

Influenza accounts for approximately 110,000 hospital admissions and 20,000 deaths each winter in the United States. The best prevention against influenzas A and B is immunization at the beginning of the influenza season each year.

Influenza A has an attack rate of 10–20%. It is highly contagious from the day before symptoms begin through approximately 5 days of illness. Droplet and airborne transmission occur. Increasing age, residential care, and chronic cardiovascular disease, respiratory disease, diabetes mellitus, and immunosuppression increase the morbidity and mortality of influenza. Among community-dwelling adults older than 60 years, influenza vaccination is 58% effective against respiratory disease and decreases hospitalization for pneumonia by 30–70%. For institutionalized patients older than 60 years, vaccination is 30–40% effective in preventing influenza, 50–60% effec-

tive in preventing hospitalization, and 80% effective in preventing death.

Vaccination with both inactivated and live attenuated vaccine (Flumist) induces an immune response. It takes 2 weeks for a person to mount the immune response after vaccination. Antivirals may be indicated for prophylaxis and treatment if a patient is exposed to influenza before their immune system has had adequate time to produce sufficient antibodies.

Antiviral drugs for prophylaxis and treatment of influenza are shown in Table 72-1. Two major classes of antiviral agents for influenza have been developed: the ion channel M2 blockers and the neuraminidase inhibitors. The ion channel inhibitors, amantadine and rimantadine, are used only with influenza A in anyone older than 1 year. They may be used orally for prophylaxis starting before exposure and continuing for up to

**TABLE 72-1.** Antiviral Drugs for Prophylaxis and Treatment of Influenza

| Drug | Adult Dosage* | | Cost ($)† |
| | Prophylaxis | Treatment | |
| --- | --- | --- | --- |
| *Influenza A* | | | |
| Amantadine‡–average generic | 100 mg by mouth twice daily or 200 mg once daily§ | Same | 5.80 |
| Symmetrel | | | 12.90 |
| Rimantadine–average generic | 100 mg by mouth twice daily or 200 mg once daily‖ | Same | 16.10 |
| *Influenza A and B* | | | |
| Oseltamivir (Tamiflu)‡ | 75 mg by mouth once daily¶ | 75 mg by mouth twice daily¶ | 72.10 |
| Zanamivir (Relenza) | 10 mg by inhalation# once daily | 10 mg by inhalation# twice daily | 57.00 |

*For prophylaxis of exposures in institutions, the drug should be taken for at least 2 weeks, and must be continued for 1 week after the end of the outbreak. For postexposure prophylaxis in households, shorter courses (7–10 days) may be effective. For treatment of infection, the duration is usually 5 days (3–5 days with amantadine or rimantadine to reduce emergence of resistance).

†Cost for 5 days' treatment at adult dosage, according to August 31, 2004, data from retail pharmacies nationwide available from NDCHealth, a health care information services company.

‡Also available as a liquid formulation.

§Dosage should be decreased to 100 mg/d in patients with diminished renal function (CrCl less than 50 mL/min) and in patients older than 65 years.

‖Lower dosage (100 mg/d) is recommended for older nursing home residents, patients older than 65 years, and patients with severe hepatic dysfunction or CrCl less than 10 mL/min.

¶The interval between doses should be every other day for prophylaxis and once daily for treatment in patients with CrCl 10–30 mL/min.

# Taken as two 5-mg inhalations using Rotadisk inhaler. Not FDA-approved for prophylaxis.

Modified from Antiviral drugs for prophylaxis and treatment of influenza. Med Lett Drugs Ther 2004;46:85–7.

6–8 weeks. Resistance can develop when used for prolonged times, and transmission of the resistant strains can cause prophylaxis failures. Treatment of infected patients shortens the duration of symptoms. Amantadine use is limited by side effects, including insomnia, nervousness, lightheadedness, delirium, difficulty concentrating, and seizures. Anticholinergics and older antihistamines with anticholinergic effects potentiate these side effects. Rimantadine has less frequent neurologic adverse effects.

The neuraminidase inhibitors, oseltamivir (Tamiflu) and zanamivir (Relenza), are effective for prophylaxis both before and after exposure to influenzas A and B. Seasonal prophylaxis with the neuraminidase inhibitors has been shown to decrease the odds of developing influenza by 70–90%. When the neuroaminidase inhibitors are started within 36–48 hours of illness, the severity and duration of symptoms also are reduced. Resistance rarely develops. Influenza A strains resistant

to the ion channel blockers remain sensitive to the neuraminidase inhibitors. Oseltamivir lowers the incidence of lower respiratory tract complications and hospitalizations. It is given orally. Zanamivir decreases symptoms by 1–2.5 days, and reduces complications by 45%. It is not approved for prophylaxis in the United States. Zanamivir is given by oral inhalation and may exacerbate cough and nasal and throat discomfort, induce bronchospasm, and decrease pulmonary function. It should not be used in patients with chronic obstructive pulmonary disease (COPD) and asthma. In the patient described, who has asthma and exposure to influenza B, the best antiviral medication is oseltamivir.

Other antiviral drugs are available to treat specific viral infections. Ribavirin works against hepatitis C when combined with pegylated interferon and has activity against arenaviruses and respiratory syncytial virus. Acyclovir acts against herpesviruses causing varicella zoster infections and HSV-1 and HSV-2 infections. These antiviral drugs show no benefit against influenza viruses.

Antiviral drugs for prophylaxis and treatment of influenza. Med Lett Drugs Ther 2004;46:85–7.

Brooks MJ, Sasadeusz JJ, Tannock GA. Antiviral chemotherapeutic agents against respiratory viruses: where are we now and what's in the pipeline? Curr Opin Pulm Med 2004;10:197–203.

Cooper NJ, Sutton AJ, Abrams KR, Wailoo A, Turner D, Nicholson KG.

Effectiveness of neuraminidase inhibitors in treatment and prevention of influenza A and B: systematic review and meta-analyses of randomised controlled trials. BMJ 2003;326:1235–41.

High levels of adamantane resistance among influenza A (H3N2) viruses and interim guidelines for use of antiviral agents—United States, 2005–06 influenza season. Centers for Disease Control and Prevention. MMWR Morb Mortal Wkly Rep 2006;55:44–6.

# 73

## Living will

A 67-year-old woman is scheduled for a hysterectomy for complex atypical endometrial hyperplasia. She has chronic hypertension and diabetes mellitus, complicated by moderate renal insufficiency. In your discussion with her of the risks of surgery, she is concerned about the possibility of becoming incapacitated and on life support. She indicates that she has very specific desires should she become incapacitated and wishes to make clear her desires regarding further health care. The best method of communicating the patient's desires if such a circumstance should occur is for the patient to

        (A) secure a health care power of attorney
        (B) sign a right-to-refuse-treatment document
        (C) sign the consent form for surgery
*    (D) complete a living will document
        (E) discuss the matter with her husband

The Self Determination Act of 1990 requires all hospitals that receive federal Medicare and Medicaid money to create a formal procedure to inform patients regarding their rights under state law in regard to health care decision making. This includes the right to refuse treatment and to provide advance directives. Advance directives generally involve a living will or a health care power of attorney (also known as a health care proxy) or both. Every state and the District of Columbia have laws that govern what an advance directive may contain and when and how it is followed. Some national hospice and palliative care organizations make available living will forms for each state.

For a patient with a terminal illness or the incapacitated patient who is unable to make health care decisions for herself, a living will gives health care providers guidance on health care issues, on what the patient would accept or refuse. Several issues are typically addressed:

- Life-sustaining treatments including cardiopulmonary resuscitation and ventilators

- Artificial nutrition and hydration as the main treatment to keep patients alive

- Degree of pain relief

- Major surgery

Health care directives such as the living will are important to put in writing. The living will gives the patient an opportunity to define the issues important to her and, if there is a designated proxy, provides better guidance for this person. It is also important for legal reasons because, without a living will, some state courts require "clear and convincing" evidence that a patient would have refused treatment before such treatment can be withheld or withdrawn. Discussing with a spouse or other designated health care proxy is helpful, but may be limiting in the types of decisions available to such a surrogate.

A health care durable power of attorney or a health care proxy involves the patient's authorization to a health care agent to make medical decisions for her. However, it should be noted that the agent is not required to comply with these wishes. The more involved the proxy is with the construction of the living will, the more informed will be the possible decisions. Within the power of attorney, the patient may specify issues about which the agent is authorized to make decisions, such as power to choose physicians, the right to decide whether to hospitalize, and the right to accept or refuse treatment. Signing the right-to-refuse-treatment document and the consent form does not address the issues that may occur when she is no longer capable of providing informed consent.

Living wills and health care proxies. Advance directives help families and loved ones make difficult decisions. Harv Health Lett 2005 Jun;30(8):1–3.

Gillick MR. Advance care planning. N Engl J Med 2004;350:7–8.

Patient care. In: American College of Obstetricians and Gynecologists. Guidelines for women's health care. 2nd ed. Washington, DC: ACOG; 2002. p. 185–7.

# 74

## Abnormal bleeding

A 12-year-old girl has been admitted to the pediatric hematology service with acute lymphocytic leukemia. Chemotherapy was prescribed and resulted in leukopenia and thrombocytopenia. Clinically, the patient reports bleeding from her gums and heavy vaginal bleeding since her platelet count fell below 20,000/mm$^3$. Her hemoglobin is declining. Her gynecologic history includes a normal pubertal course with menarche at age 11 years and regular menses every 28–30 days, lasting 4–5 days, with mild to moderate flow and occasional dysmenorrhea. Ultrasonography reveals a thin endometrial stripe of 3 mm. Your initial step in management should be

* (A) gonadotropin-releasing hormone (GnRH) agonist
* (B) platelet transfusion
* (C) combination oral contraceptives
* (D) depot medroxyprogesterone acetate
* (E) intravenous estrogen

Normal blood coagulation is achieved by three main components:

1. The vascular endothelium
2. Coagulation proteins
3. Platelets

Normal liver function is required for normal coagulation because all coagulation proteins except factor VIII are synthesized in the liver. Hepatic insufficiency or vitamin K deficiency leads to defects in the extrinsic clotting pathway and prothrombin time. Defects in the intrinsic clotting pathway manifest via a prolonged partial thromboplastin time.

Thrombocytopenia may be caused by increased platelet destruction or decreased platelet production. Drugs, including chemotherapy, are a common cause of thrombocytopenia. Some medications result in platelet destruction via induction of platelet antibody formation or alteration of bone marrow function. Platelet antibodies bind weakly and reversibly to platelets. Platelet transfusions are helpful when platelet counts are less than 50,000/mm$^3$, especially in the setting of clinically abnormal bleeding. Thus, platelet transfusion should be the first step in care of this patient.

In the uterus, adequate platelet numbers and function along with myometrial contractions produce hemostasis. In normal menstrual bleeding, vasoconstrictive activity of the spiral arterioles and collapsing endometrium result in endometrial blanching, ischemia, and stasis. Thrombin-platelet plugs appear in superficial vessels. These events result in an orderly menstrual flow.

Before initiating chemotherapy, a GnRH agonist may be administered to maximize preservation of future ovarian activity and assist with bleeding management. Oral contraceptives and depot medroxyprogesterone acetate also may be used to manage uterine bleeding once acute bleeding is controlled.

Desmopressin (DDAVP) also may help manage bleeding in patients with abnormal platelet function tests. Other pharmacologic treatments useful in platelet dysfunction include tranexamic acid, aprotinin, or intravenous estrogen. For low platelet counts, however, platelet transfusion is the treatment of choice. Dilation and curettage is contraindicated and potentially harmful.

Use of intravenous estrogen may arrest acute bleeding when hemorrhage has left little residual endometrial tissue. Doses of 25 mg of conjugated estrogen intravenously are prescribed every 4 hours for 24 hours or until bleeding decreases. One suggested mechanism for action of conjugated estrogen is that it might stimulate clotting at the capillary level. Progestin therapy usually is started at the same time, most commonly in a contraceptive formulation.

Armas-Loughran B, Kalra R, Carson JL. Evaluation and management of anemia and bleeding disorders in surgical patients. Med Clin North Am 2003;87:229–42.

Leung PL, Ng PS, Lok IH, Yuen PM. Puberty menorrhagia secondary to inherited bleeding disorders. Acta Obstet Gynecol Scand 2005; 84:921–2.

Philipp CS, Faiz A, Dowling N, Dilley A, Michaels LA, Ayers C, et al. Age and the prevalence of bleeding disorders in women with menorrhagia. Obstet Gynecol 2005;105:61–6.

# 75

## Low back pain

A 32-year-old woman is referred for evaluation of chronic pelvic pain for approximately 1 year. She has left lower quadrant pain "near her ovary" and mild low back pain. She describes the pain as stretching near the groin and left lower abdomen, and says that it is exacerbated around her menses and with prolonged sitting. She also has occasional dyspareunia, but denies any urinary urgency, frequency, or dysuria. She denies any history of abuse or trauma except a horseback riding fall as a young girl. She tried oral contraceptives without improvement. Three months ago, she underwent a diagnostic laparoscopy that showed normal pelvic anatomy, no adhesions, no endometriosis, normal appendix and small bowel, and no evidence of hernia. Your physical examination shows no costovertebral tenderness, but she has mild tenderness in her back over the sacroiliac joints. The abdominal examination shows subjective tenderness in the lower abdomen on the left greater that the right. The straight leg raise is negative for pain with an adequate range of motion in the lower extremities and mild pain with flexion of left knee toward the chest. Strength is symmetric and +5 / +5 in the lower extremities. Sensation is intact to light touch and pinprick, and deep tendon reflexes are normal. The bimanual examination shows an anteverted mobile uterus with mild tenderness in the left adnexal region but no cervical motion tenderness. The most appropriate next step is

      (A) trial of tricyclic antidepressants
      (B) cystoscopy of the bladder
\*    (C) referral to physical therapist
      (D) magnetic resonance imaging (MRI) of lumbosacral spine
      (E) referral to psychiatry

Chronic pelvic pain and low back pain are common problems and almost every structure in the abdomen and pelvis can have a role in the etiology of chronic pelvic pain. It is essential for the practitioner to think beyond the organs of the upper genital tract when determining the cause of the pain and to consider the peripheral and central nervous system, the muscles and fascia of the abdominal wall, the low back, the pelvic floor, the urologic system, and the gastrointestinal tract. The complexity is compounded by the psychologic and behavioral factors known to contribute to the experience of pain. A complete history is the most valuable tool in the evaluation of chronic pelvic pain.

Written pain questionnaires are useful in the evaluation of women with chronic pelvic pain, but there is also great benefit in the patient telling her story and the clinician listening to establish rapport. Crucial information includes medical and surgical history, obstetric and gynecologic history, psychosocial history, and history of abuse. It is

also beneficial for the patient to be able to mark the location(s) of her pain on a pain map (Box 75-1 and Fig. 75-1). Pain maps frequently show that the patient has other areas of pain; up to 90% of patients with chronic pelvic pain also have backaches. In addition to the locations of the pain, the history must include the severity, quality, and timing of the pain, the relationship to menses, and the factors that exacerbate or relieve the pain. The physical examination is then used to try to detect the exact anatomic location of pain or tenderness that can emanate from any system such as the musculoskeletal, gastrointestinal, urinary, psychoneurologic, or reproductive tract.

This patient presents with many factors that are associated with musculoskeletal dysfunction. Musculoskeletal pain often is diffuse and can be accompanied by autonomic complaints. Pain frequently is altered by positional changes, including relief with rest or aggravation with sitting or standing. Musculoskeletal dysfunction tends to worsen with stress and does not typically respond to

**Questions to Ask of Women With Chronic Pelvic Pain**

1. How old are you?
2. How many pregnancies have you had?
3. Where does it hurt?
4. How much does it hurt?
5. What is the quality or character of your pain?
6. Do you have pain with your periods?
7. Does your pain worsen with menses or just before menses?
8. Is there any cyclic pattern to your pain? Is it the same 24 hours a day, 7 days a week?
9. Is your pain constant or intermittent?
10. When and how did your pain start and how has it changed?
11. Did pain start initially as menstrual cramps (dysmenorrhea)?
12. What makes your pain better?
13. What makes your pain worse?
14. Do you have pain with deep penetration during intercourse? If so, does it continue afterwards?
15. Have you ever had or been treated for a sexually transmitted disease or pelvic inflammatory disease?
16. What form of birth control do you use and have you used in the past?
17. Have you ever had any kind of surgery?
18. What prior evaluations or treatments have you had for your pain? Have any of the previous treatments helped?
19. How has the pain affected your quality of life?
20. Are you depressed or anxious?
21. Are you taking any drugs?
22. Have you been or are you now being abused physically or sexually? Are you safe?
23. What other symptoms or health problems do you have?
24. What do you believe or fear is the cause of your pain?

Howard FM. Chronic pelvic pain. Obstet Gynecol 2003; 101:596.

| Sharp | Dull | Numb | Prickly |
|-------|------|------|---------|
| X X X | O O O | # # # | / / / |

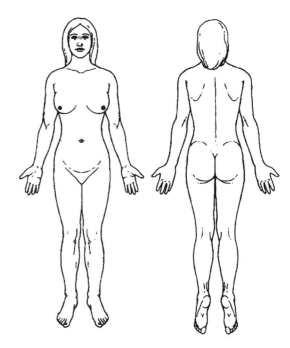

**FIG. 75-1.** Pain map that may be used by women with chronic pelvic pain. Instruction to patient: "Please mark the areas where you feel pain. Put E if external, or I if internal, near the areas you mark. Put EI if both external and internal." (Howard FM. Chronic pelvic pain. Obstet Gynecol 2003;101:596.)

interventions focused on other systems. There is often a history of stress or trauma that preceded or exacerbated the pelvic or back pain. The timing of the event (ie, occurred in childhood) is less important than the event itself. Because patients frequently do not consider the incidents relevant, direct questioning is important. Falls on the hip, pelvis, coccyx, or low back should alert the clinician to examine the musculoskeletal system. Previous injuries can be responsible for perpetuating pain or dysfunction due to weakening of muscles or spasm due to strain over time. Structural observations such as unilateral standing habits, slouched sitting, obesity, or scoliosis raise suspicions for musculoskeletal causes. Tenderness to palpation in the lower back, trigger points in the abdominal muscular wall, and tenderness to palpation of

pelvic floor muscles may help to determine the causes of pelvic pain. Because of the overlapping innervation of the musculoskeletal system in the pelvis, identifying the exact etiology of the pain can be difficult even with a detailed examination. A multidisciplinary approach is recommended, and the establishment of an accurate diagnosis should be the first step in treatment.

For a complete evaluation, many authorities have suggested performing detailed examinations in the standing, sitting, supine, and lithotomy positions. The examination is time consuming and is best performed by someone with expertise in physical therapy. This patient would be found to have low back dysfunction. Treatment with an individually designed exercise program for strengthening and stretching is effective. Other treatment measures such as reassurance and analgesics assist in modifying pain and improving function.

Tricyclic antidepressants have been used to treat a number of chronic pain syndromes. They are thought to improve pain tolerance, to restore sleep patterns, and to reduce depressive symptoms. Although this patient may receive some benefit from these medications, a more detailed evaluation for diagnosis would be a better step toward successful management.

A number of tests can help diagnose chronic pelvic pain. However, the diagnostic test of choice is best determined by history and physical examination. The test should be used if it is likely to change the diagnosis, to help in further evaluation of a suspected cause, or to change the treatment. For example, cystoscopy has been advocated as a criterion to diagnose interstitial cystitis by seeing glomerulations in the bladder. This patient is unlikely to have interstitial cystitis because of an absence of irritative voiding symptoms. Instead, objective evidence suggests that another disorder is causing her symptoms.

Magnetic resonance imaging (MRI) of the lower back can be performed, but the yield is low. Radiography early in the course of low back pain does not improve clinical outcomes or reduce the cost of care. Imaging is best used to rule out the possibility of impending neurologic injury, infection, or tumors. Additional indications for an MRI in patients with low back pain include associated neurologic signs or symptoms or persistent pain without improvement despite appropriate treatment for 6–8 weeks.

Psychologic evaluation by a professional who specializes in pain psychology frequently is part of the evaluation and treatment of chronic pelvic pain. Most women with chronic pelvic pain have psychosocial problems that need attention. Such problems include histories of sexual abuse, marital discord, personality disorders, relationship problems, and dysfunctional family backgrounds. If there is any question or need, referral to a counselor is appropriate.

Carragee EJ. Clinical practice. Persistent low back pain. N Engl J Med 2005;352:1891–8.

Hayden JA, van Tulder MW, Tomlinson G. Systematic review: strategies for using exercise therapy to improve outcomes in chronic low back pain. Ann Intern Med 2005;142:776–85.

Howard FM. Chronic pelvic pain. Obstet Gynecol 2003;101:594–611.

Prendergast SA, Weiss JM. Screening for musculoskeletal causes of pelvic pain. Clin Obstet Gynecol 2003;46:773–82.

Sharp HT. Myofascial pain syndrome of the abdominal wall for the busy clinician. Clin Obstet Gynecol 2003;46:783–8.

# 76

## Syphilis in a pregnant patient with penicillin allergy

A 28-year-old pregnant woman at 16 weeks of gestation has a positive screening test result by the rapid plasma reagin (RPR) test for syphilis. The confirmatory test, the fluorescent treponemal antibody absorption (FTA–ABS) test result, is also positive. She denies any known history of genital lesions and does not have any known exposures. The patient has a history of a penicillin allergy. The most appropriate next step is

     (A)  no further intervention
     (B)  delay treatment until postpartum
     (C)  treat with benzathine penicillin G in a single dose
     (D)  treat with ceftriaxone sodium (Rocephin) as a single dose
\*    (E)  skin testing for penicillin G

Syphilis is an infectious disease with systemic manifestations caused by *Treponema pallidum*. It has several phases. Primary infections manifest an ulcer or chancre at the infection site. Secondary infection manifestations include skin rash, mucocutaneous lesions, and lymphadenopathy. Tertiary infection includes cardiac and ophthalmic abnormalities, auditory lesions, and gummas. Some patients infected with *T pallidum* lack any clinical manifestations; such cases are termed latent infections. These infections can be confirmed only by serologic testing. Early latent syphilis is acquired within a year of the diagnosis. Infections acquired prior to a year before diagnosis are called late latent syphilis, as are infections for which the duration is unknown.

Serologic tests for syphilis include nontreponemal tests, such as the Venereal Disease Research Laboratories (VDRL) and RPR tests, and the treponemal tests, such as the FTA–ABS and *T pallidum* particle agglutination (TP–PA) tests. A syphilis antibody test, immunoglobulin (Ig) M and IgG tests, is available at some institutions as an alternative to the other treponemal tests. These tests may help determine acute infection or prior exposure when combined with a positive nontreponemal test result.

Nontreponemal tests have a significant false-positive rate because of various medical conditions (eg, vascular disease and pregnancy) and, therefore, treponemal tests must be done to confirm the diagnosis of syphilis. Current recommendations for testing in pregnancy include that all patients should be screened serologically at the first prenatal visit. Typically this is accomplished with a nontreponemal test. Given the false-positive rate of nontreponemal tests, a treponemal test is then performed for positive results to confirm the diagnosis.

Penicillin G is the treatment of choice for all cases and stages of syphilis. The dose and duration of treatment change based on the circumstances and time from diagnosis. In nonpregnant patients who report an allergy to penicillin, some efficacy has been demonstrated for doxycycline, tetracycline, ceftriaxone sodium, and azithromycin dihydrate (Zithromax). Erythromycin also shows some efficacy; however, it has a cure rate of 90% in nonpregnant patients with only early syphilis and does not cross the placenta adequately to treat the fetus in pregnant patients. Tetracycline and doxycycline are contraindicated in pregnancy. Data are insufficient in the use of ceftriaxone or azithromycin in pregnancy. Thus, parenteral penicillin G is the only therapy with documented efficacy for syphilis during pregnancy.

Fifty years of data and clinical experience have demonstrated that the appropriate intervention for a pregnant woman with syphilis at any stage who is allergic to penicillin consists of skin testing and desensitization for positive results followed by penicillin therapy appropriate to the stage of infection. In the U.S. population, up to 10% of adults have some level of allergic reaction to penicillin. It is known that most patients who have a severe reaction will stop expressing penicillin-specific IgE over time. These individuals can be safely treated with penicillin. Of the patients that report a severe allergic reaction to penicillin, 10% will remain allergic. Skin testing with the major determinant and penicillin G identifies 90–97% of the currently allergic patients. Addition of the minor determinant will reveal the remaining allergic patients. Thus, in pregnant patients who report a penicillin allergy, skin testing with the full battery of reagents is necessary.

In patients with a negative skin test result, conventional penicillin G therapy can be given. Patients with a positive skin test result should be desensitized. In some cases, only the major determinant and penicillin G are available. Many argue that those with a negative skin test result with this panel should still be desensitized because 3–10% of allergic patients will be missed. Others recommend test dosing with oral penicillin in a monitored setting where treatment for anaphylaxis is available.

Desensitization can be done orally or intravenously. Oral desensitization is safer and easier to perform and is thus more common (Table 76-1). Usually this process can be accomplished in 4 hours and should be done in a hospital setting in case the patient has an allergic reaction.

The patient described is pregnant and reports an allergy to penicillin. Given that her serologic test result was positive and she denies any history of clinical manifestations, the diagnosis is late latent syphilis of unknown duration. There is no evidence of efficacy of any other antibiotic than penicillin in this scenario and thus the patient should receive skin testing with desensitization for a positive result. Ceftriaxone, similar to other antibiotics that have shown some efficacy in nonpregnant patients, is not effective in pregnant women and therefore is not appropriate for this patient.

Syphilis in pregnancy additionally puts the fetus at risk. Thus, treatment is always required even in the absence of clinical manifestations. Because of the risks to the fetus of spontaneous abortion and congenital syphilis, it would not be appropriate to delay therapy in this patient until after delivery. Empirically treating the patient with a report of penicillin allergy would put her at risk of anaphylaxis. Excellent protocols exist for desensitization in the small percentage of patients who would be at risk. Treatment with penicillin without first using such a protocol offers excessive risk and is inappropriate. In addition, in a patient with latent syphilis of unknown duration, therapy would require penicillin G in three doses at weekly intervals (Box 76-1). A single dose even after desensitization would not be considered adequate in this patient.

**TABLE 76-1.** Oral Desensitization Protocol for Patients With a Positive Skin Test Result for Syphilis*

| Penicillin V Suspension Dose[†] | Amount[‡] (Units/mL) | mL | Units | Cumulative Dose (Units) |
|---|---|---|---|---|
| 1 | 1,000 | 0.1 | 100 | 100 |
| 2 | 1,000 | 0.2 | 200 | 300 |
| 3 | 1,000 | 0.4 | 400 | 700 |
| 4 | 1,000 | 0.8 | 800 | 1,500 |
| 5 | 1,000 | 1.6 | 1,600 | 3,100 |
| 6 | 1,000 | 3.2 | 3,200 | 6,300 |
| 7 | 1,000 | 6.4 | 6,400 | 12,700 |
| 8 | 10,000 | 1.2 | 12,000 | 24,700 |
| 9 | 10,000 | 2.4 | 24,000 | 48,700 |
| 10 | 10,000 | 4.8 | 48,000 | 96,700 |
| 11 | 80,000 | 1.0 | 80,000 | 176,700 |
| 12 | 80,000 | 2.0 | 160,000 | 336,700 |
| 13 | 80,000 | 4.0 | 320,000 | 656,700 |
| 14 | 80,000 | 8.0 | 640,000 | 1,296,700 |

*Observation period: 30 minutes before parenteral administration of penicillin.

[†]Interval between doses, 15 minutes; elapsed time, 3 hours and 45 minutes; cumulative dose, 1.3 million units.

[‡]The specific amount of drug was diluted in approximately 30 mL of water then administered orally.

Gadde J, Spence M, Wheeler B, Adkinson NF Jr. Clinical experience with penicillin skin testing in a large inner-city STD clinic. JAMA 1993;270:2456–63.

Sexually transmitted diseases treatment guidelines, 2006. Centers for Disease Control and Prevention [published erratum appears in MMWR Recomm Rep 2006;55(36):997]. MMWR Recomm Rep 2006;55 (RR-11):1–94.

Wendel GD Jr, Stark BJ, Jamison RB, Molina RD, Sullivan TJ. Penicillin allergy and desensitization in serious infections during pregnancy. N Engl J Med 1985;312:1229–32.

---

**BOX 76-1**

**Recommended Regimens for Treating Syphilis in Adults**

*Early Latent Syphilis*: Benzathine penicillin G 2.4 million units intramuscularly in a single dose
*Late Latent Syphilis or Latent Syphilis of Unknown Duration*: Benzathine penicillin G 7.2 million units total, administered as three doses of 2.4 million units intramuscularly each at 1-week intervals

---

Sexually transmitted diseases treatment guidelines, 2006. Centers for Disease Control and Prevention [published erratum appears in MMWR Recomm Rep 2006;55 (36):997]. MMWR Recomm Rep 2006;55(RR-11):1–94.

---

# 77

## Treatment of patient with premenstrual disorder

A 39-year-old woman who smokes cigarettes consults you with regard to severe irritability and poor concentration. A prospective symptom calendar kept for the previous three menstrual cycles indicates these symptoms are cyclic, occurring approximately 10 days before the onset of menstrual flow and resolving within 2 days after the onset of bleeding. The patient is concerned that her moods and cognitive changes interfere with her performance at work and have not responded to caffeine restriction, exercise, or dietary supplements. The most appropriate pharmacologic management for this patient is

    (A) buspirone hydrochloride (BuSpar) in the luteal phase
    (B) depot medroxyprogesterone acetate injections
    (C) gonadotropin-releasing hormone (GnRH) agonist therapy
\*   (D) selective serotonin reuptake inhibitor (SSRI) in the luteal phase
    (E) spironolactone (Aldactone) in the luteal phase

More than one third of menstruating women experience bothersome luteal phase symptoms. In 3–5% of menstruating women, these symptoms are severe enough to impair activities of daily living. Often such symptoms represent a mixture of physical, mood, and cognitive phenomena. Following ovulation, a reduction in serotonergic function occurs. A number of well-controlled clinical trials have demonstrated the efficacy of agents that inhibit serotonin uptake or suppress ovulation to improve symptoms. Although the American Psychiatric Association distinguishes premenstrual dysphoric disorder (PMDD) from premenstrual syndrome (PMS), it is clinically appropriate to consider PMS symptoms as mild, moderate, or severe. When the PMS symptoms are severe and cause functional impairment, a diagnosis of PMDD can be used.

Although menstruating women of any age can have symptoms, most women with PMS–PMDD are older than 30 years. Even though symptoms tend to resolve in the postmenopausal years, perimenopausal symptoms may be more severe in women with a history of PMS–PMDD. A diagnosis of PMS–PMDD can be made when symptoms are:

- Limited to the luteal phase
- Characteristic of PMS–PMDD
- Causing problems (or, in the case of PMDD, impairment) for the patient
- Not explained by a better diagnosis (eg, thyroid disease)

Symptoms characteristic of PMS–PMDD are shown in Box 77-1. Prospective charting of these symptoms, along with menstruation, is critical in establishing the diagnosis of PMS–PMDD. Symptoms can begin at any time during

---

**BOX 77-1**

---

**Symptoms Characteristic of Premenstrual Syndrome–Premenstrual Dysphoric Disorder**

Mood symptoms
- Irritability
- Depression
- Anxiety

Physical symptoms
- Bloating
- Breast tenderness
- Vasomotor symptoms
- Appetite changes
- Headache
- Fatigue

Cognitive symptoms
- Memory problems
- Confusion
- Poor concentration

---

the 2 weeks before the onset of menses and subside within 1–2 days after menses onset. For many women who suffer from PMS–PMDD, symptom charting is not only helpful diagnostically, but it also proves useful in that the onset of symptoms can be predicted. For some women, such anticipation improves the ability to cope with symptoms, and no pharmacologic therapy will be needed.

In the case described, prospective symptom charting confirmed that the patient's mood and cognitive symptoms were indeed premenstrual. Checking sex steroid or gonadotropin levels is not useful in making the diagnosis of PMS–PMDD. If no recent thyroid function testing has been performed, however, checking the thyroid-stimulating hormone (TSH) level is appropriate because thyroid disease can cause symptoms that mimic PMS–PMDD.

When pharmacologic therapy is indicated, combination oral contraceptive therapy may help with physical symptoms such as cramps and breast tenderness, but existing oral contraceptive formulations have not been found to consistently help with mood or cognitive symptoms. In fact, the progestin component in oral contraceptives may exacerbate mood symptoms in women with PMS–PMDD. An oral contraceptive formulation with 24 tablets combining 20 mcg ethinyl estradiol, 3 mg drospirenone, and 4 inert tablets has been effective in the treatment of physical and mood-related PMS symptoms. However, because this patient smokes cigarettes, she is not a candidate for combination oral contraceptives. Although spironolactone may be effective for premenstrual bloating or breast tenderness, few data suggest this agent's efficacy in treating mood or cognitive symptoms.

For women with PMS–PMDD who require pharmacologic therapy, abundant well-controlled data support the efficacy of SSRI therapy. In contrast to SSRI therapy for depression, onset of SSRI efficacy is rapid with PMS. Accordingly, cyclic therapy beginning 2 weeks before the anticipated onset of menses can be considered. Usually, low doses of the SSRI are adequate. Therapy with SSRIs often improves physical as well as mood and cognitive symptoms. If cyclic luteal phase therapy does not prove satisfactory, continuous SSRI therapy should be tried. Venlafaxine, which inhibits the intake of serotonin and norepinephrine, also represents effective therapy for PMS. When SSRI therapy is continuous and long-term, abrupt discontinuation can cause withdrawal symptoms. Therefore, SSRI therapy should be tapered in this setting rather than abruptly discontinued.

Although only limited data support the efficacy of anxiolytic agents, they may be helpful in some women with PMS–PMDD when SSRIs have not proven effective. Because buspirone is less addictive and has fewer side effects, its use is preferred to benzodiazepines. Buspirone is initiated during the luteal phase and discontinued with the onset of menses.

When the previously mentioned measures have not proven useful, ovulation suppression therapy can be considered for PMS–PMDD. Although GnRH agonist therapy is effective in this context, cost and long-term safety concerns related to hypoestrogenism limit use of these agents for PMS–PMDD. Because of their safety and lower cost, some experts use high-dose oral or injectable progestin formulations, such as depot medroxyprogesterone acetate, before trying GnRH agonist therapy.

Cohen LS, Miner C, Brown EW, Freeman E, Halbreich U, Sundell K, et al. Premenstrual daily fluoxetine for premenstrual dysphoric disorder: a placebo-controlled, clinical trial using computerized diaries. Obstet Gynecol 2002;100:435–44.

Johnson SR. Premenstrual syndrome, premenstrual dysphoric disorder, and beyond: a clinical primer for practitioners. Obstet Gynecol 2004; 104:845–59.

Muse KN, Cetel NS, Futterman LA, Yen SC. The premenstrual syndrome. Effects of "medical ovariectomy." N Engl J Med 1984;311: 1345–9.

Yonkers KA, Brown C, Pearlstein TB, Foegh M, Sampson-Landers C, Rapkin A. Efficacy of a new low-dose oral contraceptive with drospirenone in premenstrual dysphoric disorder. Obstet Gynecol 2005; 106:492–501.

# 78

## Apathetic hypothyroidism in the elderly

A 71-year-old woman is seen for an annual gynecologic examination. She has been a patient of your practice for the past 7 years. Over the past 2–3 years, she has become more listless, less energetic, and her voice is more gravelly and deeper. Her daughter notes that she seems more dull. Other physicians have seen her for various other problems including hypertension, hypercholesterolemia, constipation, and arthritis. Her current medications include an angiotensin-converting enzyme (ACE) inhibitor, a 3-hydroxy-3-methylglutaryl coenzyme A (HMG Co-A) reductase inhibitor ("statin"), a nonsteroidal antiinflammatory agent, and a gastrointestinal bulking agent. On examination, she is oriented to time, place, and person. Her blood pressure is 138/82 mm Hg in the sitting position. The dermatologic examination is normal. The gynecologic examination is unremarkable. The condition that should be evaluated first is

* (A) hypothyroidism
  (B) Addison's disease
  (C) pheochromocytoma
  (D) depression

The symptoms described are consistent with hypothyroidism. The prevalence of undiagnosed hypothyroidism was estimated to be 4.6% in the third National Health and Nutrition Examination Survey (NHANES III), a cross-sectional survey in a population of 17,353 individuals older than 12 years. The majority (4.2%) had mild or subclinical hypothyroidism, defined as elevated thyroid-stimulating hormone (TSH) levels but normal total thyroxine ($T_4$) level. However, the remaining 0.3% had biochemical evidence of clinical hypothyroidism (ie, elevated TSH level and low thyroxine level).

Aging and female sex are risk factors associated with a higher risk of hypothyroidism. There is a direct correlation between an increase in levels of TSH and aging with a higher prevalence of elevated TSH levels in women than in men. The prevalence for mild or subclinical hypothyroidism is as high as 12–22% in women aged 55 years and older, compared to a prevalence of 4–6% in women aged 44 years and younger. In the elderly, clinical hypothyroidism may be difficult to detect, because the symptoms often develop insidiously over a lengthy period and with multiple different presentations. More common symptoms such as fatigue, constipation, and cognitive loss may be attributed to the aging process. Certainly, aging and hypothyroidism share a number of symptoms (Box 78-1).

Routine screening for asymptomatic hypothyroidism has been advocated by some organizations including the American College of Physicians and American Association of Clinical Endocrinologists. However, the U.S. Preventive Services Task Force finds insufficient evidence to recommend for or against screening. The American College of Obstetricians and Gynecologists recommends

screening every 5 years patients older than 60 years who have strong family histories or autoimmune diseases, because subclinical hypothyroidism may be related to unfavorable lipid profiles. In this patient, who has suggestive symptoms (and who is thus not truly asymptomatic) and abnormal cholesterol, screening for thyroid disease with TSH is warranted.

Profound hypothyroidism is uncommon. Patients may present with myriad symptoms including evidence of hypometabolism and other symptoms as noted in Box 78-1. Physical findings may include coarse skin, puffy eyelids, bradycardia, and a delayed ankle jerk relaxation phase. Patients who exhibit stupor, confusion, somno-

---

**BOX 78-1**

**Signs and Symptoms Characteristic of Aging and Hypothyroidism**

- Anorexia
- Cognitive decline
- Cold intolerance
- Constipation
- Dry skin
- Fatigue
- Hearing loss
- Hoarseness
- Paresthesias
- Slowed reflexes
- Weakness

Mohandas R, Gupta KL. Managing thyroid dysfunction in the elderly. Answers to seven common questions. Postgrad Med 2003;113:54–6, 65–8, 100.

lence, hypothermia, bradycardia, and hypoventilation require intensive monitoring for likely myxedema coma.

The impact of untreated hypothyroidism is not yet clearly defined but possibilities include increased risks of cardiovascular disease and osteoporosis. Replacement therapy with thyroxine is indicated once the diagnosis is confirmed. In the older patient starting with low doses (eg, 25 mcg once daily) and increasing by increments (25 mcg) every 4–6 weeks minimizes the risk of cardiovascular disease.

These symptoms may be compatible with depression, but thyroid illness should be investigated first. Addison's disease may present commonly with malaise, low energy, weakness, anorexia, weight loss, hyperpigmentation of the skin, and exertional fatigue that improves with rest.

Patients tend to have low blood pressure (not hypertensive as in this patient) and often have postural hypotension. Pheochromocytoma is a disease with sporadic excess catecholamine secretion; it may manifest as chronic hypertension and classically with episodic symptoms (eg, tachycardia, palpitations, and diaphoresis).

Canaris GJ, Manowitz NR, Mayor G, Ridgway C. The Colorado thyroid disease prevalence study. Arch Intern Med 2000;160:526–34.

Felz MW, Forren AC. Profound hypothyroidism—a clinical review with eight recent cases: is it right before our eyes? South Med J 2004;97:490–8.

Hollowell JG, Staehling NW, Flanders WD, Hannon WH, Gunter EW, Spencer CA, et al. Serum TSH, T(4), and thyroid antibodies in the United States population (1988 to 1994): National Health and Nutrition Examination Survey (NHANES III). J Clin Endocrinol Metab 2003;87:489–99.

# 79

## Extended cycle contraception

A 20-year-old woman, gravida 1, para 1, presents with headaches and cramps with her periods. She has been taking an oral contraceptive of 30 mcg of ethinyl estradiol for the past 4 months. On questioning, she states that the headaches occur immediately before and during her hormone-free period and are not fully controlled with over-the-counter analgesics. She denies any other problems. She also has a history of menstrual headaches and pelvic pain when she is not taking oral contraceptives. The best alternative management option for her is

    (A) transdermal contraceptive patch
    (B) contraceptive vaginal ring
\*  (C) continuous oral contraceptives
    (D) 20-mcg estrogen-containing contraceptive
    (E) levonorgestrel-containing intrauterine device (IUD)

This patient has a typical history of estrogen withdrawal menstrual headaches. During the 7-day hormone-free interval of combination oral contraceptives, contraceptive vaginal rings, and transdermal contraceptive patches, there is an abrupt decrease in estrogen. Hormone withdrawal symptoms, which include headaches, pelvic pain, breast tenderness, and bloating or swelling, have been shown to increase during the hormone-free days in the combination oral contraceptive cycle compared to the 3 weeks of taking active oral contraceptives.

Because of the timing of the headaches and their association with abrupt withdrawal of estrogen, a lower dose estrogen pill would not be expected to provide improvement in her headaches and cramps. Because the contraceptive patch and the vaginal ring also have a 7-day hormone-free interval incorporated into the regimen, using them in the standard 21-day/7-day fashion also would not be expected to improve these headaches asso-

ciated with hormone withdrawal. Because ovulation occurs in most patients with a levonorgestrel-containing IUD, improvement in symptoms would not be expected by switching to use of an IUD.

Improvement in menstrual-associated headaches and other symptoms has been documented with extended regimens of combination oral contraceptives along with high levels of satisfaction and continuation of the extended regimen. Patients have several options when using an extended regimen of combination oral contraceptives. In patients who have symptoms associated with the hormone-free intervals, limiting the number of hormone-free days and the number of hormone-free intervals per year has been shown to be beneficial. In prospective studies, a significant reduction in menstrual headaches has been seen in patients extending their combination oral contraceptives compared to the standard 21-day/7-day regimen.

Sulak PJ, Carl J, Gopalakrishnan I, Coffee A, Kuehl JJ. Outcomes of extended oral contraceptive regimens with a shortened hormone-free interval to manage breakthrough bleeding. Contraception 2004;70: 281–7.

Sulak PJ, Kuehl TJ, Ortiz M, Shull BL. Acceptance of altering the standard 21-day/7-day oral contraceptive regimen to delay menses and reduce hormone withdrawal symptoms. Am J Obstet Gynecol 2002; 186:1142–9.

Sulak PJ, Scow RD, Preece C, Riggs MW, Kuehl TJ. Hormone withdrawal symptoms in oral contraceptive users. Obstet Gynecol 2000; 95:261–6.

Vercellini P, Frontino G, De Giorgi O, Pietropaolo G, Pasin R, Crosignani PG. Continuous use of an oral contraceptive for endometriosis-associated recurrent dysmenorrhea that does not respond to a cyclic pill regimen. Fertil Steril 2003;80:560–3.

# 80

## Breast cancer screening

A 40-year-old woman has concerns about her risk for breast cancer. She states that recently breast cancer was diagnosed in her 69-year-old mother. She also has a paternal aunt who died from breast cancer at age 42 years. Her maternal great-grandmother died of endometrial cancer. The patient underwent hysterectomy with salpingo-oophorectomy for endometriosis at age 31 years and has been taking estrogen therapy for the past 9 years. She is of Eastern European Jewish descent. Her risk factor that poses the greatest risk of *BRCA1* and *BRCA2* gene mutations is

      (A) family history of breast cancer
      (B) family member with onset of breast cancer before age 50 years
      (C) family history of endometrial cancer
\*   (D) Eastern European (Ashkenazi) Jewish descent

Hereditary breast cancer accounts for only 5–7% of all breast cancers, but for the women who carry these genes, the personal risk of developing breast cancer is quite high. Mutations of the *BRCA1* and *BRCA2* genes are not common but account for approximately 80% of all hereditary breast and ovarian cancers. Depending on the subpopulation studied, carrier rates in the United States can range from 1 in 200 to 1 in 800. Individuals of Ashkenazi Jewish descent carry a 2% risk (ie, two individuals in 100 have the risk). Women with a *BRCA* gene mutation have a 73–87% chance of developing breast cancer by age 70 years, and almost 50% of cancers appear before age 50 years.

When counseling patients for hereditary breast cancer risk, it is important to take a careful personal medical history and a complete multigenerational family history, including second- and third-degree relatives. The *BRCA1* and *BRCA2* gene mutations are passed as an autosomal dominant trait and, as a result, women have an equal chance of receiving the gene from the maternal or paternal genes. It is vital to develop a complete pedigree from both sides of the patient's family and not just the maternal side. Special consideration should be given to eliciting the patient's ethnic background and the number, age, and sex of all relatives with breast cancer. Because hereditary breast cancers tend to occur at a younger age and are more

likely to be bilateral, it is important to obtain the age at onset of breast cancer in any family member and whether the opposite breast was involved. Hereditary breast cancer has been associated with other cancers (eg, ovarian, colon, and endometrial cancer), and, therefore, the presence of any other cancer types in the family should be noted.

When reviewing this woman's history, it becomes apparent that she may have several risk factors for a *BRCA1* or *BRCA2* gene mutation. Her mother's recent diagnosis of breast cancer is of concern, but the age at onset lessens the likelihood of a *BRCA* gene involvement. The paternal aunt who died of breast cancer is significant and increases this patient's risk; however, there is no other history of breast cancer from her paternal side and she herself has never had breast cancer. Endometrial cancer is associated with hereditary nonpolyposis colorectal cancer (HNPCC) and mutations of the *MLH1* and *MSH2* genes. Her history of eastern European (Ashkenazi) Jewish descent carries the greatest risk for her of harboring a *BRCA1* or *BRCA2* gene mutation. Even if she had not been of Ashkenazi background, she may have been at some risk, but adding in her Ashkenazi heritage significantly increases her chance of carrying one of the gene mutations. Ashkenazi descent places her in a higher risk category from the beginning (Box 80-1).

BOX 80-1

**Risk Factors for Carrying a *BRCA1* or *BRCA2* Gene Mutation**

*Non-Ashkenazi ancestry*

- Family history of *BRCA1* or *BRCA2* mutation
- Personal or first-degree relative history of breast and ovarian cancer in one individual
- Personal history of breast cancer *and*
  —One first- or second-degree relative with breast cancer who is younger than 50 years
  —One first- or second-degree relative with bilateral breast cancer at any age
  —Two first- or second-degree relatives with breast cancer
  —One first- or second-degree relative with ovarian cancer at any age
  —Two first- or second-degree relatives with ovarian cancer
  —Two first- or second-degree relatives with breast cancer, one cancer diagnosed when the relative was younger than 50 years or one relative with bilateral breast disease
  —Personal or first-degree relative with male breast cancer

*Ashkenazi ancestry*

- One or more family member with breast cancer younger than 50 years
- One first-degree or two second-degree family members with breast cancer at any age

Khoury-Collado F, Bombard AT. Hereditary breast and ovarian cancer: what the primary care physician should know. Obstet Gynecol Surv 2004;59:539.

Frank TS, Critchfield GC. Inherited risk of women's cancers: what's changed for the practicing physician? Clin Obstet Gynecol 2002;45:671–83; discussion 730–2.

Gemignani ML. Breast cancer treatment and continuing care. Clin Update Womens Health Care 2005;4:1-61.

Khoury-Collado F, Bombard AT. Hereditary breast and ovarian cancer: what the primary care physician should know. Obstet Gynecol Surv 2004;59:537–42.

# 81

## Unruptured ectopic pregnancy

A 43-year-old woman presents to the emergency room with profuse vaginal bleeding and an open cervical os at 6 weeks of gestation. Her serum β-hCG titer on presentation was 220 mIU/mL. Suction curettage was performed and decidualized endometrium was found. Repeat β-hCG titer performed 3 days after the curettage is 190 mIU/mL and the hemoglobin level is 12 g/dL. Transvaginal ultrasonography reveals no evidence of an ectopic pregnancy or other abnormalities. The next step in care is

(A) laparoscopy
(B) measure serum progesterone
(C) culdocentesis
(D) repeat suction curettage
* (E) measure β-hCG titer in 3 days

Expectant management of ectopic pregnancy remains a controversial topic. The management of ectopic pregnancy has evolved from laparotomy to laparoscopy to medical therapy with methotrexate. Given the potential life-threatening nature of the condition, expectant management would not be an acceptable option for many practitioners.

Available data suggest that no therapy is required for patients with ectopic pregnancy who are hemodynamically stable with a β-hCG titer below 200 mIU/mL. Management in such a case should include measuring β-hCG at regular intervals until it reaches undetectable levels. A plateau or increase in β-hCG levels may indicate a viable trophoblast and therapy should be instituted. Methotrexate could be used if no contraindications to its use exist. Signs or symptoms of impending rupture (eg, acute pelvic pain, shoulder pain, syncope, rebound tenderness) should prompt surgical intervention. Patients who are good candidates for expectant management include those with early small tubal gestations and low β-hCG levels. Those with β-hCG levels below 200 mIU/mL will have spontaneous resolution in 88% of cases. Patients should be counseled that a risk of rupture is still present.

Laparoscopy remains a viable option for treatment of ectopic pregnancy. Salpingectomy or salpingostomy may be accomplished with laparoscopy. After salpingostomy, measuring serial β-hCG titers is required to document that the gestation was completely removed. An increase or plateau of the β-hCG titer after a salpingostomy indicates the need for further treatment with methotrexate or salpingectomy. With low β-hCG titers and hemodynamic stability, laparoscopy would be an aggressive approach to treatment in this case. Although β-hCG is not always correlated with the site of ectopic pregnancy, it is likely in this case that the site of the ectopic pregnancy may not be visible at surgery given the low titers.

Serum progesterone has been studied in the evaluation of early pregnancy failure and ectopic pregnancy. Low serum progesterone (less than 5 ng/mL) indicates either a nonviable intrauterine or ectopic pregnancy in almost all cases. High serum progesterone levels (greater than 25 ng/mL) predict a viable intrauterine pregnancy and the chance of ectopic pregnancy is reduced to 2%; 52% of women with ectopic pregnancies have progesterone levels between 10 and 20 ng/mL, which is an indeterminate range. Thus, measurement of serum progesterone is of limited utility in the evaluation of ectopic pregnancy.

Culdocentesis potentially provides information regarding the presence of free intraperitoneal blood. Aspiration of nonclotting blood is indicative of intraperitoneal hemorrhage. The finding of nonclotting blood can be due to ectopic pregnancy, ruptured corpus luteum cysts, or an upper abdominal bleeding source. Transvaginal ultrasonography offers an accurate and less invasive method for evaluating the presence of posterior cul-de-sac fluid. The presence of a significant amount of free fluid in the pelvis, particularly if it is echogenic, is indicative of intraperitoneal hemorrhage. Therefore, ultrasonography often obviates the need for culdocentesis in most cases.

Initially, suction curettage was performed on this patient to rule out an unresolved spontaneous abortion. Suction curettage is preferred to endometrial biopsy for determination of presence of villi, and the procedure remains an important step in the diagnosis of ectopic pregnancy. Ruling out a nonviable intrauterine pregnancy may help confirm the presence of an ectopic pregnancy and provides a clear indication for expectant management or medical therapy. It is possible that this patient had a spontaneous abortion before the suction curettage.

Presumptively treating with methotrexate in cases without definitive evidence of ectopic pregnancy will lead to misdiagnosis 40% of the time. Repeat of the suction curettage in this case, particularly with the transvaginal ultrasonography findings demonstrating no intrauterine pregnancy, would be unnecessary and expose the patient to the risk of a second procedure.

American College of Obstetricians and Gynecologists. Medical management of tubal pregnancy. ACOG Practice Bulletin 3. Washington, DC: ACOG; 1998.

Barnhart KT, Katz I, Hummel A, Gracia CR. Presumed diagnosis of ectopic pregnancy. Obstet Gynecol 2002;100:505–10.

Korhonen J, Stenman UH, Ylostalo P. Serum human chorionic gonadotropin dynamics during spontaneous resolution of ectopic pregnancy. Fertil Steril 1994;61:632–6.

Shalev E, Peleg D, Tsabari A, Romano S, Bustan M. Spontaneous resolution of ectopic tubal pregnancy: natural history. Fertil Steril 1995;63:15–9.

# 82

## Safety of breastfeeding with hepatitis C viremia

A 30-year-old nurse, gravida 1, at 30 weeks of gestation has a history of remote occupational exposure to hepatitis C virus (HCV). She knows she is HCV antibody-positive and HCV RNA-positive. Her alanine aminotransferase is normal. She is not currently being treated for HCV. Her human immunodeficiency virus (HIV) screen is negative. She wants to breastfeed, but is concerned about transmission of hepatitis C to her baby. Your best advice about breastfeeding for this patient is that it is allowed

* (A) if desired by the mother
  (B) when the maternal viral load is undetectable
  (C) with HCV genotypes 2 and 3
  (D) if maternal HCV load is less than 1 million copies per milliliter

Hepatitis C virus causes a chronic infection with persistent viremia in the majority of infected individuals. It is an RNA virus with six known genotypes. Genotype 1a and 1b cause approximately 75% of infections in the United States, with genotypes 2 and 3 accounting for the remainder. Hepatitis C infects 2.3–4.5% of women of childbearing age.

The transmission of HCV is most often by percutaneous exposure to blood. More than 90% of seronegative recipients who receive blood products from an HCV-antibody-positive donor will become infected. Illicit drug use paraphernalia causes HCV infections in 50–95% of individuals who report drug use. Tattooing has been associated with an increased risk of HCV infection. Transmission to health care workers after accidental needlestick exposures to HCV-infected patients is approximately 0.5%. Sexual transmission does occur, with the risk low in monogamous couples and higher in drug users.

The rate of HCV transmission from an infected mother to her neonate is 2.4–11.9%. Maternal viral load is a risk factor for vertical transmission but, because of overlap in studies, the relative risk is unknown. Although elective cesarean delivery before labor may decrease vertical transmission, no data are available from large studies to make recommendations on route of delivery. Co-infection with HIV increases the risk of vertical transmission of HCV threefold.

According to the American Academy of Pediatrics' Section on Breastfeeding, mothers infected with HCV may breastfeed. Hepatitis C RNA has been detected in breast milk, but in most studies the risk of transmission is similar in breast-fed and bottle-fed infants. Hepatitis C viral load, genotype, and liver function tests are not used as determinates of safety with breastfeeding.

Mothers with HIV, with or without HCV co-infection, should not breastfeed if they live in the United States. In some areas of the world with unsafe water supplies, the risks of other infectious diseases and nutritional deficiencies associated with artificial feeding may outweigh the risk of HIV infection acquired postnatally in breastfed infants.

Patients usually are treated for HCV infection when there is a detectable viral load and persistently elevated alanine aminotransferase (ALT). Liver biopsy findings of fibrosis, moderate inflammation, or cirrhosis support the decision to initiate therapy, but are not required. It may take some time after the initial infection for the ALT to be persistently elevated. Therefore, patients with known HCV may be monitored and just observed for a long time before beginning treatment.

Patients who present with acute HCV infection also may have elimination of virus if immediately treated with interferon α-2b or pegylated interferon. However, clinical presentation with acute HCV infection is rare; such acute infection may be detected with screening after a needle-stick exposure. Hepatitis C is detected in breast milk, but the risk of transmission is very low and breastfeeding is not contraindicated.

The patient described is infected with the hepatitis C virus and wants to breastfeed. There are no data to suggest enhanced transmission from mother to baby through breast milk. Her HCV genotype and viral load are not germane to safety of lactation. Breastfeeding is allowed for this patient and is not contraindicated in this situation. However, breastfeeding should be discontinued if nipples are cracked or bleeding.

Berger A, Preiser W. Viral genome quantification as a tool for improving patient management: the example of HIV, HBV, HCV and CMV. J Antimicrob Chemother 2002;49:713–21.

Colgan R, Michocki R, Greisman L, Moore TA. Antiviral drugs in the immunocompetent host: part I. treatment of hepatitis, cytomegalovirus, and herpes infections. Am Fam Phys 2003;67:757–62.

Gartner LM, Morton J, Lawrence RA, Naylor AJ, O'Hare D, Schanler RJ, et al. Breastfeeding and the use of human milk. American Academy of Pediatrics Section on Breastfeeding. Pediatrics 2005;115:496–506.

Hupertz VF, Wyllie R. Perinatal hepatitis C infection. Pediatr Infect Dis J 2003;22:369–72.

# 83

## Weight-bearing exercise in the elderly

A 72-year-old woman with osteoporosis of the hip ($T$-score of $-2.6$) has been prescribed bisphosphonate therapy. She asks what she can do to further decrease her fracture risk. You advise her that the major effect of weight-bearing exercises will be to increase

      (A) risk of hip fracture
      (B) risk of falls
\*    (C) muscle tone
      (D) body mass index
      (E) bone mass

Physical activity may prevent hip fractures through enhanced balance, reaction time, coordination, mobility, and muscle strength. Exercise also may enhance bone mineral density (BMD) or structural integrity of bone, reducing the likelihood of fracture in the event of a fall. Exercise has beneficial effects on BMD in premenopausal and postmenopausal women. Aerobics, weight-bearing exercises, and resistance exercises are all effective in increasing spinal BMD in postmenopausal women. Walking can help increase BMD of the spine and hip. Aerobic exercise can increase BMD of the wrist.

Exercise has been associated with a reduced risk of hip fracture in older women. Women who walk 4 hours or more per week have a 41% lower risk of hip fracture than those who walked up to 1 hour per week. After controlling for age, body mass index, use of hormone therapy (HT), smoking, and dietary intake, risk of hip fracture was lowered by 6% for each increase of 3 metabolic equivalent (MET)-hours per week of activity (equivalent to 1 hour per week of walking at an average pace). Active women with at least 24 MET-hours per week had a 55% lower risk of hip fracture compared with sedentary women with less than 3 MET-hours per week. Even women with a lower risk of hip fracture due to higher body weight experienced a further reduction in risk with higher levels of activity. Risk of hip fracture decreased linearly with increasing levels of activity among women who were not on HT, although no reduction in risk was observed among women who were on HT.

Among older community-dwelling women, physical activity is associated with a reduced risk for hip fracture but not wrist or vertebral fracture. Higher levels of leisure time, sports activity, and household chores and fewer hours of sitting daily were associated with a significantly reduced relative risk for hip fracture after adjustment for age, dietary factors, falls at baseline, and functional and health status. Very active women had a statistically significant 36% reduction in hip fractures compared with the least active women. Intensity of physical activity also was related to fracture risk. Moderately to vigorously active women compared with inactive women had statistically significant reductions of 42% and 33% in risk for hip and vertebral fractures, respectively.

Enjoyment of the exercise regimen is important. The benefits of exercise are quickly lost after the woman stops exercising, thus, women should pick a regular weight-bearing exercise regimen that they enjoy to facilitate long-term compliance. Women with osteoporosis (or who are seeking to prevent it) should exercise prudently for at least 30 minutes three times per week, because exercise has been associated with improvements in bone density and a reduced risk of hip fracture. Any weight-bearing exercise regimen, including walking, should be prescribed.

In older, postmenopausal women, weight-bearing exercise led to significant increases above baseline in bone mineral content; these increases were maintained with continued training. With reduced weight-bearing exercise, bone mass reverted to baseline levels. Nevertheless, in older women, except for vigorous regimens, the beneficial effect of exercise on reducing fractures is small; any decrease in fractures is probably the result of increased muscular strength. A major factor in the reduction of falls may be increased muscle tone with continued exercise.

Bonaiuti D, Shea B, Iovine R, Negrini S, Robinson V, Kemper HC, et al. Exercise for preventing and treating osteoporosis in postmenopausal women. The Cochrane Database of Systematic Reviews 2002, Issue 2. Art. No.: CD000333. DOI: 10.1002/14651858.CD000333.

Dalsky GP, Stocke KS, Ehsani AA, Slatopolsky E, Lee WC, Birge SJ Jr. Weight-bearing exercise training and lumbar bone mineral content in postmenopausal women. Ann Intern Med 1988;108:824–8.

Feskanich D, Willett W, Colditz G. Walking and leisure-time activity and risk of hip fracture in postmenopausal women. JAMA 2002; 288:2300–6.

Friedlander AL, Genant HK, Sadowsky S, Byl NN, Gluer CC. A two-year program of aerobics and weight training enhances bone mineral density of young women. J Bone Miner Res 1995;10:574–85.

Gregg EW, Cauley JA, Seeley DG, Ensrud KE, Bauer DC. Physical activity and osteoporotic fracture risk in older women. Study of Osteoporotic Fractures Research Group. Ann Intern Med 1998;129: 81–8.

# 84

## Hormone therapy in patients with breast cancer

A healthy 64-year-old woman previously treated for stage I breast cancer has begun a new relationship and notes severe vaginal dryness and discomfort during sexual intercourse. Use of over-the-counter lubricants has not provided adequate relief. Examination reveals severe genital atrophy. The most appropriate initial treatment for this patient would be

    (A) venlafaxine hydrochloride (Effexor)
    (B) isoflavone dietary supplements
    (C) gabapentin (Neurontin)
\*   (D) vaginal estrogen
    (E) oral estrogen

Along with vasomotor symptoms, changes that result from genital atrophy represent the most common symptoms related to postmenopausal hypoestrogenism. As the vaginal mucosa loses its rugae, the lining becomes thin, translucent, and friable. The maturation index shifts in the direction of basal and parabasal cells and the pH increases, allowing the growth of pathogenic organisms. Symptoms caused by genital atrophy include vaginal dryness, dyspareunia, pruritus, burning, and bleeding or spotting. Because sexual intercourse precipitates symptoms in many women with genital atrophy, use of water-based lubricants during sexual contact reduces discomfort in many women. When these nonprescription remedies do not provide adequate relief, systemic as well as vaginal estrogen therapy has consistently been found to improve symptoms in well-controlled clinical trials.

Some 2 million–3 million breast cancer survivors in the United States are postmenopausal. Accordingly, obstetrician–gynecologists frequently are called on to treat symptomatic genital atrophy in this population. Two recent randomized trials assessed the safety of systemic hormone therapy (HT) in postmenopausal breast cancer survivors. The multicountry European study was halted prematurely because of an observed elevated recurrence risk with HT. A Swedish trial, in contrast, found no such increase. Of note, the HT regimen in the Swedish study used less progestin in women with an intact uterus than that used in the multicountry European study. A substantial number of other studies suggest that HT does not increase recurrence risk in breast cancer survivors (some studies assessed only systemic HT whereas others assessed vaginal as well as systemic therapy). Although the observational nature of these reports raises concerns regarding selection bias (eg, HT may have been disproportionately prescribed to survivors with a better prognosis), the volume of reassuring observations suggests that if systemic HT does increase recurrence risk in breast cancer survivors, the magnitude of any such increase is likely to be modest. Because vaginal estrogen therapy is associated with lower systemic estrogen levels, it can be speculated that it would have even less impact, if any, on recurrence risk.

The American College of Obstetricians and Gynecologists' Task Force on Hormone Therapy recommended that, for breast cancer survivors, alternatives to HT should be considered for the treatment of menopausal symptoms. Clinicians and women should be aware that the package labeling for all estrogens, including vaginally administered formulations, states that a personal history of breast cancer is a contraindication to use. The routine use of combination HT in women who have had breast cancer is not recommended. Nonetheless, obstetrician–gynecologists and their patients should recognize that use of vaginal estrogen therapy may be appropriate in well-counseled breast cancer survivors with bothersome symptoms of genital atrophy that have not responded to the nonprescription measures previously discussed. In addition, clinicians should be aware that use of vaginal estrogen tablets (Vagifem) has less systemic estrogenic absorption than does vaginal estrogen cream, whereas the 3-month vaginal ring containing estradiol (Estring) has less systemic estrogen than either vaginal tablets or cream. Accordingly, in selected well-counseled, motivated breast cancer survivors, use of vaginal estrogen offers effective, appropriate therapy.

Isoflavones are found in soybeans. Nonprescription remedies containing isoflavones are commonly used for the treatment of menopausal vasomotor symptoms. Controlled clinical trials have not consistently found isoflavone supplements to be more effective than placebo in treating vasomotor symptoms. Neither of these treatments is known to be effective in treating symptoms of genital atrophy. The mixed selective serotonin reuptake inhibitor and serotonin noradrenergic reuptake inhibitor venlafaxine has been found to be more effective than placebo in the treatment of menopausal vasomotor symptoms. This antidepressant medication has not, however, been found effective in the treatment of symptomatic genital atrophy.

Breast cancer. American College of Obstetricians and Gynecologists. Obstet Gynecol 2004;104 suppl:11S–16S.

Holmberg L, Anderson H. HABITS (hormonal replacement therapy after breast cancer—is it safe?), a randomised comparison: trial stopped. HABITS Steering and Data Monitoring Committees. Lancet 2004;363:453–5.

Notelovitz M, Funk S, Nanavati N, Mazzeo M. Estradiol absorption from vaginal tablets in postmenopausal women. Obstet Gynecol 2002; 99:556–62.

O'Meara ES, Rossing MA, Daling JR, Elmore JG, Barlow WE, Weiss NS. Hormone replacement therapy after a diagnosis of breast cancer in relation to recurrence and mortality. J Natl Cancer Inst 2001;93:754–62.

Rioux JE, Devlin C, Gelfand MM, Steinberg WM, Hepburn DS. 17beta-estradiol vaginal tablet versus conjugated equine estrogen vaginal cream to relieve menopausal atrophic vaginitis. Menopause 2000;7: 156–61.

Vasomotor symptoms. American College of Obstetricians and Gynecologists. Obstet Gynecol 2004;104 suppl:106S–117S.

von Schoultz E, Rutqvist LE. Menopausal hormone therapy after breast cancer: the Stockholm randomized trial. Stockholm Breast Cancer Study Group. J Natl Cancer Inst 2005;97:533–5.

# 85
## Smoking cessation strategies

The transtheoretical model for stages of change can be used to evaluate the behavior of cigarette smokers. The phase that best describes a smoker who indicates that they are thinking about quitting in the next month is

* (A) precontemplation
* (B) contemplation
* (C) preparation
* (D) maintenance
* (E) relapse

Cigarette smoking is the number one preventable cause of disease and death in the United States. The many reproductive health consequences of cigarette smoking in women include an increased risk for low-birth-weight delivery, preterm premature rupture of membranes, sudden infant death syndrome, and stillbirth as well as decreased fertility and early menopause.

Interventions to decrease the rate of smoking include such useful measures as tobacco taxes, public health measures, advertising bans, and school-based and media-sponsored antismoking campaigns targeted to adolescents. Tobacco use can be approached as a chronic, sometimes relapsing condition. Office-based intervention is one of the most effective methods to help smokers quit. However, only about 2% of established smokers quit annually. A physician's recommendation to quit is associated with cessation rates of 9–12% per year. Pharmacologic intervention with nicotine replacement or bupropion plus behavioral counseling has 1-year smoking cessation rates of approximately 25% among those who initially quit smoking.

The U.S. Public Health Service (USPHS) practice guidelines for treating tobacco use and dependence provide evidence about treatment effectiveness. Before prescribing therapy, however, physicians should assess the patient's readiness to give up smoking.

The USPHS guidelines suggest the use of the "5A's" to deliver brief interventions:

* ASK about tobacco use
* ADVISE smokers to quit
* ASSESS willingness to quit
* ASSIST with quitting
* ARRANGE follow-up

Setting goals and being empathetic are important. Quitting does not necessarily mean "cold turkey," but can be gradual, deliberate, and staged.

In the transtheoretical model of change, the phase that best describes a smoker who is thinking about quitting in the next month is the contemplative stage. Identification of the behavioral state of the patient with the model allows the busy clinician and staff to focus efforts on patients who are ready to receive help. Asking the question, "Are you planning to quit smoking in the next 6 months?" differentiates precontemplative and contemplative patients. Contemplators should then be asked, "Are you planning to quit smoking in the next month?" Those who say yes are in preparation. Following a relapse or resumption of smoking, patients may move back and forth between stages.

Randomized clinical trials also have reported that nicotine delivered by gum or a transdermal patch have similar short-term abstinence rates in the range of 16–27%. Individual counseling and behavioral counseling are associated with abstinence rates in the range of 15%. Most authorities recommend combination therapy with a pharmacologic agent plus behavioral counseling. Table 85-1 shows messages and goals to tailor to achieve stage-specific change in smoking behavior, and Table 85-2 shows a comparison of drugs used to treat tobacco use.

Swartz SH, Hays JT. Office-based intervention for tobacco dependence. Med Clin North Am 2004;88:1623–41, xii–xiii.

U.S. Public Health Service. Treating tobacco use and dependence. Clinical practice guideline. Rockville (MD): USPHS; 2000.

**TABLE 85-1.** Tailoring Messages and Goals to Patient's Stage of Change

| If Patient Reports. . . | Goals for This Patient | Examples of Messages |
|---|---|---|
| Not ready to quit smoking | Think about quitting<br>• Praise prior attempts<br>• Examine reasons for smoking | "Quitting smoking can be difficult."<br>"What do you like about smoking?"<br>"Is there any reason you might think about quitting in the future?"<br>"It sounds like you are not thinking about quitting right now. If you want to talk about your smoking any time, please let me know." |
| Wants to quit but is not ready right now | Enhance desire to quit<br><br>• Praise prior attempts<br><br>• Help her to identify benefits to quitting<br>• Legitimize the challenge | "Tell me about any time in the past you tried to quit smoking."<br>"It's understandable that you have mixed feelings about smoking."<br>"Is there anything in particular that might motivate you to try to quit?"<br>"There are better methods to help you quit now than ever before." |
| Ready to quit now | Develop treatment plan<br>• Set a quit date<br><br><br>• Counsel briefly<br><br>• Offer medication<br><br>• Refer for intensive counseling if appropriate<br>• Follow-up | "It's important to set a quit date."<br>"Getting added help, such as medications or counseling, can really increase your success."<br>"What are your plans if you get cravings for cigarettes?"<br>"We need to talk or meet again, I want to see how you're doing." |
| Recently quit | Maintain abstinence<br>• Review ways to avoid slips<br>• Identify social supports | "You should feel proud of yourself."<br>"Are others supporting your efforts?"<br>"If there is anything you're ready to try again, we are ready to help you." |
| Recently relapsed | Reassess motivation<br><br>• Praise attempt at quitting<br><br>• Turn feeling of failure into small success | "You should feel good about trying to quit."<br>"Any time you're ready to try again, we are ready to help you."<br>"What might you do different next time?" |

Reprinted from Swartz SH, Hays JT. Office-based intervention for tobacco dependence. Med Clin North Am 2004;88:1623–41, xii–xiii, with permission from Elsevier. Copyright © 2004 Elsevier.

**TABLE 85-2.** Comparison of Drugs Used to Treat Tobacco Use

| Product | Sales Method | Recommended Daily Dose* |
|---|---|---|
| *Nicotine replacement therapy* | | |
| Transdermal patch (21 mg, 14 mg, 7 mg) | OTC | 1 patch for 24 hours |
| Nicotrol (15 mg) | OTC | 1 patch for 16 hours |
| Private label† (22 mg, 11 mg; 21 mg, 14 mg, 7 mg) | OTC | 1 patch for 24 hours |
| Gum (Nicorette, 2 mg, 4 mg) | OTC | 1 piece per hour, 12 pieces per day |
| Inhaler (Nicotrol inhaler) | Rx | 6–16 cartridges per day |
| Nasal spray (Nicotrol NS) | Rx | 1–2 doses per hour, 12–14 doses per day |
| *Nonnicotine drug therapy* | | |
| Bupropion (Zyban, Wellbutrin) | Rx | 150 mg twice daily |
| Nortriptyline | Rx | 75 mg per day |

OTC, over-the-counter; Rx, prescription only.

*Adapted and expanded from Pharmacotherapy for the Treatment of Nicotine Dependence, Massachusetts Tobacco Control Program

†Private label is similar to a generic product.

Modified from Rigotti NA. A 36-year-old woman who smokes cigarettes. JAMA 2000;284:746.

# 86

## Contraception advice for patients with systemic lupus

A 31-year-old woman comes to your office for a periodic health examination. She is getting married and requests information about contraceptive options, particularly combination (estrogen and progesterone) oral contraceptives. Two years ago, lupus erythematosus was diagnosed. Her disease is currently stable with no recent history of flare. Her family history is positive for hypertension and gestational diabetes mellitus in her sister and a previous deep vein thrombosis (DVT) in an aunt. Her weight is 83.9 kg (185 lb), height 1.65 m (65 in.), blood pressure 120/70 mm Hg, and pulse 75 beats per minute. Recent laboratory results show a serum creatinine level of 1.4 mg/dL, a positive lupus anticoagulant level, and a total cholesterol level of 224 mg/dL. In this patient with known lupus erythematosus, the most important reason to avoid using combination oral contraceptives is

    (A) family history of hypertension
    (B) family history of DVT
*   (C) positive lupus anticoagulant level
    (D) hyperlipidemia
    (E) obesity

Women with systemic lupus erythematosus may have a wide range of medical factors, which complicate the disease process itself, coexist with it, or are a result of longstanding disease. Systemic vascular disease or uncontrolled hypertension represent contraindications to combination oral contraceptives. However, recent data indicate that women with this disorder can use combination oral contraceptives safely if their disease is mild or moderate in severity. However, because this patient has a lupus anticoagulant, this places her at increased risk for thromboembolism, and the condition is a contraindication to combination oral contraceptives. A family history of DVT, without documentation of thrombophilia, may slightly increase her risk while she is using combination oral contraceptives, but does not represent an absolute contraindication.

Many women with systemic lupus erythematosus will develop hypertension and vascular disease, and, in such women, the use of an estrogen-containing hormonal oral contraceptive may increase the risk of cardiovascular complications. Well-controlled hypertension alone in the presence of lupus erythematosus does not represent a contraindication to estrogen-containing hormonal contraceptive regimens, but close follow-up of blood pressure and exclusion of end-organ disease is required. A family history of hypertension is not a contraindication.

Hyperlipidemia may be associated with an increased risk of cardiovascular disease but this factor in itself does not contraindicate the use of combination oral contraceptives. Obesity also poses a slightly increased risk for thromboembolic disease, but is not a contraindication for oral contraceptive use.

A number of other contraception options should be considered for women with systemic lupus erythematosus. Progestin-only methods are satisfactory choices for such women. These women do not appear to have any increased side effects from the progestin-only methods.

Barrier contraceptives are also an excellent choice for patients regardless of the severity of systemic lupus erythematosus. Patient compliance and correct use may be reduced in some patient populations using barriers alone. To any patient using a barrier contraception, the availability of emergency contraception should be communicated.

Bermas BL. Oral contraceptives in systemic lupus erythematosus—a tough pill to swallow? [Editorial.] N Engl J Med 2005;353:2602–4.

Petri M, Kim MY, Kalunian KC, Grossman J, Hahn BH, Sammaritano LR, et al. Combined oral contraceptives in women with systemic lupus erythematosus. OC-SELENA Trial. N Engl J Med 2005;353:2550–8.

Sánchez-Guerrero J, Uribe AG, Jiménez-Santana L, Mestanza-Peralta M, Lara-Reyes P, Seuc AH, et al. A trial of contraceptive methods in women with systemic lupus erythematosus. N Engl J Med 2005; 353:2539–49.

# 87

## Ultrasonographic findings in adnexal torsion

A 17-year-old adolescent reports acute onset of right lower quadrant pain in the past 24 hours. Abdominal examination reveals rebound tenderness in the right lower quadrant with guarding. Bimanual examination reveals tenderness in the right lower quadrant. Her white blood cell count is slightly elevated and her temperature is 38.1°C (100.6°F). Ultrasonography reveals a uterus with normal dimensions and an 11-mm homogeneous endometrial stripe. The left ovary measures 2.3 × 2.5 × 2.4 cm and contains several small follicles. The right ovary measures 5.3 × 6.1 × 6.4 cm with a central echo dense area surrounded by multiple peripheral follicles. No free fluid is seen in the cul-de-sac. Based on these findings, the patient is most likely to have

     (A) an ovarian corpus luteum cyst
     (B) a tuboovarian abscess
\*   (C) an ovarian torsion
     (D) an ovarian physiologic cyst

Adnexal torsion is initially suspected based on clinical presentation. It may occur in women of all ages, including female fetuses prior to birth. In utero, torsion may result in auto-amputation and subsequent absence of the adnexa. In infants and young children, failure to diagnose and treat may result in eventual necrosis of an ovary or adnexa and loss of the ovary and possibly the fallopian tube.

The clinical presentation of ovarian torsion may mimic an acute abdominal process. The right adnexa is more commonly involved than the left, and torsion may involve the ovary, the fallopian tube, or both. Torsion may occur in an adnexa in which the ovary contains a cyst. The presence of this cyst or neoplasm may result in adnexal movement with daily activities and eventual twisting of the adnexa. Most adnexal findings are benign, with the most frequent diagnoses being corpus luteum cysts and benign teratomas. The corpus luteum cyst will be seen around and after puberty and menarche, although benign teratomas may occur at any age.

The clinical findings include abdominal pain, rebound, and other signs of peritonitis. The torsion may be intermittent or persistent, and if intermittent, there may be periods when the persistent signs and symptoms completely resolve. Alternatively, the patient may present with signs and symptoms of an acute abdomen. A high index of suspicion for ovarian torsion is necessary in order to make the correct diagnosis.

Diagnostic testing may include ultrasonography, computed tomography, or magnetic resonance imaging to rule out appendicitis. The classical observation is an enlarged ovary with echo dense areas. Ultrasound diagnoses may be enhanced by Doppler flow studies. Initial torsion involves the venous and lymphatic drainage first, followed by occlusion of the arterial supply. This results in an early

increase in the size of the ovary. Findings on ultrasonography or other imaging studies may be those of a homogeneous echo dense mass. This consists of the normal ovarian tissue, the cyst or neoplasm, and vascular engorgement with stromal edema. If the torsion is intermittent, these anatomic findings may regress. In older women, the mass is located within the pelvis. In younger children, it may be abdominopelvic according to the age and normal placement of the adnexa.

Close inspection of the adnexa on imaging of the torsion may reveal normal-appearing follicles along the periphery of the ovary. Free fluid may be present in the pelvis due to hemorrhage or an exudative process. Although the differential diagnosis includes nongynecologic disorders, such as appendicitis, the suspicion of torsion must be high in order to make the diagnosis in a timely fashion. Although there may be mild elevations of the temperature and white blood cell count, markedly increased levels traditionally seen with peritonitis, salpingitis, and abscess are not customarily observed.

The therapy involves surgical intervention, with laparoscopy preferred to an open laparotomy procedure. In young patients, detorsion and preservation of the adnexa is important. Following detorsion, removal of the cyst is required.

The findings in this patient are compatible with an ovarian torsion. If calcifications are noted, they may represent a cyst within the ovary, such as a benign teratoma, which will require removal at the time of surgery.

Although a corpus luteum cyst may mimic other ovarian findings and occasionally result in adnexal torsion, it often contains flow within it or is associated with free fluid in the cul-de-sac. A tuboovarian abscess is a homogeneous mass in the adnexa without evidence of flow. It often has thickened walls and rarely is associated with torsion. A physiologic cyst is a thin-walled fluid-filled area within the ovary and is likely to regress if less than 6 cm. It contains no excrescences or papillations.

Breech LL, Hillard PJ. Adnexal torsion in pediatric and adolescent girls. [Review.] Curr Opin Obstet Gynecol 2005;17:483–9.

Graif M, Itzchak Y. Sonographic evaluation of ovarian torsion in childhood and adolescence. AJR Am J Roentgenol 1988;150:647–9.

Grant EJ. Benign conditions of the ovaries in transvaginal ultrasound. In: Nyberg DA, Hill MN, Böhm-Vélez M, Mendelson EB, editors. Transvaginal ultrasound. St. Louis (MO): Mosby-Year Book; 1992. p. 194–5.

Meyer JS, Harmon CM, Harty MP, Markowitz RI, Hubbard AM, Bellah RD. Ovarian torsion: clinical and imaging presentation in children. J Pediatr Surg 1995;30:1433–6.

# 88

## Testing for chlamydia

An 18-year-old nulligravid adolescent, who is taking oral contraceptives, tests positive for cervical chlamydia on a nucleic acid amplification test. She is treated with azithromycin, 1 g orally. She is instructed to ask her boyfriend to seek treatment and told to refrain from sexual intercourse for the next week. Repeat testing for chlamydia should next be performed in

      (A) 1 week
      (B) 2–3 weeks
\*    (C) 3–4 months
      (D) 1 year

In the United States, *Chlamydia trachomatis* infection is the most commonly reported notifiable disease with 877,478 cases reported to the Centers for Disease Control and Prevention (CDC) in 2003. Approximately 72% of reported cases occurred among teenagers and young adults aged 15–24 years (Table 88-1). Most cases are not reported, however, and the estimated incidence is actually 2.8 million, which results in an anticipated tangible cost of $2.4 billion annually in the United States.

Most females (75%) and approximately 50% of males with chlamydia are asymptomatic. Up to 40% of women with untreated chlamydia or gonorrhea will develop pelvic inflammatory disease (PID). Of those women, 20% will become infertile, 18% will experience debilitating chronic pelvic pain, and 9% will have a tubal pregnancy. Because the cervix of teenage girls and young women is not fully matured, they are at particularly high risk for infection if sexually active and exposed to chlamydia.

Treatment with azithromycin, 1 g single oral dose, or doxycycline, 100 mg orally twice a day for 7 days, is equally effective, but often the single dose of azithromycin is a better treatment option if the physician is concerned about patient compliance. Patients also should be counseled about the importance of referring their sexual partners for evaluation, testing, and treatment. Chlamydia-infected individuals should abstain from sexual intercourse until they and their sexual partners have completed treatment; otherwise, reinfection is possible.

Chlamydia testing at less than 3 weeks after completion of therapy with a nucleic acid amplification test (NAAT) can result in a false-positive result. This test is designed to amplify nucleic acid sequences that are specific to the organism being detected and do not require viable organisms. The improved sensitivity of NAATs is due to their ability to produce a positive signal from a single copy of the target DNA or RNA.

**TABLE 88-1.** Chlamydia—Reported Cases and Rates by Age and Sex, United States, 2003

| Age Group (Years) | No. of Cases | | |
|---|---|---|---|
| | Total | Male | Female |
| 10–14 | 14,911 | 1,061 | 13,849 |
| 15–19 | 310,505 | 44,331 | 266,175 |
| 20–24 | 324,411 | 71,476 | 252,936 |
| 25–29 | 124,890 | 34,916 | 89,974 |
| 30–34 | 53,572 | 17,810 | 35,762 |
| 35–39 | 24,658 | 9,772 | 14,886 |
| 40–44 | 12,287 | 5,675 | 6,612 |
| 45–54 | 8,214 | 4,012 | 4,202 |
| 55–64 | 1,653 | 883 | 770 |
| 65+ | 776 | 323 | 453 |
| Total | 877,478 | 190,723 | 686,755 |

Centers for Disease Control and Prevention. Sexually transmitted disease surveillance, 2003. Atlanta, GA: US Department of Health and Human Services, Centers for Disease Control and Prevention; September 2003. Available at: http://www.cdc.gov/std/stats/toc2003.htm. Retrieved June 20, 2005.

Women whose sexual partners have not been appropriately treated are at high risk for reinfection. A greater occurrence of chlamydia is found in women who have had a previous chlamydial infection in the preceding several months. Having multiple infections increases a woman's risk of serious reproductive health problems, including infertility. Although an immediate test of cure is not recommended, repeat screening is recommended by CDC for women, especially adolescents, 3–4 months after treatment is completed to rule out reinfection. This is especially true if a woman does not know if her sex partner received treatment. Sexually transmitted disease (STD) treatment guidelines issued by CDC indicate that sexually active adolescent women should be screened for chlamydia at least annually, even if symptoms are not present. Rescreening is distinct from retesting to detect therapeutic failure (test of cure). Except in pregnant women, test of cure is not recommended for individuals treated with recommended regimens unless therapeutic compliance is a question.

American College of Obstetricians and Gynecologists. Sexually transmitted diseases in adolescents. ACOG Committee Opinion No. 301. Washington, DC: ACOG; 2004.

Centers for Disease Control and Prevention. Sexually transmitted disease surveillance, 2003. Atlanta, GA: US Department of Health and Human Services, Centers for Disease Control and Prevention; September 2003. Available at: http://www.cdc.gov/std/stats/toc2003.htm. Retrieved June 20, 2005.

Hopkins RS, Jajosky RA, Hall PA, Adams DA, Connor FJ, Sharp P, et al. Summary of notifiable diseases—United States, 2003. Centers for Disease Control and Prevention. MMWR Morb Mortal Wkly Rep 2005;52:1–85.

Johnson RE, Newhall WJ, Papp JR, Knapp JS, Black CM, Gift TL, et al. Screening tests to detect Chlamydia trachomatis and Neisseria gonorrhoeae infections—2002. Centers for Disease Control and Prevention. MMWR Recomm Rep 2002;51(RR-15):1–38; quiz CE 1–4.

Sexually transmitted diseases treatment guidelines, 2006. Centers for Disease Control and Prevention [published erratum appears in MMWR Recomm Rep 2006;55(36):997]. MMWR Recomm Rep 2006;55(RR-11):1–94.

Weinstock H, Berman S, Cates W Jr. Sexually transmitted diseases among American youth: incidence and prevalence estimates, 2000. Perspect Sex Reprod Health 2004;36:6–10.

# 89

## Determine the correct coding for a short office visit

A 27-year-old woman comes to your office for evaluation of vaginitis. Her last visit with you was 4 years ago. She now lives in a different state, where she receives her medical care. She is visiting her parents for 2 weeks. You note her chief complaint, take a brief history and a problem-pertinent review of systems (ROS), perform a pelvic examination and wet mount, and diagnose yeast vaginitis. The total time for the visit is approximately 20 minutes. When you complete your billing voucher, the Current Procedural Terminology (CPT) code for this patient should be

    (A) 99201 New Patient, problem-focused
\*   (B) 99202 New Patient, expanded problem-focused
    (C) 99212 Established Patient, problem-focused
    (D) 99213 Established Patient, expanded problem-focused

A good understanding of medical coding is necessary for proper billing of physician services. Evaluation and management codes (E/M) are used for patient encounters in which the provider performs three key components: history, examination, and medical decision making. Several E/M codes have been developed for different situations including inpatient and outpatient services, problem oriented or preventive visits, consultations, and counseling encounters. Each of these categories has certain requirements that must be documented in order to use the correct code. Outpatient codes can reflect whether the visit is for a new patient or an established patient. A new patient has never been provided services by you or a physician of the same specialty in your practice, or has not been seen in the practice for at least 3 years. An established patient has received care from you or an associate of the same specialty in your practice within the past 3 years and reflects an ongoing relationship with the patient.

New patient codes require documentation of all three of the key components (ie, history, examination, and medical decision making); established patient codes require only two of the three components. Problem-focused visits differ from preventive and other types of visits in that the patient has presented with a specific problem for which she desires diagnosis and treatment. Problem-focused visits can be simple, expanded, detailed, and comprehensive to reflect differing levels of history taking, physical examination, medical decision making, and time. Each level of service requires specific documentation (see Table 89-1).

Because the woman in this example was last seen 4 years ago, she clearly qualifies for a new patient code. By documenting a chief complaint, brief history of present illness (HPI), a problem-pertinent review of systems (ROS), and six elements from the CPT genitourinary single system examination (Table 89-2), the E/M code 99202, "New Patient, expanded problem-focused" can correctly be applied.

**TABLE 89-1**. Current Procedural Terminology (CPT) Coding for Brief Office Visits for New Patients

| Element | CPT Code No. | | | |
| --- | --- | --- | --- | --- |
| | 99201 | 99202 | 99203 | 99204 |
| Level | Problem-focused | Expanded problem-focused | Detailed | Comprehensive |
| Chief complaint (CC) | Required | Required | Required | Required |
| History of present illness (HPI) | Brief | Brief | Extended | Extended |
| Review of systems (ROS) | N/A | Problem pertinent | Extended | Complete |
| Past, family, or social | N/A | N/A | Pertinent | Complete history (PFSH) |
| Examination | One to five elements | At least six elements | At least 12 elements | Complete system examination |
| Decision making | Straightforward | Straightforward | Low | Moderate to high |
| Time | 10 minutes | 20 minutes | 30 minutes | 45+ minutes |

N/A, not applicable.

American College of Obstetricians and Gynecologists. CPT coding in obstetrics and gynecology 2006. Washington, DC: ACOG; 2006.

**TABLE 89-2.** Genitourinary Single System Examination

| System/Body Area | Elements of Examination |
|---|---|
| Constitutional | • Recording of any three of the following vital signs: 1) sitting or standing blood pressure, 2) supine blood pressure, 3) pulse rate and regularity, 5) temperature, 6) height, 7) weight (May be measured and recorded by ancillary staff)<br>• General appearance of patient (eg, development, nutrition, body habitus, deformities, attention to grooming) |
| Neck | • Examination of thyroid (eg, enlargement, tenderness, mass)<br>• Examination of neck (eg, masses, overall appearance, symmetry, tracheal position, crepitus) |
| Respiratory | • Assessment of respiratory effort (eg, intercostal refractions, use of accessory muscles, diaphragmatic movement)<br>• Auscultation of lungs (eg, breath sounds, adventitious sounds, rubs) |
| Cardiovascular | • Auscultation of the heart with rotation of sounds, abnormal sounds, and murmurs<br>• Examination of peripheral vascular system by observation (eg, swelling, varicosities) and palpation (eg, pulses, temperature, edema, tenderness) |
| Chest (Breast) | • See genitourinary (female). |
| Lymphatic | • Palpation of lymph nodes in neck, axillae and groin, and other locations |
| Skin | • Inspection and palpation of skin and subcutaneous tissue (eg, rashes, lesions, ulcers) |
| Neurologic/ Psychiatric | • Brief assessment of mental status, including:<br>—Orientation (ie, time, place, and person) and<br>—Mood and affect (eg, depression, anxiety, agitation) |
| Gastrointestinal (Abdomen) | • Examination of abdomen with rotation of presence of masses and tenderness<br>• Examination of liver and spleen<br>• Obtain stool sample for occult blood test, when indicated<br>• Examination for presence of absence of hernia |
| Genitourinary | • Inspection and palpation of breasts (eg, masses or lumps, tenderness, symmetry, nipple discharge)<br>• Digital rectal examination, including sphincter tone, presence of hemorrhoids, rectal masses<br>• Pelvic examination (with or without specimen collection for smears and cultures) of:<br>—External genitalia (eg, general appearance, hair distribution, lesions)<br>—Urethral meatus (eg, size, location, lesions, prolapse)<br>—Urethra (eg, masses, tenderness, scarring)<br>—Bladder (eg, fullness, masses, tenderness)<br>—Vagina (eg, general appearance, estrogen effect, discharge, lesions, pelvic support, cystocele, rectocele)<br>—Cervix (eg, general appearance, lesions, discharge)<br>—Uterus (eg, size, contour, position, mobility, tenderness, consistency, descent or support)<br>—Adnexa/parametria (eg, masses, tenderness, organomegaly, nodularity)<br>—Anus and perineum |

American College of Obstetricians and Gynecologists. CPT coding in obstetrics and gynecology 2006. Washington, DC: ACOG; 2006.

American Medical Association. Current procedural terminology—2004. Chicago (IL): AMA; 2004.

# 90

## Suppression of herpes simplex virus in pregnancy

A 26-year-old antenatal woman, gravida 2, para 1, comes to your office for a routine obstetric visit at 32 weeks of gestation. Her partner has recurrent genital herpes. Antenatal laboratory test results reveal a positive titer to herpes simplex virus type 2 (HSV-2) with a glycoprotein G-based test and a negative titer to herpes simplex virus type 1 (HSV-1). She had one outbreak of genital herpes earlier in pregnancy. The next step in care is

* (A) prophylactic antiviral drugs after 36 weeks, allow vaginal delivery
  (B) planned cesarean delivery at 39 weeks
  (C) initiate prophylactic antiviral drugs now
  (D) initiate prophylactic antivirals now, plan cesarean delivery at 39 weeks
  (E) expectant management

Genital herpesvirus infection is one of the most common sexually transmitted diseases (STDs). Based on serology and clinical evidence, 45 million adolescents and adults in the United States are infected; 30% of women have antibodies to HSV-2, the most common agent in genital herpes infections.

Vertical transmission and perinatal morbidity and mortality are a significant health concern among women infected with HSV. Because of the risks to both the mother and fetus, appropriate forms of close monitoring and management of infection in pregnancy have been studied.

Serology and clinical presentation have demonstrated that there are three stages of HSV infection:

• Primary infections, ie, presence of lesions but no antibodies to either HSV-1 or HSV-2

• Nonprimary first episode, ie, presence of antibodies to either HSV-1 or HSV-2 when clinical presentation of the other HSV type occurs

• Recurrent HSV, ie, recurrent lesions with antibodies to the same type present

Vertical transmission of genital HSV is related to the gestational age at time of exposure and stage of infection (primary vs nonprimary first episode vs recurrent infection). At delivery, vertical transmission in women with recurrent infection is very low (0–3%); transmission after primary infection is approximately 50%. Recurrent outbreaks can be symptomatic or subclinical, either of which are capable of vertical transmission. It is known that primary infection later in pregnancy (late second or third trimester) is much more likely to result in neonatal transmission.

In pregnant patients who have a primary outbreak of HSV, antiviral therapy is strongly recommended to reduce viral shedding. It is impossible to distinguish a primary infection from nonprimary first outbreak without sero-

logic testing. Given that primary infection in pregnancy is at significantly higher risk for vertical transmission, serologic testing is routinely recommended in the antenatal period. Serologic assays that are not glycoprotein G-based have a high false-positive rate (14–88%) for HSV-2 antibodies in sera positive for HSV-1. Therefore, only glycoprotein G-based testing is recommended.

The experience of rare outbreaks during pregnancy does not eliminate the risk of asymptomatic shedding at the time of delivery. Most perinatal infections occur from contact with infected maternal secretions from asymptomatic mothers without identified lesions. Although the risk of vertical transmission from recurrent HSV is much lower than primary infections, because recurrent HSV is more common than primary HSV, the overall proportion of perinatal HSV infections related to recurrent HSV is high. Thus, prevention of neonatal herpes involves not only prevention of new primary infections but also prevention of exposure of the neonate to the virus from recurrent lesions during delivery.

Research has focused on the use of suppressive therapy in pregnancy and whether it decreases viral shedding, the need for cesarean delivery, and the incidence of neonatal herpes. More than one randomized study has shown the efficacy of antiviral suppression from 36 weeks of gestation through delivery to prevent active infection in the neonate and reduce the need for cesarean delivery. Current research is being carried out to determine the extent to which suppressive therapy will prevent vertical transmission. A randomized study specifically to assess acyclovir in the last 4 weeks of gestation showed a reduction in recurrences and a concomitant reduced need for cesarean delivery. Suppressive therapy reduces but does not eliminate subclinical viral shedding, and thus it is not yet clear to what extent suppressive therapy will prevent vertical transmission.

According to the U.S. Food and Drug Administration (FDA), acyclovir is a class C drug in pregnancy and valacyclovir is class B. In 1984, the Centers for Disease Control and Prevention (CDC) established a registry to track the clinical outcome of acyclovir use in pregnancy. To date, there has been no evidence of increased risk of birth defects in neonates exposed to acyclovir in utero. Pharmacokinetic studies have indicated that in late pregnancy there is a requirement for slightly higher doses to maintain steady state peak and trough levels (Table 90-1).

Based on this information, the American College of Obstetricians and Gynecologists recommends antiviral therapy for pregnant women who experience a primary HSV outbreak and consideration of suppression therapy beyond 36 weeks for pregnant women who have recurrent HSV.

The patient described has known recurrent HSV, that is, she is at risk for recurrent lesions and asymptomatic shedding at term. The vertical transmission rate for recurrent HSV is low. Current research suggests that it can be even lower with antiviral therapy initiated at 36 weeks of gestation. Cesarean delivery for recurrent HSV is recommended at term if clinical evidence of an outbreak is present. Planned cesarean delivery in the absence of clinical evidence of active HSV is not supported by the literature. The benefits of cesarean delivery in such a setting do not outweigh the potential risks.

The use of antivirals to reduce recurrence rate and neonatal transmission, and the need for cesarean delivery, is not supported by the literature until 36 weeks of gestation. The patient is asymptomatic at this time and her gestational age is too early to achieve this benefit. Thus, starting antiviral medications now is not recommended. Use of antiviral medications can be delayed until 36 weeks of gestation or when clinical evidence or symptoms of lesions appear.

**TABLE 90-1.** Antiviral Treatment for Herpes Simplex Virus

| Indication | Dosage | | |
| | Valacyclovir | Acyclovir | Famciclovir |
| --- | --- | --- | --- |
| First clinical episode | 1,000 mg twice daily for 7–10 days | 200 mg five times daily or 400 mg three times daily for 7–10 days | 250 mg three times daily for 7–10 days |
| Recurrent episodes | 500 mg twice daily for 5 days | 400 mg three times daily for 5 days | 125 mg twice daily for 5 days |
| Daily suppressive therapy | 500 mg once daily (up to nine recurrences per year) or 1,000 mg once daily | 400 mg twice daily | 250 mg twice daily |

Sexually transmitted diseases treatment guidelines, 2006. Centers for Disease Control and Prevention [published erratum appears in MMWR Recomm Rep 2006;55(36):997]. MMWR Recomm Rep 2006;55(RR-11):1–94.

American College of Obstetricians and Gynecologists. Management of herpes in pregnancy. Practice Bulletin 8. Washington, DC: ACOG; 1999.

Brocklehurst P, Kinghorn G, Carney O, Helsen K, Ross E, Ellis E, et al. A randomised placebo controlled trial of suppressive acyclovir in late pregnancy in women with recurrent genital herpes infection. Br J Obstet Gynaecol 1998;105:275–80.

Kimberlin DF, Weller S, Whitley RJ, Andrews WW, Hauth JC, Lakeman F, et al. Pharmacokinetics of valacyclovir and acyclovir in late pregnancy. Am J Obstet Gynecol 1998;179:846–51.

Morrow RA, Brown ZA. Common use of inaccurate antibody assays to identify infection status with herpes simplex virus type 2. Am J Obstet Gynecol 2005;193:361–2.

Scott LL, Sanchez PJ, Jackson GL, Zeray F, Wendel GD Jr. Acyclovir suppression to prevent cesarean delivery after first-episode genital herpes. Obstet Gynecol 1996;87:69–73.

Sexually transmitted diseases treatment guidelines, 2006. Centers for Disease Control and Prevention [published erratum appears in MMWR Recomm Rep 2006;55(36):997]. MMWR Recomm Rep 2006;55 (RR-11):1–94.

# 91

## Transcervical hysteroscopic sterilization

A 44-year-old woman, gravida 4, para 3, abortus 1, requests transcervical hysteroscopic sterilization. Her history is significant for a unicornuate uterus and chlamydial cervicitis treated 2 years ago. Her weight is 113.4 kg (250 lb) and pelvic examination reveals a uterus the size of 10 weeks of gestation. A right adnexal mass is palpable; ultrasonography reveals a 4-cm simple cyst arising from the right ovary. The major contraindication for her request for transcervical hysteroscopic sterilization is

       (A) history of chlamydial infection
       (B) uterine enlargement
\*    (C) unicornuate uterus
       (D) ovarian cyst
       (E) obesity

Sterilization represents the most commonly used method of contraception in the age group 15–44 years. Among women and their partners in this age range, 39% use sterilization, with two thirds of these couples using tubal sterilization and the remainder using vasectomy. In the United States, until 2002, tubal sterilization operations in women were performed either by means of minilaparotomy, laparoscopy, or colpotomy. In November 2002, the U.S. Food and Drug Administration (FDA) approved the first transcervical method for tubal sterilization (Essure).

The procedure is performed via hysteroscopy, placing coils made of nickel titanium alloy in the cornual ostia. The coils surround polyethylene terephthalate fibers, which induce a tissue reaction that causes tissue ingrowth and occlusion of the fallopian tubes over the course of 3 months. After placement of the devices, women must use a back-up contraceptive method for 3 months until hysterosalpingography demonstrates tubal occlusion. In the phase 3 trial that preceded FDA approval of the device, 92% of patients had occlusion of both tubes after 3 months. All of the women with tubal patency at 3 months had tubal occlusion 6 months after the device was inserted.

Several conditions contraindicate the procedure, particularly those conditions in which both ostia cannot be accessed or are occluded. Specifically, women with known or suspected tubal occlusion and those with unicornuate uteri are not recommended to have the procedure. Other contraindications include nickel allergy (due to the nickel content of the device), known allergy to contrast media (secondary to the need for hysterosalpingography), and active pelvic infection. As is the case for tubal sterilization performed by other methods, pregnancy should be excluded preoperatively.

In the case described, the presence of a unicornuate uterus would preclude use of the procedure. However, other methods of sterilization, such as the laparoscopic approach, would be possible and would allow for confirmation of tubal anatomy. The option to offer her partner a vasectomy is part of the informed consent process for tubal sterilization, especially given that sterilization in males has lower morbidity. Prior pelvic chlamydial infection is a risk factor for tubal adhesions and tubal factor infertility, possibly leading to occlusion. Active chlamydial infection is a contraindication to transcervical sterilization because placement of a foreign body into infected tissue might make treatment of the infection more difficult. The patient's history of chlamydia is not a contraindication to the procedure, although device placement may be more challenging if proximal tubal occlusion or scarring is present. Many clinicians would consider screening for chlamydia before performing the procedure, particularly in those at high risk for infection.

Uterine enlargement may create difficulty with endometrial cavity distention during hysteroscopic placement of the tubal sterilization devices. However, no limit on uterine size exists for transcervical sterilization using this method. The presence of an ovarian cyst does not interfere with the procedure. A persistent complex ovarian mass that requires surgical evaluation in a patient who desires permanent sterilization might make concomitant laparoscopic sterilization a better choice. Obesity is not a contraindication to the procedure. Abdominal surgical approaches to sterilization are more difficult and of higher morbidity in obese women than in nonobese women. Thus, the transcervical approach may prove useful for sterilization in the obese patient.

Other transcervical sterilization procedures are under development, including several hysteroscopically based procedures. Transcervical placement of quinacrine hydrochloride (mepacrine hydrochloride) pellets in the uterus is another method under investigation in the United States that may hold promise as an office-based nonhysteroscopic method of sterilization. Quinacrine, an antimalarial chemotherapy widely available in the United States and in other countries, induces scarring at the cornua of the uterus. Insertion is accomplished using an intrauterine device applicator, followed by repeat application 1 month later. The failure rate was 1.2% in a study of 300 women in China. Currently, quinacrine is not approved for sterilization in the United States.

Benefits and risks of sterilization. ACOG Practice Bulletin No. 46. American College of Obstetricians and Gynecologists. Obstet Gynecol 2003;102:647–58.

Cooper JM, Carignan CS, Cher D, Kerin JF. Microinsert nonincisional hysteroscopic sterilization. Selective Tubal Occlusion Procedure 2000 Investigators Group. Obstet Gynecol 2003;102:59–67.

Essure: instructions for use. U.S. Food and Drug Administration, November 2002. Available at: http://www.fda.gov/cdrh/pdf2/p020014c.pdf. Retrieved September 7, 2005.

Lu W, Zhu J, Zhong C, Zhao Y. A comparison of quinacrine sterilization (QS) and surgical sterilization (TL) in 60 women in Guizhou Province, China. Int J Gynaecol Obstet 2003;83(suppl 2):S51–8.

# 92

## Body weight as a factor in contraceptive method failure

A 44-year-old woman uses the contraceptive patch. Her only other medication is St. John's wort. She uses the sauna regularly and applies the patch to her buttocks. Physical examination is remarkable for a weight of 92.1 kg (203 lb). Given her medical history and physical examination, the characteristic that is associated with an increased risk of contraceptive method failure is

* (A) weight
(B) patch location
(C) use of St. John's wort
(D) sauna use
(E) age

The contraceptive patch is a convenient alternative to the standard combination oral contraceptive. Within the patch available in the United States is ethinyl estradiol, the same estrogenic compound in most oral contraceptives. The progestin in the patch is norelgestromin, the primary active metabolite of norgestimate, which is also contained in several marketed oral contraceptives. The patch is worn weekly for 3 weeks, followed by a patch-free week. Analysis of data from three multicenter open-label contraceptive studies showed a failure rate of 0.9% for the patch. Compliance with the patch appears to be greater than that for oral contraceptives when compared in clinical trials. Clinicians should counsel patients about factors that have the potential to decrease efficacy as well as overall effectiveness with all contraceptive methods.

Using the data from the three large multicenter studies, the investigators retrospectively examined the possible predictors of contraceptive patch failure. Race and age were not associated with an increased risk of pregnancy while using the patch. A significant association was seen between body weight and method failure. During the research, 15 women conceived while on the patch, and five of these women weighed 90 kg (198 lb) or more. In women less than 90 kg, there was no association between body weight and pregnancy, and the pregnancy rates were uniform across body weight deciles. The decreased efficacy in women 90 kg or more was not entirely explained by differences in pharmacokinetics.

Subsequent case–control studies have been performed to examine the effects of body weight on oral contraceptive failure. Among women with a body mass index (weight in kilograms divided by height in meters squared [$kg/m^2$]) greater than 27.3, the risk of oral contraceptive failure was more than double the risk in women with a lower body mass index. Using weight alone, women who weighed more than 74.8 kg (165 lb) have a 70% higher risk of pregnancy.

The patch may be worn on the buttock, abdomen, upper outer arm, or upper torso but not on the breasts. It should not be applied to irritated or nonintact skin. Creams, lotions, or other cosmetic products should not be used on the skin to which the patch is applied.

There have been some case reports of intermenstrual bleeding in patients who have used oral contraceptives along with St. John's wort. The mechanism of the interaction may be from induction of cytochromes responsible for steroid metabolism by St. John's wort. No data exist to suggest decreased efficacy of oral contraceptives or the contraceptive patch in St. John's wort users.

In all drugs delivered by transdermal patch, adherence of the patch to the skin is a vital characteristic of the delivery system. Investigators have found that contraceptive patches became detached in nearly 5% of users. In one study, the risk of detachment was studied in 30 women under exercise conditions using a crossover design. Women participated in six different activities on separate days while wearing the patch (ie, normal activity including bathing, normal activity excluding bathing, sauna, whirlpool, treadmill, cool-water immersion, or a combination of activities). No differences were observed in patch detachment during the various activities. The authors also examined pooled data from 3,319 women, analyzed patch detachment risk as a function of warm and humid climates, and did not find a difference based on ambient conditions.

Burkman RT. The transdermal contraceptive system. Am J Obstet Gynecol 2004;190 suppl:S49–S53.

Holt VL, Scholes D, Wicklund KG, Cushing-Haugen KL, Daling JR. Body mass index, weight, and oral contraceptive failure risk. Obstet Gynecol 2005;105:46–52.

Yue QY, Bergquist C, Gerden B. Safety of St. John's wort (Hypericum perforatum). Lancet 2000;355:576–7.

Zacur HA, Hedon B, Mansour D, Shangold GA, Fisher AC, Creasy GW. Integrated summary of Ortho Evra/Evra contraceptive patch adhesion in varied climates and conditions. Fertil Steril 2002;77(suppl 2):S32–5.

Zieman M, Guillebaud J, Weisberg E, Shangold GA, Fisher AC, Creasy GW. Contraceptive efficacy and cycle control with the Ortho Evra/Evra transdermal system: the analysis of pooled data. Fertil Steril 2002;77(suppl 2):S13–8.

# 93

## Management of condylomata in the pregnant patient

A 26-year-old woman, gravida 1, comes to your office for routine antenatal care at 32 weeks of gestation. She has a history of genital condylomata, and the condylomata have recurred during her pregnancy. On examination, you find 5–7 small (less than 5 mm) condylomata scattered across the labia majora, posterior fourchette, and perianal region. She inquires about the risk of passing the condylomata to her fetus and wonders if this will have an impact on her hopes of a vaginal birth. The most appropriate care for this patient is

      (A) cesarean delivery at term
      (B) laser ablative therapy of condylomata
      (C) trichloroacetic acid (TCA)
      (D) topical podophyllin (Podocon-25) therapy
\*   (E) no intervention necessary, allow spontaneous labor

It is not uncommon for genital condylomata to first appear or enlarge during pregnancy. Because pregnancy is a relative immunosuppressed state, women who have never had condylomata may first develop them during this time. Given the high recurrence rate, small asymptomatic lesions do not warrant treatment during pregnancy. A high chance of resolution is probable in the postpartum period, and persistent lesions can be treated after pregnancy if necessary.

Vertical transmission of the two most common types of human papillomavirus (HPV), 6 and 11, can cause neonatal laryngeal papillomatosis. This rare infection of the neonatal larynx is the most serious result of HPV vertical transmission and is responsible for significant childhood morbidity and occasional mortality. Juvenile laryngeal papillomas result in hoarseness, chronic cough, recurrent respiratory infections, and sometimes life-threatening airway obstruction. Treatment is available but recurrence is common and there is no cure. Children with cry changes should be evaluated by their pediatricians for laryngeal papillomatosis.

Juvenile laryngeal papillomatosis may occur in infancy or well into childhood. The overwhelming majority of cases are associated with mothers who exhibit genital condyloma. The remaining cases are presumed to be secondary to maternal subclinical infections with HPV types

6 and 11. The route of transmission has not been clearly demonstrated, however, and could occur transplacentally (HPV has been documented in the placenta of pregnant women), perinatally, or postpartum. Based on the rate of HPV infection in the United States, it is estimated that 2–5% of all births are at risk for neonatal HPV exposure. Despite this, there is a very low rate of laryngeal papillomatosis (approximately 1,550 cases per 3.6 million annual births in the United States). This conveys a 0.04% risk of laryngeal infection in each neonate born vaginally. Given this exceedingly low risk, cesarean delivery is not considered an option for patients just because they have an HPV infection. Cesarean delivery may be considered in cases where genital warts obstruct the pelvic outlet or where vaginal birth may result in tearing of friable condylomata and excessive bleeding.

This patient has small condylomata that are otherwise asymptomatic, and she is at very low risk for vertical transmission or other HPV-associated risk. Therefore, no further intervention is warranted at this time. It is safe to allow spontaneous labor and vaginal birth. Ablative treatment (medical or surgical) for small asymptomatic condylomata in pregnancy is not necessary because recurrence is high. No evidence exists that treatment of

genital condylomata will decrease the rate of vertical transmission. Juvenile laryngeal papillomatosis has occurred in which the mother did not have visible lesions.

Podophyllin (Podocon-25) therapy is contraindicated in pregnancy. Imiquimod therapy (Aldara) has not been approved for use in pregnancy and in any case significant side effects of localized pain preclude its use for asymptomatic condylomata. Topical ablative therapy including TCA and imiquimod can be considered in pregnant patients with small, symptomatic condylomata. Surgical ablative therapy, including laser use, is more appropriate for larger symptomatic condylomata.

Human papillomavirus. ACOG Practice Bulletin No. 61. American College of Obstetricians and Gynecologists. Obstet Gynecol 2005; 105:905–18.

Beutner KR, Wiley DJ, Douglas JM, Tyring SK, Fife K, Trofatter K, et al. Genital warts and their treatment. Clin Infect Dis 1999;28 (suppl):S37–S56.

Sexually transmitted diseases treatment guidelines, 2006. Centers for Disease Control and Prevention [published erratum appears in MMWR Recomm Rep 2006;55(36):997]. MMWR Recomm Rep 2006;55 (RR-11):1–94.

Silverberg MJ, Thorsen P, Lindeberg H, Grant LA, Shah KV. Condyloma in pregnancy is strongly predictive of juvenile-onset recurrent respiratory papillomatosis. Obstet Gynecol 2003;101:645–52.

# 94

## Practice patterns to decrease legal risk

You receive a subpoena from a law firm with a signed release requesting all office records on a patient whom you last saw 10 months ago. In reviewing the chart, you notice an unfinished entry on the obstetrics flow sheet from 2 years earlier. The correct course of action would be to

* (A) send the records as they are
  (B) complete the entry, then send the records
  (C) refrain from sending incomplete records
  (D) call the patient's lawyer to inquire about the situation
  (E) hold an office meeting to discuss the situation

The medical record is the official account of all of your interactions with your patient. Maintenance of accurate, timely, and legible records is critically important, not only for provision of quality care, but also to protect yourself from allegations of malpractice. Being served with a lawsuit or having your records subpoenaed can be an emotional and disruptive experience. If the record is incomplete or contains mistakes, it may be tempting to redress those errors before providing access to the file. However, alteration of the medical record is never advisable.

In most states, medical records constitute legal documents, and intentionally altering the records may qualify as a misdemeanor. Moreover, many insurance carriers may not advance coverage if there is clear evidence that the record has been tampered with. Many times the plaintiff's attorney already has a copy of the record from another source and any discrepancies will be easily noted. An altered record belies your credibility and may be viewed as an obvious attempt to cover up or mislead the jury.

The medical record is a confidential document and is subject to certain privacy and security laws. In most instances, you are not permitted to release requested information without written authorization signed by the patient or a valid subpoena. It may be advisable in many situations to notify your insurance carrier when records have been released; however, in the absence of an actual lawsuit this may not be necessary. Many times records are requested not in anticipation of litigation, but rather to contest insurance coverage or other situations (eg, workmen's compensation and labor disputes).

It may be tempting to contact the patient's lawyer to inquire about the situation and set your mind at rest. In most cases, this is inadvisable because you may only be providing information and knowledge that could lead to further litigation or be damaging to your case should a suit be filed against you. In addition, most lawyers will advise against discussing a lawsuit or potential lawsuit with anyone except your legal counsel because such discussions may be discoverable and admitted as evidence in court.

American College of Obstetricians and Gynecologists. Professional liability and risk management. An essential guide for obstetrician–gynecologists. Washington, DC: ACOG; 2005.

Culley CA Jr, Spisak LJ. So you're being sued: do's and don'ts for the defendant. Cleve Clin J Med 2002;69:752, 755–6, 759–60.

Hoffman PJ, Plump JD, Courtney MA. The defense counsel's perspective. Clin Orthop Relat Res 2005;433:15–25.

Johnson LJ. Don't "polish" your records. Med Econ 2002;79(12):74.

Kern SI. You just received a subpoena. Now what? Med Econ 2002 Nov;79:43–4, 49.

# 95

## Thyroid disease

A 26-year-old woman, gravida 1, at 12 weeks of gestation returns for follow-up of nausea and vomiting in pregnancy. Two weeks ago, she presented to the emergency room with vomiting and dehydration that was treated with intravenous fluids and promethazine. Laboratory evaluation showed normal electrolytes but a low thyroid-stimulating hormone (TSH) level of 0.2 µU/mL. Since that time, she has still vomited 2–3 times a day, but is drinking fluids and eating frequent small meals. Her medical history is unremarkable. Her examination reveals a blood pressure reading of 112/66 mm Hg, pulse rate of 96 beats per minute, and no change in prepregnancy weight of 61.7 kg (136 lb). She seems tired, but her eyes appear normal, and she has moist mucous membranes. A neck examination shows a nontender, symmetric thyroid gland with each lobe measuring $3 \times 4$ cm. Her lungs are clear to auscultation with cardiac examination showing dynamic first and second heart sounds with a suspected fourth heart sound present. She has no pretibial edema. The uterus is approximately 12 weeks in size and fetal heart tones are 160 beats per minute. Laboratory test results ordered today show a free thyroxine ($T_4$) level of 2.1 ng/dL, a free triiodothyronine ($T_3$) level of 180 ng/dL, and a negative test for thyroid-stimulating immunoglobulins. The next step in management is

    (A) prescribe iodine supplementation
    (B) prescribe propylthiouracil
    (C) prescribe levothyroxine sodium (Synthroid)
    (D) prescribe methimazole (Tapazole)
\*    (E) repeat laboratory work in 6–8 weeks

In pregnancy, there is an increase in metabolic rate, iodine uptake, and thyroid gland size due to hyperplasia and increased vascularity. The normal thyroid is approximately 2 cm thick with each lobe measuring $4–5$ cm $\times$ $2–3$ cm. With the availability of a sensitive assay for TSH, important insights have been gained to better define the pattern of serum TSH during pregnancy. Due to a corresponding increase in human chorionic gonadotropin (hCG), TSH transiently decreases in the first trimester in a normal pregnancy. The TSH activity found in the serum of pregnant women is correlated with serum hCG levels and can be explained on the basis of molecular homologies between the hCG and TSH molecules and between the receptors for these hormones. This concept is confirmed in pathologic conditions such as trophoblastic disease where the elevated hCG can induce hyperthyroidism. Therefore, as hCG increases in the first trimester, the TSH is decreased and the thyroid increases hormonal output. This results in a linear relationship between hCG and free $T_4$ concentrations during early pregnancy (Fig. 95-1).

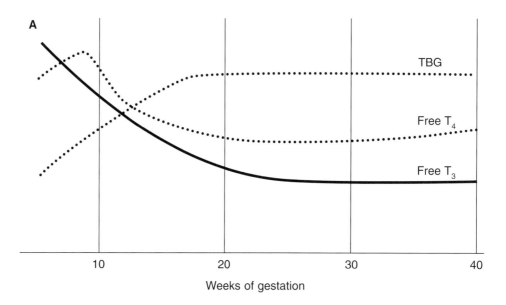

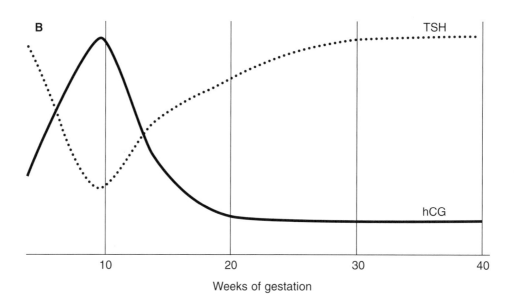

**FIG. 95-1.** Comparisons of **(A)** maternal thyroid hormones and **(B)** maternal thyroid-stimulating hormone (TSH) and human chorionic gonadotropin (hCG). $T_4$, thyroxine; $T_3$, triiodothyronine; TBG, $T_4$-binding globulin. (Speroff L, Fritz MA, editors. Clinical gynecologic endocrinology and infertility. 7th ed. Philadelphia (PA): Lippincott Williams & Wilkins; 2005. p. 816.)

At the time of the peak hCG levels in normal pregnancy, serum TSH levels decrease and bear a mirror image to the peak of hCG. The increase in hCG most likely causes an increased secretion of free $T_4$ and free $T_3$. This is difficult to establish with certainty because of the increased level of thyroxin-binding globulin in pregnancy. In surveys of pregnant patients in the first trimester, approximately 20% of patients will have transient subnormal TSH levels, and a significant number of these patients will have elevated free thyroxin levels above the normal range. This increase usually is transient because the hCG peak is maintained only briefly and the stimulatory effects of hCG on the thyroid should be minor. Most of these patients have no symptoms of hyperthyroidism.

Many reports exist of series of patients with hyperemesis gravidarum who have abnormal thyroid stimulation. Hyperemesis is characterized by prolonged and severe nausea and vomiting in early pregnancy sufficient to produce weight loss, dehydration, alkalosis, and hypokalemia. A correlation has been observed between the degree of vomiting and the serum hCG level. The etiology of hyperemesis gravidarum is unknown, but it may be related to the high hCG level and possibly some action of hCG that is still unclear. The increased thyroid function or clinical hyperthyroidism is attributed to the effect of hCG on the TSH receptor.

This patient presents with nausea and vomiting in pregnancy with laboratory values showing hyperthyroidism. This clinical picture is consistent with a diagnosis of transient hyperthyroidism or gestational hyperthyroidism. Such a diagnosis should be considered in any woman who has biochemical evidence of hyperthyroidism in early pregnancy. The syndrome is characterized by an association with hyperemesis, possible thyrotoxic symptoms, circulating hCG with high biologic activity, increases in free $T_4$ and free $T_3$, absence of a goiter, and negative thyroid-stimulating antibodies. Most patients will have spontaneous remission of the increased thyroid function when the vomiting stops in several weeks.

The prevalence of gestational hyperthyroidism is thought to be 2–3% although the clinical manifestations will not always be detected. Gestational hyperthyroidism is not autoimmune in origin and differs from Graves' disease in that it occurs in women without a history of Graves' disease and without detectable thyroid stimulating antibodies. Symptoms of hyperthyroidism such as weight loss or absence of weight gain, tachycardia, and tremulousness are present in a small portion of the patients. The syndrome is characterized by a slightly enlarged thyroid gland as assessed by ultrasonography, a transiently suppressed TSH level, and supranormal $T_4$ concentrations. Most women require no treatment, although some patients with noticeable symptoms can be treated with β-adrenergic blockers or rarely with antithyroid drugs. Monitoring the patient clinically and with laboratory tests as needed is appropriate. Hyperemesis is associated with the most severe thyrotoxic cases, and therefore obstetricians should be aware of the disorder to check thyroid function in women with significant gestational emesis.

In pregnancy, iodine clearance by the kidney increases, resulting in increasing incidence of goiter in iodine deficient areas. Pregnancy increases the risk of iodine deficiency in many parts of the world where iodine is not sufficiently available. This is not a problem in the United States; any goiter diagnosed in a patient in this country should be considered pathologic.

The antithyroid drugs propylthiouracil and methimazole (Tapazole) are used to treat hyperthyroidism in pregnancy. Propylthiouracil is favored in the United States because of the possible association of methimazole with the development of aplasia cutis. Because this patient has only laboratory evidence of hyperthyroidism, the use of antithyroid medicines is not necessary. Levothyroxine sodium (Synthroid) is used sometimes as a supplement with antithyroid drugs when treating hyperthyroidism or thyroiditis, but it has no value in this setting.

Glinoer D. The regulation of thyroid function in pregnancy: pathways of endocrine adaptation from physiology to pathology. Endocr Rev 1997;18:404–33.

Hershman JM. Physiological and pathological aspects of the effect of human chorionic gonadotropin on the thyroid. Best Pract Res Clin Endocrinol Metab 2004;18:249–65.

Rodien P, Jordan N, Lefevre A, Royer J, Vasseur C, Savagner F, et al. Abnormal stimulation of the thyrotrophin receptor during gestation. Hum Reprod Update 2004;10:95–105.

Speroff L, Fritz MA, editors. Clinical gynecologic endocrinology and infertility. 7th ed. Philadelphia (PA): Lippincott Williams & Wilkins; 2005. p. 805–23.

# 96

## Neuropathic pain

A 72-year-old woman tells you that she has a steady burning pain along the lower left portion of her back and flank that is made worse by light touch and clothing. Two months ago, she had an outbreak of shingles in the same area; the rash has resolved but the pain has continued. She is otherwise healthy, but she takes medication for glaucoma. The agent that would be most effective for the treatment of her symptoms is

      (A) capsaicin
      (B) amitriptyline
      (C) acyclovir (Zovirax)
      (D) topical lidocaine
  *   (E) gabapentin (Neurontin)

Postherpetic neuralgia is a common complication of herpes zoster in the elderly; more than two thirds of cases occur in people older than 70 years. The varicella zoster virus usually is acquired in childhood as chickenpox and lies dormant in the dorsal root ganglia of the spine. Reactivation of this latent viral infection later in life results in herpes zoster or shingles. The classic rash of herpes zoster is distinguished by an erythematous vesicular eruption along the dermatomal pattern of an infected dorsal nerve root and is associated with an intense burning and stinging sensation that can be aggravated by the slightest stimuli. The pain of an acute shingles infection is constant and at times can be debilitating. In most cases, the eruption will begin to resolve spontaneously in 7–10 days. Postherpetic neuralgia is a common complication that occurs in approximately 20% of cases and is distinguished by persistent pain 1 month or more after resolution of the herpes zoster skin lesions. The pain usually will subside over time and the patient will have resolution of discomfort within 6–12 months. However, in a few cases, the pain may become long term or even permanent. Postherpetic neuralgia is thought to represent a neuropathic pain syndrome. Neuropathic pain is a consequence of injury to sensory somatic nerves and results in an accentuated perception of pain at both the central and peripheral levels with minimal stimuli. It can be difficult to manage and usually fails to respond to common analgesic treatments.

A variety of topical and oral agents are available for treatment of postherpetic neuralgia and neuropathic pain. Capsaicin, an extract of chili peppers, can be applied to the affected area three to five times daily and has been shown to be an effective analgesic agent. Local skin irritation and an initial worsening of the condition coupled with the need to reapply several times daily limit its use. Lidocaine preparations, when applied topically, have low systemic absorption and can provide effective pain relief. As with capsaicin, the use of lidocaine is limited by its temporary effect. Lidocaine is best reserved as an adjunct to more effective treatments for local relief. Acyclovir (Zovirax), when started within 72 hours of the onset of an acute herpes zoster eruption, will decrease the incidence of postherpetic neuralgia. It is, however, an antiviral agent and ineffective for the treatment of neuropathic pain.

Tricyclic antidepressant agents can be very effective in the treatment of postherpetic neuralgia and are thought to work by inhibiting the reuptake of serotonin and norepinephrine. In general, the tricyclic antidepressant agents are more effective than the selective serotonin reuptake inhibitors in the treatment of neuropathic pain syndromes. Amitriptyline usually is started at a low dose and the dose is increased weekly until a therapeutic effect is achieved, side effects become intolerable, or maximum dose is reached. A therapeutic trial of amitriptyline should last 6–8 weeks. Adverse effects of tricyclic antidepressants can be significant and may include dry mouth, drowsiness, constipation, and urinary retention. The use of amitriptyline is contraindicated in patients with glaucoma. Other tricyclic agents that may be useful in the treatment of neuropathic pain include nortriptyline hydrochloride (Pamelor), desipramine hydrochloride (Norpramin), and imipramine hydrochloride.

The anticonvulsant gabapentin (Neurontin) is approved by the U.S. Food and Drug Administration for the treatment of postherpetic neuralgia. The exact mechanism of action of gabapentin is unknown, but recent trials have shown it to be as effective as amitriptyline in the treatment of neuropathic pain. Like amitriptyline, gabapentin is started at a low dose and the dose is gradually increased every 3–7 days until a therapeutic effect is achieved, side effects become intolerable, or maximum dose is reached. Side effects of gabapentin may include drowsiness, tremor, and incoordination. In general, however, gabapentin is tolerated very well by most patients even at high doses and has a better safety profile than amitriptyline. Thus, it provides the best option for the treatment of this patient's postherpetic neuralgia.

A recent randomized, double-blind, placebo-controlled trial examined use of varicella zoster vaccine for the prevention of herpes zoster and postherpetic neuralgia. More than 19,000 subjects were given live attenuated varicella zoster vaccine. Results showed a 51.3% reduction in the incidence of herpes zoster and a 66.5% reduction in the incidence of postherpetic neuralgia at 3 years. Such findings raise the possibility that, in the future, vaccination against varicella will provide immunity from herpes zoster and subsequent postherpetic neuralgia.

Bennett GJ. Neuropathic pain: new insights, new interventions. Hosp Pract (Minneap) 1998;33:95–8, 101–4, 107–10, passim.

Chen H, Lamer TJ, Rho RH, Marshall KA, Sitzman BT, Ghazi SM, et al. Contemporary management of neuropathic pain for the primary care physician. Mayo Clin Proc 2004;79:1533–45.

Oxman MN, Levin MJ, Johnson GR, Schmader KE, Straus SE, Gelb LD, et al. A vaccine to prevent herpes zoster and postherpetic neuralgia in older adults. Shingles Prevention Study Group. N Engl J Med 2005;352:2271–84.

Stankus SJ, Dlugopolski M, Packer D. Management of herpes zoster (shingles) and postherpetic neuralgia. Am Fam Physician 2000;61: 2437–44, 2447–8.

# 97

## Care of a patient treated for syphilis

A 33-year-old woman comes to your office for a routine gynecologic examination. Her last such examination was 18 months ago, when a vulvar lesion was diagnosed as syphilitic chancre. At diagnosis, she had a Venereal Disease Research Laboratories (VDRL) test result of 1:32. She received a single dose of antibiotics at that time and the lesion resolved. The result of a follow-up VDRL test at 6 months was 1:4. Cervical cytologic screening has been normal. The best next step in care is

    (A) no further follow-up
*   (B) repeat serologic testing
    (C) lumbar puncture for cerebrospinal fluid (CSF) testing
    (D) benzathine penicillin G
    (E) ceftriaxone sodium (Rocephin)

Syphilis is an infectious disease with systemic manifestations caused by *Treponema pallidum*. It has several phases. Primary infection manifests as an ulcer or chancre at the infection site. Secondary infection symptoms include skin rash, mucocutaneous lesions, and lymphadenopathy. Tertiary infection is characterized by cardiac and ophthalmic abnormalities, auditory lesions, and gummas. Some patients infected with *T pallidum* lack any clinical manifestations; such infections are termed latent infections. Such asymptomatic infections must be confirmed by serologic testing. Early latent syphilis is acquired within a year of the diagnosis; syphilis infections that are acquired prior to a year before diagnosis or that are of unknown duration are called late latent syphilis.

Serologic tests for syphilis include the nontreponemal tests, such as the VDRL and rapid plasma reagin tests, and the treponemal tests, including the fluorescent treponemal antibody absorption screen and *T pallidum* particle agglutination (TP–PA) tests. A syphilis antibody test, immunoglobulin (Ig) M and IgG test, is available at some institutions as an alternative to the other treponemal tests. These tests may help determine acute infection or prior exposure when combined with a positive nontreponemal test result.

Nontreponemal tests have a significant false-positive rate because of various medical conditions (eg, vascular disease and pregnancy). Thus, both types of tests must be used to reach an accurate diagnosis. Nontreponemal antibody titers usually correlate with disease status, and results of these tests should be reported quantitatively. Nontreponemal tests typically become nonreactive over time after therapy and thus can be used to follow patients for treatment response. A fourfold decrease in titer equivalent to a change of two dilutions is considered necessary to demonstrate effective therapy. Ideally for accurate comparison, sequential serologic test results in a patient should be obtained with the same testing method (ie, VDRL or rapid plasma reagin). Although the tests constitute equally reliable assays, the quantitative results of each cannot be compared with the other.

Treponemal antibody tests, such as fluorescent treponemal antibody absorption screen, remain positive for life once converted. Therefore, these tests are not useful in follow-up of treatment efficacy. Nor do they establish a diagnosis of syphilis on their own, because they could be present from an earlier infection.

Penicillin G has been historically the treatment of choice for all stages of syphilis. The duration and dose of therapy depend on the stage and duration of infection. Treatment for latent syphilis and tertiary syphilis may require longer therapy as the organisms at that point are dividing more slowly. Parenteral benzathine penicillin G is effective for primary syphilis in a single dose of 2.4 million units to achieve resolution of clinical symptoms, prevent sexual transmission, and prevent late sequelae. Treatment failure can occur with this regimen. No definitive criteria exist for cure or failure because the rate of decline of antibody titers is somewhat variable. The Centers for Disease Control and Prevention (CDC) recommends clinical and serologic follow-up for patients at 6 and 12 months after therapy. In patients whose symptoms persist or recur or who have a fourfold increase in nontreponemal antibody titer, failure of treatment or reinfection can be assumed. These patients should be retreated and tested for human immunodeficiency virus (HIV). In addition, CSF analysis should be performed in such patients because it is often difficult to distinguish between treatment failure and reinfection.

Failure of the nontreponemal test titers to decrease fourfold within 6 months of therapy for primary syphilis indicates treatment failure. Patients whose titers do not fall should be retreated. The CDC recommends that patients who are retreated should receive benzathine peni-

cillin G in weekly dosages of 2.4 million units for 3 weeks. Patients should then be followed serologically in at least 6-month intervals to ensure decline of nontreponemal antibody titers. Follow-up is important for several reasons: cure is documented by a return to negative titer, a baseline is then documented should the same patient later again reveal a reactive titer, and failure to respond or an increasing titer demonstrates a need for further treatment. Repeated tests to document a trend are recommended because some variability exists among laboratories and test kits; twofold to fourfold differences are not uncommon in the absence of any change in disease status.

This patient had a lesion consistent with primary syphilis. The standard treatment would be a single dose of benzathine penicillin G (Table 97-1). She reports taking a single dose of antibiotics, which is consistent with the appropriate treatment. She had inadequate follow-up to confirm effective cure. Subsequent (12-month) serologic follow-up is needed to confirm effective therapy. If a nontreponemal antibody test result is negative, cure is confirmed and no further intervention would be warranted.

Failure of therapy in primary syphilis has been reported. Therefore, serologic follow-up is recommended in all cases of syphilis to confirm effective cure and reassure the patient that they are not at risk for systemic disease. Because the patient has not had adequate serologic follow-up, her ability to transmit the infection sexually cannot be ruled out. The CSF test would be necessary only if therapy has failed and antibody titers are increasing, if a patient is HIV-positive with latent syphilis, or if neurosyphilis is present.

Additional therapy for this patient with the standard treatment (ie, benzathine penicillin G) is not warranted without confirmed treatment failure. Ceftriaxone sodium, which does not have demonstrated efficacy in treatment of syphilis, would not be recommended.

**TABLE 97-1.** Syphilis Treatment Guidelines

| | Treatment | |
| --- | --- | --- |
| **Syphilis Stage** | **Non–Penicillin-Allergic Patients** | **Penicillin-Allergic Patients** |
| Primary, secondary, and early latent syphilis* | Benzathine penicillin G 50,000 units/kg intramuscularly, up to the adult dose of 2.4 million units in one dose | Doxycycline 100 mg orally twice daily for 14 days *or* tetracycline 500 mg orally four times a day for 14 days |
| Late latent† and late syphilis | Benzathine penicillin G 50,000 units/kg intramuscularly, up to the adult dose of 2.4 million units, administered as three doses at 1-week intervals | Doxycycline 100 mg orally twice daily for 28 days *or* tetracycline 500 mg orally four times a day for 28 days |
| Neurosyphilis | Aqueous crystalline penicillin G 3 million–4 million units intravenously every 4 hours for 10–14 days *or* procaine penicillin 2.4 million units intramuscularly daily *plus* probenecid 500 mg orally four times a day for 10–14 days | Desensitization to penicillin, followed by penicillin therapy |
| Pregnant patients | Penicillin regimen appropriate for the stage of syphilis as above | Desensitization to penicillin, followed by penicillin therapy |
| Congenital syphilis | | |
|   Neonatal | Aqueous crystalline penicillin G 50,000 units/kg intravenously every 12 hours during the first 7 days of life and every 8 hours thereafter for a total of 10 days *or* procaine penicillin G 50,000 units/kg intramuscularly daily for 10 days | Desensitization to penicillin, followed by penicillin therapy |
|   Postneonatal | Benzathine penicillin G 50,000 units/kg intramuscularly if cerebrospinal fluid examination is negative | |
|   Neurosyphilis | Aqueous crystalline penicillin G 50,000 units/kg intravenously every 4–6 hours for 10–14 days | |

*Some experts recommend additional treatments (eg, benzathine penicillin G administered at 1-week intervals for 3 weeks, as recommended for late syphilis) for patients with human immunodeficiency virus coinfection.

†Patients with latent syphilis of unknown duration should be treated as those with late syphilis.

Zeltser R, Kurban AK. Syphilis. Clin Dermatol 2004;22:467.

Sexually transmitted diseases treatment guidelines, 2006. Centers for Disease Control and Prevention [published erratum appears in MMWR Recomm Rep 2006;55(36):997]. MMWR Recomm Rep 2006;55 (RR-11):1–94.

Zeltser R, Kurban AK. Syphilis. Clin Dermatol 2004;22:461–8.

# 98
## Headache

A 42-year-old woman comes to your office and reports a long history of unilateral throbbing headaches with photophobia and visual aura. The headaches usually occur within 2 days of her menses and at no other time in her cycle. She has used sumatriptan succinate (Imitrex) with some success for treatment of acute headache, but is now interested in short-term prophylaxis. The most cost-effective prophylaxis for intermittent headache for this patient would be

* (A) nonsteroidal antiinflammatory drugs (NSAIDs)
  (B) methylergonovine
  (C) danazol (Danocrine)
  (D) transdermal estrogen
  (E) frovatriptan (Frova)

The incidence of migraine headache in childhood is roughly equal between the sexes. However, around the time of puberty and menarche, an abrupt increase is seen in the number of migraine headaches reported by girls. This increase in migraines continues during the reproductive years, peaking in the fourth and fifth decades of life. Approximately 25% of the female population experience migraine headache at some point in their lives. The percentage of female migraineurs in adulthood is 16% with women outnumbering men 3:1. Most women report an increase in headache activity each month around the time of their menses. It is important, however, to differentiate women with menstrually related migraine from women with true menstrual migraine. Women with menstrually related migraine experience headache with greater frequency during their menses but also may have migraine headaches at other times of the month. It is estimated that up to 70% of migraineurs experience menstrually related migraine. True menstrual migraine, suggested by this woman's history, is a rare condition characterized by migraine headaches that occur only from 2 days before to 3 days after the onset of menses. Women with true menstrual migraine will typically not have attacks at any other time in their cycles. It is believed that falling levels of estradiol in the late luteal phase act as the trigger for the migraine headache, which can be with or without aura. Women whose migraines usually are not preceded by aura have a 66% greater incidence of true menstrual migraine.

Acute attacks of migraine headache can be treated successfully with several different medications including narcotics, NSAIDs, ergot derivatives, and triptans. Likewise, a number of different treatments for long-term prophylaxis and prevention of migraines have been developed. True menstrual migraine is unique in that the absolute predictability of the headache makes the prospect of short-term prophylaxis in the luteal phase of the cycle alone feasible. Drugs such as aspirin, naproxen sodium, ibuprofen, and mefenamic acid can provide effective prophylaxis for menstrual migraine when taken for several days before and after the onset of menses. Because NSAIDs are inexpensive, easy to obtain, safe, and well tolerated by most women, they represent the best initial choice for short-term prophylaxis of menstrual migraine.

The ergot derivatives, methylergonovine and dihydroergotamine, given for 2 days before expected menses and 5 days after menses, have been shown to decrease the incidence of menstrual migraine and may be a good choice for second-line prophylaxis. Although the ergot derivatives are relatively safe when used for short periods of time, the possibility of significant side effects and a category X classification in pregnancy may limit their use in some populations.

Because of its antiestrogenic activity, danazol (Danocrine) given before the expected menses also can be used to prevent menstrual migraine. However, danazol has significant androgenic activity that can lead to undesirable side effects for most women. Transdermal estrogen given during the luteal phase may prevent menstrual migraine by prolonging the interval to estrogen withdrawal. Results reported in the literature have been mixed. For many women, transdermal estrogen may only delay the time to onset of headache, and in some women its use may interfere with the normal menstrual cycle. Frovatriptan (Frova) given for 6 days premenstrually has been shown in a randomized trial to be an effective agent for intermittent prevention. Triptans show great promise for the short-term prophylaxis of menstrual migraine; however, the significant cost of these medications may limit their clinical usefulness.

Chavanu KJ, O'Donnell DC. Hormonal interventions for menstrual migraines. Pharmacotherapy 2002;22:1442–57.

Fettes I. Menstrual migraine. Methods of prevention and control. Postgrad Med 1997;101:67–70, 73–7.

Granella F, Sances G, Messa G, de Marinis M, Manzoni GC. Treatment of menstrual migraine. Cephalalgia 1997;17:35–8.

Loder E, MacGregor A. Menstrual migraine. In: Loder E, Marcus DA, editors. Migraine in women. Hamilton (ON): BC Decker; 2004. p. 102–11.

MacGregor EA, Hackshaw A. Prevalence of migraine on each day of the natural menstrual cycle. Neurology 2004;63:351–3.

Rasmussen MK, Binzer M. Non-steroidal anti-inflammatory drugs in the treatment of migraine. Curr Med Res Opin 2001;17(suppl 1):S26–9.

Silberstein SD, Capobianco DJ, Dodick DW. Migraine in special populations. Neurology 2003;60(suppl 2):S50–S57.

Silberstein SD, Elkind AH, Schreiber C, Keywood C. A randomized trial of frovatriptan for the intermittent prevention of menstrual migraine. Neurology 2004;63:261–9.

Silberstein SD, Freitag FG. Preventive treatment of migraine. Neurology 2003;60(suppl 2):S38–S44.

# 99

## Treatment of vulvodynia

A 52-year-old woman presents with a 2-year history of vulvar burning and pain. The pain is constant and unprovoked, and it encompasses the perineum. Physical examination reveals a normal appearing vulva, vestibule, and perineum. Wet mount test results are negative for vaginitis. Light touches with a cotton-tipped swab reveal diffuse burning and tenderness throughout the perineum. The most appropriate treatment for her is

(A) vestibulectomy
(B) topical high-potency steroid cream
\* (C) oral amitriptyline
(D) low oxalate diet
(E) biofeedback therapy

The vulvar pain syndromes represent a difficult and frustrating diagnosis for both the patient and the practitioner. Localized vulvar dysesthesia or vestibulitis most commonly occurs in younger women and is characterized by a discrete area of tenderness in the vestibule and fourchette and frequently is associated with erythema. The pain is intermittent and present only with touch or pressure. Vestibulitis usually can be tied to an inciting event such as childbirth, physical trauma, or infection. Generalized vulvar dysesthesia or vulvodynia usually occurs in older white women and is characterized by a vague and constant burning pain that encompasses the entire perineum. Unlike vestibulitis, the pain of vulvodynia is unremitting and not related to touch or an inciting event. Physical examination usually reveals no specific findings. Several theories have been proposed to explain the etiology of vulvodynia, including excess urinary oxalates and genetic, autoimmune, and infectious causes. Most likely vulvodynia represents a neuropathic pain syndrome as is seen in other conditions with dysesthesia and hyperalgesia.

Many suggested treatments for vulvodynia are only marginally effective, anecdotal, or not supported by well-controlled studies reported in the medical literature. Frequently a trial and error method of treatment is necessary. Oral tricyclic antidepressant agents such as amitriptyline have been shown to be effective first-line treatments for neuropathic pain syndromes, including vulvodynia. A low starting dose of amitriptyline is given to minimize side effects such as drowsiness, dry mouth, and tinnitus. The dose can then be titrated up until a therapeutic response is obtained, which can take up to 6 months. Treatment should then be maintained for 4–6 weeks, after which it can be tapered slowly. In one study, amitriptyline was effective in treating vulvodynia with 47% of patients reporting a complete response to treatment. Anticonvulsants such as gabapentin (Neurontin) can be effective for treatment of neuropathic pain in patients who cannot take amitriptyline, but such drugs are less well studied than amitriptyline.

Biofeedback therapy can provide an effective adjunct in treating vulvodynia and has been shown to be successful in 34.6% of patients. However, cost, time, and patient commitment to biofeedback can provide barriers to successful treatment. Placing the patient on a low oxalate diet with calcium citrate supplementation has been proposed to decrease the symptoms of vulvodynia by decreasing the levels of calcium oxalate crystals in the urine. This treatment has not been definitively proven to be effective in the literature. Vestibulectomy is an effective treatment for vestibulitis but not for vulvodynia. Surgery can be a serious undertaking, though, and should be considered only in women with severe and refractory pain. Other treatments for vulvodynia, including topical anesthetics, estrogen, capsaicin, acupuncture, and interferon, may provide only temporary or limited relief. Topical high-potency steroid preparations, such as clobetasol propi-

onate (Cormax, Temovate), have not been shown to be effective in treating vulvodynia.

Edwards L. New concepts in vulvodynia. Am J Obstet Gynecol 2003; 189 suppl:S24–S30.

Gaunt G, Good A, Stanhope CR. Vestibulectomy for vulvar vestibulitis. J Reprod Med 2003;48:591–5.

Haefner HK, Collins ME, Davis GD, Edwards L, Foster DC, Hartmann ED, et al. The vulvodynia guideline. J Low Genit Tract Dis 2005;9: 40–51.

McKay M. Dysesthetic ("essential") vulvodynia. Treatment with amitriptyline. J Reprod Med 1993;38:9–13.

Wall JW. Vulvar dysesthesia. Mo Med 2004;101:51–3.

# 100

## Contraception following thrombosis

A 31-year-old woman experienced a pulmonary embolism shortly after giving birth 2 years ago. Although she currently desires contraception, she tells you she may wish to conceive within the next 6–12 months. Her husband does not like to use condoms. The most appropriate contraceptive for this couple is

    (A) combination oral contraception
    (B) transdermal contraception
    (C) contraceptive vaginal ring
\*    (D) progestin-only oral contraception

Combination oral contraceptives increase the risk of venous thromboembolism in users. Although no epidemiologic data have assessed venous thromboembolism risk with use of the contraceptive ring or patch, clinicians should prescribe the newer combination oral contraceptives with the assumption that use of these combination formulations likewise increase venous thromboembolism risk.

Unlike combination estrogen–progestin oral contraceptives, progestin-only oral contraceptives have not been found to increase the risk of thromboembolism. Clinicians should be aware that package labeling for depot medroxyprogesterone acetate and certain brands of progestin-only oral contraceptives inappropriately indicates that a history of venous thromboembolism contraindicates use of these progestin-only methods.

Although use of depot medroxyprogesterone acetate would be safe for the patient described, return to ovulation does not occur for a mean of 9–10 months from the last injection. Given her future fertility desires, depot medroxyprogesterone acetate would therefore not be appropriate for this patient.

Women with a documented history of unexplained venous thromboembolism or venous thromboembolism

associated with pregnancy or exogenous estrogen use should not use combination estrogen-progestin oral contraceptives unless they currently take anticoagulants. A woman who had experienced a single episode of venous thromboembolism years earlier, associated with a nonrecurring risk factor (eg, venous thromboembolism that occurs during immobilization following a motor vehicle accident) may not currently be at increased risk for venous thromboembolism. Accordingly, the decision to initiate combination hormonal contraception can be individualized in such a candidate. Procoagulant changes induced by combination hormonal method use do not appear to resolve until 6 weeks or more following oral contraceptive discontinuation. Accordingly, the risks associated with stopping combination oral contraceptives 1 month or more before major surgery should be balanced against the risks of an unintended pregnancy. Because of the low risk of venous thromboembolism associated with laparoscopic sterilization, discontinuation of combination oral contraceptives is not necessary before this or other brief surgical procedures.

Postpartum women remain in a hypercoagulable state for weeks after childbirth. Product labeling for combination oral contraceptives advises women who are not breastfeeding to defer use of combination oral contraceptives until 4 weeks postpartum. Because first ovulation can occur in as little as 25 days in such women, some clinicians initiate the use of combination oral contraceptives in nonbreastfeeding women as early as 2 weeks postpartum, although no data are available on the safety of this approach. Progestin-only contraceptives can be initiated safely immediately postpartum.

Women with factor V Leiden who use oral contraceptives experience a risk of venous thromboembolism many times higher than oral contraceptive users who are not carriers of this mutation. Therefore, some have queried whether, before initiating combination hormonal contraception, candidates should be screened for this hereditary condition, which occurs in approximately 5% of U.S. women. Most women identified as having factor V Leiden through screening will never experience venous thromboembolism, even if they use combination oral contraceptives. Given the rarity of fatal venous thromboembolism, one group of investigators concluded that screening more than one million candidates for thrombophilic markers would, at best, prevent two combination oral contraceptives-associated deaths. Such routine screening, therefore, is not recommended before initiating combination contraceptive use.

Cardiovascular disease and steroid hormone contraception. Report of a WHO Scientific Group. World Health Organ Tech Rep Ser 1998; 877:i–vii,1–89.

Kaunitz AM. Injectable long-acting contraception. Clin Obstet Gynecol 2001;44:73–91.

Sidney S, Petitti DB, Soff GA, Cundiff GA, Tolan DL, Quesenberry CP Jr. Venous thromboembolic disease in users of low-estrogen combined estrogen-progestin oral contraceptives. Contraception 2004;70:3–10.

Use of hormonal contraception in women with coexisting medical conditions. ACOG Practice Bulletin No. 73. American College of Obstetricians and Gynecologists. Obstet Gynecol 2006;107:1453–72.

---

# 101

## Breast cancer prophylaxis

---

At her periodic health examination, a healthy 33-year-old woman with a history of hysterectomy for uterine leiomyomata indicates that breast cancer was diagnosed in her mother at age 44 years and in a sister at age 41 years. Testing indicated that the sister carries the *BRCA1* mutation. The patient does not wish to have genetic testing. She is anxious about her risk for breast cancer and asks what she can do to lower her risk. The most appropriate pharmacologic treatment for this patient is

      (A) leuprolide injections
\*    (B) tamoxifen citrate (Nolvadex)
      (C) aromatase inhibitor
      (D) nonsteroidal antiinflammatory drugs (NSAIDs)

The selective estrogen receptor modulator (SERM), tamoxifen, has demonstrated efficacy in the prevention of estrogen receptor-positive breast cancer and is approved by the U.S. Food and Drug Administration (FDA) for this indication. Overall, four trials that assessed tamoxifen's efficacy as breast cancer chemoprophylaxis found a 38% reduction in breast cancer risk ($P < .001$). Risk reduction has been found for invasive and noninvasive breast cancers.

The *BRCA1* mutation is inherited in an autosomal dominant fashion. Accordingly, there is a 50% chance that the 33-year-old woman described has this mutation, which would mean that her risks for ovarian and breast cancer are approximately 50% and 80%, respectively. In the absence of genetic testing, chemoprophylaxis with tamoxifen appears reasonable. Use of tamoxifen is associated with an increased risk of venous thromboembolic disease. Although use of tamoxifen increases the risk of endometrial polyps and neoplasia, this concern is moot for the patient in this case, given her prior hysterectomy. If, in the future, the patient is found to harbor the *BRCA1* mutation, she might consider undergoing prophylactic mastectomy and bilateral salpingo-oophorectomy, surgeries that substantially reduce invasive cancer in carriers. Given the young age at which breast cancer was diagnosed in her first-degree relatives, regular mammography would be appropriate. Another option would be magnetic resonance imaging (MRI), which is increasingly being used to screen high-risk women.

Although use of raloxifene may reduce the risk of developing breast cancer without increasing risk of endometrial disease, fewer data have assessed chemoprophylaxis with raloxifene than tamoxifen. However, a recently completed trial demonstrated the effectiveness of raloxifene as a prophylactic agent with more efficacy than tamoxifen. Use of either raloxifene or tamoxifen can increase vasomotor symptoms.

In 2004, the American Society of Clinical Oncology (ASCO) recommended that appropriate adjuvant treatment of postmenopausal women with hormone receptive-positive breast tumors should include aromatase inhibitors. Leuprolide acetate (Lupron) or other gonadotropin-releasing hormone agonists are not recommended for breast cancer chemoprophylaxis. Although NSAIDs may modestly reduce breast cancer risk, they are not recommended for chemoprophylaxis.

Breast cancer. American College of Obstetricians and Gynecologists. Obstet Gynecol 2004;104 suppl:11S–6S.

Cuzick J, Powles T, Veronesi U, Forbes J, Edwards R, Ashley S, et al. Overview of the main outcomes in breast-cancer prevention trials. Lancet 2003;361:296–300.

Haber D. Prophylactic oophorectomy to reduce the risk of ovarian and breast cancer in carriers of BRCA mutations [editorial]. N Engl J Med 2002;346:1660–2.

Hartman LC, Schaid DJ, Woods JE, Crotty TP, Myers JL, Arnold PG, et al. Efficacy of bilateral prophylactic mastectomy in women with a family history of breast cancer. N Engl J Med 1999;340:77–84.

King MC, Marks JH, Mandell JB. Breast and ovarian cancer risks due to inherited mutations in BRCA1 and BRCA2. New York Breast Cancer Study Group. Science 2003;302:643–6.

Winer EP, Hudis C, Burstein HJ, Wolff AC, Pritchard KI, Ingle JN, et al. American Society of Clinical Oncology technology assessment on the use of aromatase inhibitors as adjuvant therapy for postmenopausal women with hormone receptor-positive breast cancer: status report 2004. J Clin Oncol 2005;23:619–29.

Zhang Y, Coogan PF, Palmer JR, Strom BL, Rosenberg L. Use of nonsteroidal antiinflammatory drugs and risk of breast cancer: the Case–Control Surveillance Study revisited. Am J Epidemiol 2005; 162:165–70.

# 102

## Diverticulitis

A 42-year-old woman, gravida 2, para 2, has a 3-day history of left lower quadrant pain and fever. She reports a maximum temperature at home of 38.9°C (102°F). She reports decreased stool frequency (every 2–3 days instead of daily) and nausea without vomiting. She denies hematochezia, diarrhea, or nocturia. Office urinalysis reveals trace protein, trace leukocyte estrace, 10–15 epithelial cells, 0–3 red blood cells. Her vital signs are a temperature of 38°C (100.4°F), blood pressure 110/70 mm Hg, and pulse 75 beats per minute. Normal bowel sounds with tenderness in the left lower quadrant are noted on physical examination. Bimanual examination reveals normal findings except for tenderness in the left lower quadrant. No palpable masses are present. Some guarding is noted. The most appropriate next diagnostic study would be

    (A) complete blood count with differential
\*   (B) computed tomography (CT) scan of the abdomen and pelvis with contrast
    (C) ultrasonography of the abdomen and pelvis
    (D) barium enema
    (E) testing for gonorrhea and chlamydia

Based on the patient's history, laboratory studies may include urinalysis, electrolytes, creatinine, complete blood count, toxin screens, sexually transmitted disease evaluation, and other testing such as lipase, amylase, liver function tests, and coagulation studies. Imaging studies often begin with ultrasonography, abdominal plain films, or CT scan. The differential diagnosis includes appendicitis, adnexal torsion, bowel obstruction, incarcerated hernia, acute mesenteric ischemia, cystitis, kidney stones, ovarian cysts, pelvic inflammatory disease, neoplasms, or a leaking abdominal aortic aneurysm.

The risk of colonic diverticular disease increases with age. Most patients seek care before there is perforation

into the peritoneal cavity. Perforation of a diverticulum leads to acute abdominal findings associated with peritonitis. Pain associated with diverticulitis often originates in the hypogastrium and secondarily localizes to the left lower quadrant. Most patients have left lower quadrant pain (93–100%), fever (57–100%), and leukocytosis (69–83%). Alterations in bowel habits are frequent, and diarrhea occurs more often than constipation; 25% of patients have heme-positive stools. Urinary symptoms of dysuria or urgency may occur if the affected portion of the colon is in proximity to the bladder. Pain may be associated with nausea and vomiting or referred to the genitalia or suprapubic area.

No imaging studies are needed to diagnose the disorder if the clinical presentation is clear. However, a CT scan is helpful if the diagnosis is uncertain or if the patient's clinical condition deteriorates. In the case of the patient under discussion, a CT scan would offer the best next diagnostic step because it is both sensitive and specific for diverticular disease and it also can identify free air, abscesses, or phlegmons. Ultrasonography is useful for diagnosis of diseases of the uterus or adnexa, which is unlikely in this patient.

Laboratory studies such as a complete blood count may help in diagnosing infectious or inflammatory processes, but such studies are not specific for diverticulitis. Sex-

ually transmitted disease is not indicated in this patient due to a lack of any suggestive history. A barium enema is not indicated for this patient if perforation has not been ruled out.

Lawrimore T, Rhea JT. Computed tomography evaluation of diverticulitis. J Intensive Care Med 2004;19:194–204.

Whetstone D, Hazey J, Pofahl WE 2nd, Roth JS. Current management of diverticulitis. Curr Surg 2004;61:361–5.

Wong WD, Wexner SD, Lowry A, Vernava A 3rd, Burnstein M, Denstman F, et al. Practice parameters for the treatment of sigmoid diverticulitis—supporting documentation. The Standards Task Force. The American Society of Colon and Rectal Surgeons. Dis Colon Rectum 2000;43:290–7.

# 103

## Mammography in patient with no family history of breast cancer

A 44-year-old woman, gravida 3, para 3, comes to your office for her periodic health examination. She has regular monthly menses and is on no medications. The examination reveals no irregularities and her breast examination is normal. She does not want to have a mammogram performed because she has no family history of breast cancer. You inform her that several medical organizations have recommended mammography guidelines and all agree that screening mammography should begin at age

       (A) 35 years
   *   (B) 40 years
       (C) 45 years
       (D) 50 years
       (E) 55 years

Breast cancer remains the most frequently diagnosed cancer in women with more than 200,000 new invasive cases projected to occur among U.S. women annually. The incidence of breast cancer diagnosis increased rapidly in the 1980s as a result of improved use of mammography. Among women, breast cancer is now the second leading cause of cancer death after lung cancer, with more than 40,000 deaths from breast cancer expected each year. Mortality rates decreased 2.3% per year from 1990 to 2001 in all women, with an even greater decrease among women younger than 50 years. These decreases are attributed to increased awareness, earlier detection through screening, and improved treatment.

The earliest sign of breast cancer is usually an abnormality detected on a mammogram before it can be felt by the patient or her health care provider. Numerous studies have shown that early detection saves lives and increases treatment options. Sensitivity of mammography is lower among women who are younger than 50 years, who have denser breasts, or who are taking hormone therapy.

The American Cancer Society, the U.S. Preventive Services Task Force, the American College of Obstetricians and Gynecologists (ACOG), and the American College of Radiology recommend that women at average risk begin screening mammography at age 40 years. Beginning screening at age 40 years instead of age 50 years reduces breast cancer mortality.

Mortality reductions for women ages 40–69 years have been observed in trials that screened for breast cancer at intervals of 1–2 years. The estimated lead time between detection on mammography and when the lesion is clinically detectable for invasive breast cancer is 1.7 years. The U.S. Preventive Services Task Force concluded that mammography screening sensitivity does not differ substantially by age, although absolute benefits are lower in women younger than 50 years compared with women older than 50 years. According to the American Cancer Society, recent data have provided significant evidence that younger women will benefit more from annual screening than from screening at 2-year intervals.

Most women who develop breast cancer have no family history of the disease. Women with a family history of breast cancer in a mother or sister, with a previous breast biopsy that revealed atypical hyperplasia, or with first childbirth after age 30 years are at an increased risk for breast cancer. These high-risk patients are more likely to benefit from regular mammography. The recommendation for women to begin mammography in their 40s is strengthened for women who have one of the high-risk characteristics. The American Cancer Society guidelines suggest that women at increased risk for breast cancer may benefit from earlier initiation of screening, screening at shorter intervals, and screening with additional modalities, such as ultrasonography, magnetic resonance imaging (MRI), and digital mammography.

The potential risks of regular mammography (ie, false-positive results, unnecessary anxiety, biopsies, and costs) lessen as women age. The diagnosis of invasive breast cancer in women aged 65 years and older accounts for approximately 45% of all new breast cancer cases. Breast cancer mortality increases with increasing age, from 86 deaths per 100,000 women aged 65–69 years to 200 deaths per 100,000 women aged 85 years and older. As long as a patient is in reasonably good health and would be a candidate for treatment, she should continue to be screened with mammography. However, if an individual has severe functional limitations or multiple or severe comorbidities likely to limit life expectancy to 5 years or less, it may be appropriate to end screening.

American Cancer Society. Cancer facts and figures 2006. Atlanta (GA): American Cancer Society; 2006.

American College of Radiology. ACR practice guidelines for the performance of screening mammography. ACR Practice Guideline 2004: 245–56.

Breast cancer screening. ACOG Practice Bulletin No. 42. American College of Obstetricians and Gynecologists. Obstet Gynecol 2003; 101:821–32.

Smith RA, Cokkinides V, Eyre HJ. American Cancer Society guidelines for the early detection of cancer, 2005. CA Cancer J Clin 2005;55:31–44; quiz 55–6.

Smith RA, Saslow D, Sawyer KA, Burke W, Constanza ME, Evans WP 3rd, et al. American Cancer Society guidelines for breast cancer screening: update 2003. CA Cancer J Clin 2003;53:141–69.

U.S. Preventive Services Task Force. Screening for breast cancer: recommendations and rationale. Rockville (MD): Agency for Healthcare Research and Quality; 2002. Available at: http://www.ahrq.gov/clinic/uspstf/uspsbrca.htm. Retrieved August 19, 2005.

# 104

## Risks of untreated asymptomatic bacteriuria in pregnancy

A 19-year-old woman, gravida 1, is screened for bacteriuria at her first prenatal visit. She has no symptoms. She has greater than 100,000 *Escherichia coli* colony-forming units (cfu/mL) on urine culture. She is treated with oral cephalexin. She asks what benefits are achieved with treatment of asymptomatic bacteriuria. You tell her that the major effect of treatment of asymptomatic bacteriuria is decreased

      (A) resistance to antibiotics
      (B) risk of renal damage
      (C) risk of neonatal sepsis
\*   (D) risk of pyelonephritis
      (E) need for subsequent screening for bacteriuria in this pregnancy

Asymptomatic bacteriuria is defined as persistent bacterial colonization of the urinary tract without specific symptoms. Significant colonization generally is defined as 100,000 cfu/mL of a single organism from a midstream urine sample. Culture is still considered the best method for diagnosis. Rapid urine screening tests are not accurate enough in pregnancy because the organisms that cause infection do not always reduce nitrates to nitrites, and elevated white blood cells may be normal in pregnant women's clean catch specimens.

Asymptomatic bacteriuria occurs in approximately 5–10% of all pregnancies. The prevalence of infection is closely linked to economic status for unknown reasons. However, it occurs in all socioeconomic groups. Medical conditions associated with increased risk include sickle cell disease and trait and history of a urinary tract infection before pregnancy. The most commonly detected organism is *E coli*. Other organisms that commonly cause bacteriuria are *Klebsiella pneumoniae, Proteus mirabilis, Enterococcus, Staphylococcus* species, and group B streptococci. A patient with urinary group B streptococci is presumed to be heavily vaginally colonized. She should be treated when the bacteriuria is diagnosed, and she should be considered group B streptococci positive when labor begins.

Patients should be screened for asymptomatic bacteriuria with a urine culture at the first prenatal visit. Pyelonephritis may occur in all trimesters of pregnancy, and thus there is no need to delay screening. Asymptomatic bacteriuria should be treated with antibiotics that are safe in pregnancy and effective against the usual uropathogens. Because the patients are without symptoms, they usually are treated as outpatients with oral antibiotics. Short, 3–7-day treatments are adequate and as effective as longer term treatments. Single-dose treatments cause fewer side effects, and a World Health Organization trial of single-dose therapy in pregnancy is under way. Patients should be reassessed for recurrent infection.

The treatment of asymptomatic bacteriuria results in approximately a 75% reduction of pyelonephritis in pregnancy. From 15% to 45% of women with asymptomatic bacteriuria in pregnancy develop pyelonephritis unless given antibiotic treatment. Preterm delivery is probably reduced with the avoidance of pyelonephritis. Early studies did not look at co-infection of the vagina and cervix with other organisms, which might contribute to preterm labor. A recent Cochrane database review showed an increase in low-birth-weight infants delivered by mothers who were not treated for asymptomatic bacteriuria. This confirms a previous observation that showed an association between asymptomatic bacteriuria, pyelonephritis, preterm birth, and low birth weight (less than 2,500 g). Treatment of bacteriuria reduced preterm birth and increased birth weight in this classic study. Neonatal sepsis is not affected by treatment of asymptomatic bacteriuria.

Hill JB, Sheffield JS, McIntire DD, Wendel GD. Acute pyelonephritis in pregnancy. Obstet Gynecol 2005;105:18–23.

Kass EH. Prevention of apparently non-infectious disease by detection and treatment of infections of the urinary tract. J Chronic Dis 1962;15:665–73.

Smaill F. Antibiotics for asymptomatic bacteriuria in pregnancy. The Cochrane Database of Systematic Reviews 2001, Issue 2. Art. No.: CD000490. DOI: 10.1002/14651858.CD000490.

Villar J, Widmer M, Lydon-Rochelle MT, Gulmezoglu AM, Roganti A. Duration of treatment for asymptomatic bacteriuria during pregnancy. The Cochrane Database of Systematic Reviews 2000, Issue 2. Art. No.: CD000491. DOI: 10.1002/14651858.CD000491.

# 105

## Preoperative evaluation for hypertension

A 61-year-old woman is seen in the office before surgery is scheduled to remove an adnexal mass. She is a smoker who is sedentary but can climb two flights of stairs to her sister's apartment. Three years ago, she was admitted for congestive heart failure (CHF). On examination today, she has uncontrolled hypertension with a blood pressure reading of 154/96 mm Hg. The risk factor described that poses the highest perioperative cardiac risk for her is

  (A) age older than 60 years
  (B) uncontrolled systemic hypertension
  (C) smoking
  (D) low functional capacity
\*  (E) history of CHF

Preoperative assessment of a patient who will undergo gynecologic surgery requires a detailed history and physical examination. Despite advancing technologies and the array of available tests, history and physical examination remain the key elements to assess cardiac risk. The risk factor that poses the highest perioperative cardiac risk for the described patient is a history of CHF. Other independent predictors of major cardiac complications in noncardiac surgery include the following:

- High-risk surgery (vascular or prolonged intraperitoneal or intrathoracic procedures)
- History of ischemic heart disease
- History of cerebrovascular disease
- Preoperative treatment with insulin
- Preoperative serum creatinine level greater than 2.0 mg/dL

The American College of Cardiology and the American Heart Association have published clear guidelines for perioperative cardiac risk assessment (Box 105-1). Perioperative cardiac risk may be stratified by three major components:

1. Patient risk factors
2. Patient functional capacity
3. Intrinsic risk of the surgery

Patient risk factors are divided into major, intermediate, and minor factors. Current or known history of coronary artery disease (CAD) is the most important risk factor. Diabetes mellitus and renal insufficiency are other common conditions that are of higher risk.

Minor patient risk factors include advanced age, uncontrolled hypertension, smoking, and a low functional capacity (eg, inability to walk one flight of stairs with a bag of groceries). Advanced age has been considered by some to be an intermediate risk factor but only if the patient's physiologic age is greater than 70 years. Limited studies indicate that severe hypertension (systolic blood pressure greater than 180 mm Hg and diastolic blood pressure greater than 110 mm Hg) may increase the risk for perioperative death or myocardial infarction. This patient would be classified as having mild hypertension. Few data suggest that patients with mild to moderate hypertension have higher perioperative complications. Optimally, blood pressure should be controlled gradually over 6–8 weeks before surgery, but the discovery of hypertension just before scheduled surgery is not an absolute contraindication to proceeding.

Smoking is a definite risk factor for CAD, and it increases mortality if a myocardial infarction occurs. Smoking acts independently and synergistically with other risk factors for CAD and increases the risk of postoperative pulmonary complications. As a clinical predictor of perioperative cardiovascular events, smoking is important but is considered a minor predictor of adverse outcomes.

The patient's functional capacity or exercise tolerance, expressed in metabolic equivalent (MET) levels, is estimated from her ability to perform activities of daily living (Table 105-1). Functional capacity has been classified as excellent (greater than 10 METs), good (7–10 METs), moderate (4–7 METs), poor (less than 4 METs), or unknown.

Most gynecologic surgeries will be safe for patients who have minor or no clinical predictors of risk and moderate or excellent functional capacity (greater than 4 METs). For example, a patient with minor clinical predictors of risk who can walk up a flight of stairs or participate in moderate activities (eg, bowling or dancing) would be considered at low risk for cardiac complications.

Intrinsic risk of surgery entails the expected degree of hemodynamic stress of a selected procedure. Gyne-

## BOX 105-1

### Clinical Predictors of Increased Perioperative Cardiovascular Risk (Myocardial Infarction, Heart Failure, Death)

*Major*
Unstable coronary syndromes
- Acute or recent myocardial infarction* with evidence of important ischemic risk by clinical symptoms or noninvasive study
- Unstable or severe[†] angina (Canadian class III or IV)[‡]
- Decompensated heart failure

Significant arrhythmias
- High-grade atrioventricular block
- Symptomatic ventricular arrhythmias in the presence of underlying heart disease
- Supraventricular arrhythmias with uncontrolled ventricular rate

Severe valvular disease

*Intermediate*
Mild angina pectoris (Canadian class I or II)
Previous myocardial infarction by history or pathologic Q waves
Compensated or prior heart failure
Diabetes mellitus (type 1 diabetes mellitus)
Renal insufficiency

*Minor*
Advanced age
Abnormal electrocardiogram (left ventricular hypertrophy, left bundle-branch block, ST-T abnormalities)
Rhythm other than sinus (eg, atrial fibrillation)
Low functional capacity (eg, inability to climb one flight of stairs with a bag of groceries)
History of stroke
Uncontrolled systemic hypertension

---

*The American College of Cardiology National Database Library defines recent MI as greater than 7 days but less than or equal to 1 month (30 days); acute MI is within 7 days.

[†]May include "stable" angina in patients who are unusually sedentary.

[‡]Campeau L. Grading of angina pectoris. Circulation 1976;54:522–3.

Eagle KA, Berger PB, Calkins H, Chaitman BR, Ewy GA, Fleischmann KE, et al. ACC/AHA Guideline Update for Perioperative Cardiovascular Evaluation for Noncardiac Surgery—Executive Summary. A report of the American College of Cardiology/American Heart Association Task Force on Practice Guidelines (Committee to Update the 1996 Guidelines on Perioperative Cardiovascular Evaluation for Noncardiac Surgery). Circulation 2002;105:1261.

---

hysterectomy with significant hemorrhage) have a cardiac risk often greater than 5%.

- Intermediate-risk procedures (eg, abdominal hysterectomy) have a cardiac risk generally less than 5%.
- Low-risk procedures (eg, extraperitoneal gynecologic and brief laparoscopic procedures) have a cardiac risk usually less than 1%.

No consensus exists on cardiac risk stratification for most laparoscopic procedures. However, most would likely fall into the low- to intermediate-risk category.

**TABLE 105-1.** Estimated Energy Requirements for Various Activities*

| Energy Expended | Question Regarding Activity |
|---|---|
| 1 MET | *Can you* Take care of yourself? Eat, dress, or use the toilet? Walk indoors around the house? Walk a block or two on level ground at 2–3 mph (3.2–4.8 km/h)? Do light work around the house like dusting or washing dishes? |
| 4 METs | Climb a flight of stairs or walk up a hill? Walk on level ground at 4 mph (6.4 km/h)? Run a short distance? Do heavy work around the house like scrubbing floors or lifting or moving heavy furniture? Participate in moderate recreational activities like golf, bowling, dancing, doubles tennis, or throwing a baseball or football? |
| More than 10 METs | Participate in strenuous sports like swimming, singles tennis, football, basketball, or skiing? |

MET indicates metabolic equivalent.

*Adapted from the Duke Activity Status Index and the American Heart Association Exercise Standards.

Eagle KA, Berger PB, Calkins H, Chaitman BR, Ewy GA, Fleischmann KE, et al. ACC/AHA Guideline Update for Perioperative Cardiovascular Evaluation for Noncardiac Surgery—Executive Summary. A report of the American College of Cardiology/American Heart Association Task Force on Practice Guidelines (Committee to Update the 1996 Guidelines on Perioperative Cardiovascular Evaluation for Noncardiac Surgery). Circulation 2002;105:1261.

Chassot PG, Delabays A, Spahn DR. Preoperative evaluation of patients with, or at risk of, coronary artery disease undergoing non-cardiac surgery. Br J Anaesth 2002;89:747–59.

Eagle KA, Berger PB, Calkins H, Chaitman BR, Ewy GA, Fleischmann KE, et al. ACC/AHA Guideline Update for Perioperative Cardiovascular Evaluation for Noncardiac Surgery—Executive Summary. A report of the American College of Cardiology/American Heart Association Task Force on Practice Guidelines (Committee to Update the 1996 Guidelines on Perioperative Cardiovascular Evaluation for Noncardiac Surgery). Circulation 2002;105:1257–67.

---

cologic surgical procedures are not specifically categorized in current guidelines although inferences can be drawn from the literature:

- High-risk procedures (eg, exenteration, radical hysterectomy, ovarian cancer staging with ascites, and

Howell SJ, Sear JW, Foex P. Hypertension, hypertensive heart disease and perioperative cardiac risk. Br J Anaesth 2004;92:570–83.

Lee TH, Marcantonio ER, Mangione CM, Thomas EJ, Polanczyk CA, Cook EF, et al. Derivation and prospective validation of a simple index

for prediction of cardiac risk of major noncardiac surgery. Circulation 1999;100:1043–9.

# 106

## Criteria for a good screening test

During her postpartum care, your patient asks for your advice in regard to neonatal screening for cystic fibrosis. She states that she declined prenatal screening because of the cost. You inform her that the value of neonatal screening for cystic fibrosis is controversial because

    (A) early intervention does not improve clinical outcomes
    (B) it involves invasive testing
    (C) disease morbidity is high
    (D) the positive predictive value is high
\*   (E) disease prevalence is low

In assessing the benefit of conducting a screening test, the risks and costs associated with the test must be weighed against the potential benefits of disease identification. The disease itself should pose a substantial risk of morbidity and mortality, and effective treatment before symptom development should be available. Prevalence of the disease in the target population should be high. The test itself should be widely accessible, simple to administer, and inexpensive, and induce minimal discomfort and morbidity to the population screened. Results of the test must be valid and reproducible.

Neonatal screening for cystic fibrosis involves testing of dried blood spots already collected from infants at birth for screening of a variety of diseases and conditions. The multistage cystic fibrosis protocol results in sensitivities of 85–95%. The cost of screening is less than the cost of traditional diagnosis with the sweat chloride test. In regard to these issues, neonatal screening for cystic fibrosis is consistent with the criteria for a good screening test.

An increasing body of evidence indicates that presymptomatic interventions for cystic fibrosis lead to improvements in pulmonary and nutritional status. Neonatal screening thus meets the objective of improving clinical outcomes by allowing for therapy before the development of symptoms.

The estimated prevalence of cystic fibrosis varies from 1 in 2,500 among whites and 1 in 32,000 among Asian Americans. Because disease prevalence in the general population is low, the positive predictive value of the test is also low. In addition, false–positive screening results have been shown to influence parents' perceptions of the

health of their newborn in a negative fashion. Parents of newborns with false-positive results demonstrate increased vigilance and heightened parental anxiety. Thus, although targeted screening in specific ethnic groups is reasonable, the costs associated with screening in the general population may be unjustifiably high. Accordingly, universal neonatal screening for cystic fibrosis currently is not recommended.

Although universal neonatal screening has not been adopted as the standard of care, the obstetrician should be aware that prenatal carrier screening for cystic fibrosis is available. The American College of Obstetricians and Gynecologists recommends that carrier screening be made available to all couples presenting for preconception or prenatal care. Early diagnosis allows the patient to exercise her reproductive options if cystic fibrosis is present.

American College of Obstetricians and Gynecologists. Update on carrier screening for cystic fibrosis. ACOG Committee Opinion No. 325. Washington, DC: ACOG; 2005.

Farrell PM, Kosorok MR, Rock MJ, Laxova A, Zeng L, Lai HC, et al. Early diagnosis of cystic fibrosis through neonatal screening prevents severe malnutrition and improves long-term growth. Wisconsin Cystic Fibrosis Neonatal Screening Study Group. Pediatrics 2001;107:1–13.

Herman CR, Gill HK, Eng J, Fajardo LL. Screening for preclinical disease: test and disease characteristics. AJR Am J Roentgenol 2002; 179:825–31.

Merelle ME, Nagelkerke AF, Lees CM, Dezateux C. Newborn screening for cystic fibrosis. The Cochrane Database of Systematic Reviews 2001, Issue 3. Art. No.: CD001402. DOI: 10.1002/14651858. CD001402.

Wang SS, O'Leary LA, Fitzsimmons SC, Khoury MJ. The impact of early cystic fibrosis diagnosis on pulmonary function in children. J Pediatr 2002;141:804–10.

# 107

## Grieving after stillbirth

A couple in their mid-twenties come to your office 6 weeks after the delivery of a stillborn infant at 39 weeks of gestation. At that time, the patient presented with decreased fetal movement, and ultrasonography confirmed fetal death in utero. Labor was induced, and the stillborn infant was born with no apparent abnormalities. The couple named the baby, held it, and grieved with their extended family. The patient was discharged home on postpartum day 1. The husband is concerned because his wife is very sad and cries daily, but she denies thoughts of suicide. She seems disorganized and performs just a few of her normal daily activities. She is not sleeping well and her appetite is fair. The patient discusses the loss and hardship, and she cries in the office during the visit. She is angry that fetal monitoring was not done earlier in her pregnancy. Her husband states that she did not want to return for her follow-up appointment. The patient acknowledges feeling a little guilty, as if she could have prevented the death in utero. You review with the couple the events of the pregnancy and delivery. The best next step in care is

        (A) advise the couple to consider conceiving another pregnancy
        (B) refer to a counselor for marital therapy
        (C) start a selective serotonin reuptake inhibitor (SSRI)
\*     (D) discuss the grief process and follow up in 2 weeks

Health care providers have the opportunity to play an important role in helping parents heal from a pregnancy loss. Some studies have shown that a large number of patients judge the care that they receive from their physicians at the time of miscarriage as inadequate. Many physicians have been viewed by the bereaved couples to be insensitive because little time is provided for the parents to talk about the loss. Physicians need to respond with warmth, understanding, and support following a pregnancy loss. A clear understanding of the grieving process is essential to provide appropriate care.

Bereavement is the fact of loss through death and a bereavement reaction is any psychologic, physiologic, or behavioral response to bereavement. Grief is the feelings and associated behaviors, such as crying accompanying the awareness of an irrevocable loss. The changing affective state of the patient over time constitutes the grieving process. Manifestations of grief reflect an individual's personality, previous experiences, bonding to the infant, psychologic history, the existing social network, intercurrent events, current health, and other factors. Typically, three phases of grieving occur: shock and denial, acute anguish, and resolution (Box 107-1).

In the United States today, expectations for general bereavement after a loss are for the bereaved to return to work or school in a few weeks, to establish equilibrium within a few months, and to be capable of pursuing new relationships within 6–12 months. Ample evidence exists to indicate that the bereavement process does not end with

---

| BOX 107-1 |
| --- |

**Phases of Grief**

Shock and denial (minutes, days, weeks)
- Disbelief and numbness
- Searching behaviors: pining, yearning, protesting

Acute anguish (weeks, months)
- Waves of somatic distress
- Withdrawal
- Preoccupation
- Anger
- Guilt
- Loss of patterns of conduct
   —Restless and agitated
   —Aimless and amotivational
- Identification with the bereaved

Resolution (months, years)
- Have grieved
- Return to work
- Resume old roles
- Acquire new roles
- Reexperience pleasure
- Seek companionship and love of others

---

Zisook S, Downs NS. Death, dying and bereavement. In: Sadock BJ, Sadock VA, editors. Kaplan and Sadock's comprehensive textbook of psychiatry. 7th ed. Philadelphia (PA): Lippincott Williams & Wilkins; 2000. p. 1975.

a prescribed period of time. Certain aspects can persist indefinitely for otherwise high-functioning individuals.

Grief reactions to the loss of a baby are of the strongest magnitude. Many expectant parents have made household arrangements for the newborn long before delivery, and expectations have been built over time. With the death of the infant, parents grieve over the child's anticipated future and for the loss of their anticipated parenthood. After stillbirth, parents now face the unexpected necessity of dealing with the funeral, burial, or cremation arrangements. Later, additional grief reactions around important dates or milestones can resurface. The recovery process following the death of a child usually lasts for 1–2 years but can last longer, and some aspects of grief may endure permanently.

To discern what is needed, distinction between normal grief and depression is essential (Box 107-2). Grief is a painful yet normal reaction to the loss whereas depression is a clinical syndrome with many biologically linked symptoms that lead to a high degree of impairment. Both interfere with sleep, concentration, and appetite, but patients are at higher risk for depression if there is a history of depression, low intimacy with partner, inadequate social support, or a lack of other children at home.

---

**BOX 107-2**

**Differentiating the Depressive Symptoms Associated With Bereavement From Major Depressive Disorder**

*Depressive Symptoms of Bereavement*

Symptoms may meet syndrome criteria for major depressive episode, but survivor rarely has morbid feelings of guilt and worthlessness, suicidal ideation, or psychomotor retardation

Dysphoria often triggered by thoughts or reminder of the deceased

Onset within the first 2 months of bereavement

Duration of depressive symptoms is less than 2 months

Functional impairment is transient and mild

No family or history of major depressive disorder

*Symptoms of Major Depressive Disorder*

Any symptoms as defined by *Diagnostic and Statistical Manual of Mental Disorders, Fourth Edition.*

Dysphoria often triggered by thoughts or reminder of the deceased

Onset at any time

Depression often becomes chronic, intermittent, or episodic

Clinically significant distress or impairment

Family or personal history of major depressive disorder

---

Zisook S, Downs NS. Death, dying and bereavement. In: Sadock BJ, Sadock VA, editors. Kaplan and Sadock's comprehensive textbook of psychiatry. 7th ed. Philadelphia (PA): Lippincott Williams & Wilkins; 2000. p. 1976.

---

Women are at especially high risk for clinical depression if there is a lack of grief expressed within the first 2 weeks after the loss or for ongoing grieving with no signs of abating 6–9 months after the loss.

The grief process has been described as containing six separate but interactive processes, as follows:

1. Recognition of the loss, acknowledging the death, and understanding the ramifications

2. Reaction to the separation by going through grief

3. Recollection and reexperience of the deceased and the relationship

4. Relinquishment of attachments to the deceased and the old assumptions

5. Readjustment to the "new world" without forgetting the deceased

6. Reinvestment of the freed-up energy into a new life or identity

Ability to go through the process helps the family come to a grief resolution and to live with the loss of the child while never forgetting it.

With support, reassurance, and information, most bereaved couples will do well without pharmacologic treatment. The physician may offer prayer with the patient or a referral to the patient's spiritual leader for assistance. The goals of the health care team are to help the family experience a normal grief reaction, to actualize the loss, to acknowledge the grief, and to meet the particular needs of the family. The best antidote for patient anger and blame is the physician's willingness to be open, honest, and sympathetic as well as to acknowledge the patients' feelings and complaints. Physicians must attempt to answer questions on why the pregnancy loss occurred and whether it will happen again. Patients need encouragement to express their feelings and to ask questions. They frequently feel blame in some capacity wondering if they could have done something differently or not done something that would have prevented the stillbirth. Mothers also might believe that they have disappointed their spouses or families by failing to produce the healthy baby that was expected. Acknowledgment of these feelings and others as "normal" allows for more open expression and communication. It is important that these conversations not be rushed and allow for a full discussion. It has been suggested that after an earlier miscarriage, close follow-up within 1 week is needed, and an allotted time of 30 minutes is a minimum.

With some parents or families, a timely or complete grief resolution does not occur. When the loss is not or cannot be acknowledged openly, mourned publicly, or supported sufficiently, there is "disenfranchised grief," which increases the risk for depression, marital problems, and substance abuse. Appropriate referral to medical social workers, counselors, support groups, and psychiatrists is warranted.

It is vital to understand different manifestations of grieving between the sexes. Men tend to experience less intense or prolonged grief reactions. Husbands may respond by throwing themselves into work or spending more time with friends to avoid the expression of sadness. With a husband's controlled expression of grief, wives may misunderstand and think that the husband is not grieving. On the other hand, a man may have difficulty with his wife's crying and expressions of grief. He may believe he is unable to console her and that he only makes the problem worse by his presence. An appropriate exchange of experiences and clarification of misconceptions can be done during an office visit. Formal marriage counseling is not usually needed unless additional relational problems are present, but it is recommended that

obstetricians provide follow-up for grieving couples at regular intervals throughout the first 1–2 years after stillbirth.

Bartellas E, Van Aerde J. Bereavement support for women and their families after stillbirth. J Obstet Gynaecol Can 2003;25:131–8.

Brier N. Understanding and managing the emotional reactions to a miscarriage. Obstet Gynecol 1999;93:151–5.

Forrest GC, Standish E, Baum JD. Support after perinatal death: a study of support and counselling after perinatal bereavement. Br Med J (Clin Res Ed) 1982;285:1475–9.

Hunfeld JA, Wladimiroff JW, Passchier J. The grief of late pregnancy loss. Patient Educ Couns 1997;31:57–64.

Zisook S, Downs NS. Death, dying and bereavement. In: Sadock BJ, Sadock VA, editors. Kaplan and Sadock's comprehensive textbook of psychiatry. 7th ed. Philadelphia (PA): Lippincott Williams & Wilkins; 2000. p. 1963–80.

# 108

## Therapy to decrease risk of colon cancer

A 40-year-old woman with a family history of colon cancer asks about prevention of colorectal cancer. You tell her that the noninvasive intervention consistently associated with a decreased incidence of adenomas or colon cancer is

    (A) supplementation of dietary fiber
\*   (B) estrogen plus progestin therapy
    (C) increased fruit and vegetable consumption
    (D) magnesium supplementation

Colorectal cancer accounts for 10% of cancer mortality in the United States, or approximately 57,000 deaths per year. Screening and early intervention have contributed to the decline in mortality, but interest in dietary prevention is high. In the epidemiologic literature, colorectal cancer is associated with consumption of processed and red meat, but the strength of the relationship varies between studies, with odds ratios and relative risks ranging from 1.2 to 1.5.

Chemoprevention is defined as the use of chemical, biologic, or nutritional compounds to prevent or inhibit carcinogenesis before the development of invasive disease. Most studies on chemoprevention of colon cancer have shown negative results. Based on a meta-analysis of 18 studies, hormone therapy may reduce the risk by 20%. The estrogen plus progestin arm of the Women's Health Initiative study showed a decrease in risk of 37%. Patients should be advised that the noninvasive intervention that has been consistently associated with a decreased incidence of adenomas or colon cancer is estrogen plus progestin therapy.

Nonsteroidal antiinflammatory drugs (NSAIDs) are efficacious against colonic neoplasia related to the inhibition of one or both cyclooxygenase enzymes. The effects of dietary supplements, such as fiber, fruits, vegetables, vitamin C and E, selenium, calcium, and beta-carotene, in colorectal cancer are believed to be negligible.

Baron JA. Dietary fiber and colorectal cancer: an ongoing saga. [Editorial.] JAMA 2005;294:2904–6.

Chao A, Thun MJ, Connell CJ, McCullough ML, Jacobs EJ, Flanders WD, et al. Meat consumption and risk of colorectal cancer. JAMA 2005;293:172–82.

Hawk ET, Umar A, Richmond E, Viner JL. Prevention and therapy of colorectal cancer. Med Clin North Am 2005;89:85–110, viii.

Robertson DJ, Sandler RS, Haile R, Tosteson TD, Greenberg ER, Grau M, et al. Fat, fiber, meat and the risk of colorectal adenomas. Am J Gastroenterol 2005;100:2789–95.

Rossouw E, Anderson GL, Prentice RL, LaCroix AZ, Kooperberg C, Stefanick ML, et al. Risks and benefits of estrogen plus progestin in healthy postmenopausal women. Principal results from the Women's Health Initiative Randomized Controlled Trial. Writing Group for the Women's Health Initiative Investigators. JAMA 2002;288:321–33.

# 109

## Surgery to correct stress urinary incontinence

A 45-year-old woman has urodynamically proven stress urinary incontinence. Physical examination reveals a cystocele and urethral hypermobility. You inform her that the surgical procedure that has an equivalent cure rate to a retropubic bladder neck suspension (Burch procedure) is

    (A) anterior colporrhaphy
    (B) needle urethropexy
    (C) paravaginal repair
    (D) periurethral collagen injections
\*   (E) tension-free vaginal tape (TVT) procedure

Stress urinary incontinence is the involuntary leakage of urine during effort or exertion or during sneezing or coughing. It can be confirmed during urodynamic testing by identifying leakage from the urethra coincident with increased abdominal pressure in the absence of a bladder contraction. Stress incontinence can be addressed by non-surgical and surgical means, weight loss if the patient is obese, pessaries, urethral inserts, or bulking agents. The Cochrane Incontinence Group found that pelvic floor muscle training was consistently better than no treatment or placebo, and the addition of biofeedback did not improve outcomes. Newer medications awaiting U.S. Food and Drug Administration approval include duloxetine chloride, a selective serotonin reuptake inhibitor, which, in clinical trials, decreased the frequency of incontinence by 64% vs 41% in women on placebo. Phenyl-propanolamine was effective in decreasing the number of leak episodes compared with placebo but was withdrawn from the market because of a detected association with hemorrhagic strokes.

For patients who fail medical therapy, surgery is available. The best cure rate is reported for the Burch retropubic colposuspension and for suburethral sling procedures, as well as for the newer mid-urethral sling or TVT procedures. These procedures carry a risk of urinary retention and recurrent prolapse. Slings are prone to erosions and bladder injury, and Burch procedures may cause urge incontinence and apical prolapse. An ongoing randomized trial sponsored by the National Institutes of Health is comparing the Burch and autologous rectus fascia slings.

The American Urologic Association has published clinical guidelines that advocate Burch and sling procedures as more effective (83–84%) than transvaginal needle suspensions (67%) or anterior repairs (61%) at 48 months postprocedure. Needle suspension procedures (eg, the Pereyra, Stamey, Raz, Gittings techniques) rely on using the needle to pass a suture through the vagina and affixing it to the abdominal wall fascia. Collagen injections or other periurethral bulking agents are indicated for intrinsic sphincter deficiency in the absence of hypermobility and so would be inappropriate for this patient.

Hay-Smith EJC, Dumoulin C. Pelvic floor muscle training versus no treatment, or inactive control treatments, for urinary incontinence in women. The Cochrane Database of Systematic Reviews 2006, Issue 1. Art. No.: CD005654. DOI: 10.1002/14651858.CD005654.

Leach GE, Dmochowski RR, Appell RA, Blaivas JG, Hadley HR, Luber KM, et al. Female Stress Urinary Incontinence Clinical Guidelines Panel summary report on surgical management of female stress urinary incontinence. The American Urological Association. J Urol 1997;158: 875–80.

Nygaard IE, Heit M. Stress urinary incontinence. Obstet Gynecol 2004;104:607–20.

Nygaard IE, Kreder KJ. Pharmacologic therapy of lower urinary tract dysfunction. Clin Obstet Gynecol 2004;47:83–92.

Urinary Incontinence in Adults Guideline Update Panel. Urinary incontinence in adults. Clinical practice guideline no. 2, 1996 update. Rockville (MD): U.S. Department of Health and Human Services, Agency for Healthcare Policy and Research, 1996. (AHCPR publication no. 96-0682).

Ward KL, Hilton P. A prospective multicenter randomized trial of tension-free vaginal tape and colposuspension for primary urodynamic stress incontinence: two-year follow-up. UK and Ireland TVT Trial Group. Am J Obstet Gynecol 2004;190:324–31.

# 110

## Irritable bowel syndrome

A 32-year-old woman reports worsening pelvic pain. She has urinary frequency but denies fever, urinary symptoms, or abnormal vaginal discharge. She often notes abdominal bloating. Heavy meals occasionally are followed by acute abdominopelvic pain and diarrhea. Her abdominal discomfort is relieved by defecation. She reports more than three bowel movements a day, some containing mucus. Her family history is positive for ulcerative colitis in a first cousin. Her complete blood count (CBC) is normal. A urinalysis and a Hemoccult test obtained at rectal examination are both negative. The most likely diagnosis is

      (A) endometriosis
      (B) interstitial cystitis
      (C) diverticulitis
      (D) ulcerative colitis
*    (E) irritable bowel syndrome (IBS)

The current understanding of IBS is that it is part of a spectrum of gastrointestinal and central nervous system reactions to stimuli, both external and internal. The American Gastroenterological Association defines IBS as "a group of functional bowel disorders in which abnormal discomfort or pain is associated with defecation or a change in bowel habits and with features of disordered defecation." Controversy has surrounded the etiology of IBS as to whether the condition is functional or organic. Box 110-1 shows the Rome II diagnostic criteria for IBS.

Detailed information involving the history of signs and symptoms associated with IBS is required for best diagnosis. Diarrhea is evacuation of a liquid or mushy stool associated with rapid transit time through the bowel. Bloating is defined as both abdominal distention and tympany, although patients may associate it with borborygmus, increased flatus, and frequent eructation. Abdominal discomfort may be described by patients as a range of feelings associated with fullness, early satiety, bloating, and nausea.

The association of chronic pelvic pain with IBS may represent different etiologies. Gynecologists may use this term to describe discomfort from organs contained within the true or bony pelvis; gastroenterologists may describe the symptoms as abdominal in location. There may, however, be an association of gynecologic symptoms with IBS, menstrual exacerbations of IBS symptoms, and an array of psychosomatic disorders in women with chronic pelvic pain and IBS not present in women with IBS but no chronic pelvic pain. Hysterectomy rates have been reported to be 32% and 17%, respectively, in patients with and without physician-diagnosed IBS. Careful history and judicious testing may detect signs and symptoms most compatible with IBS and allow other possibilities in the differential diagnosis to be excluded.

Endometriosis is a leading cause of chronic pelvic pain. Patients with endometriosis usually present with dysmenorrhea or dyspareunia, thus making it an unlikely diagnosis given this patient's symptoms.

Interstitial cystitis refers to a clinical syndrome most commonly characterized by urinary urgency, urinary frequency, and pelvic pain. Associated symptoms include vulvar pain or hematuria. In patients with interstitial cys-

---

**BOX 110-1**

**Rome II Diagnostic Criteria for Irritable Bowel Syndrome (IBS)**

Abdominal discomfort or pain lasting at least 12 weeks (which need not be consecutive) in the preceding 12 months and is accompanied by at least two of the following features:
- It is relieved with defecation.
- Onset is associated with a change in frequency of stool.
- Onset is associated with a change in form (appearance) of stool.

Other symptoms that are not essential but support the diagnosis of IBS include:
- Abnormal stool frequency (more than three bowel movements per day or less than three bowel movements per week)
- Abnormal stool form (lumpy and hard or loose and watery stool)
- Abnormal stool passage (straining, urgency, or feeling of incomplete evacuation)
- Passage of mucus
- Bloating or feeling of abdominal distention

---

Longstreth GF. Definition and classification of irritable bowel syndrome: current consensus and controversies. Gastroenterol Clin North Am 2005;34:177.

titis, defecatory disorders are uncommon, making it a less likely diagnosis.

Diverticular disease is common and age dependent. The prevalence is less than 5% in patients younger than 40 years. Among patients with diverticulosis, 70% remain asymptomatic, 15–25% develop diverticulitis, and 5–15% develop diverticular bleeding. Diverticulitis results from a microscopic or macroscopic perforation of a diverticulum. The clinical presentation is relative to the severity of the underlying inflammatory process whether or not complications are present; left lower quadrant pain is the primary complaint. Other symptoms may include nausea and vomiting (20–60%), constipation (50%), diarrhea (25–35%), and urinary urgency, frequency, or dysuria (10–15%).

Ulcerative colitis is characterized by recurring episodes of inflammation of the mucosal lining of the colon. A variety of signs and symptoms may precede the diagnosis of mild disease including rectal bleeding, mucus in the stool, mild diarrhea with less than four stools per day, crampy abdominal pain, tenesmus, and constipation. More serious manifestations of the disease are associated with worsening pain, increasing number of loose stools, gastrointestinal bleeding, and anemia. The diagnosis of IBS best fits the clinical scenario of the patient presented.

Drossman DA, Camilleri M, Mayer EA, Whitehead WE. AGA technical review on irritable bowel syndrome. Gastroenterology 2002; 123:2108–31.

Longstreth GF. Definition and classification of irritable bowel syndrome: current consensus and controversies. Gastroenterol Clin North Am 2005;34:173–87.

Mertz HR. Irritable bowel syndrome. N Engl J Med 2003;349:2136–46.

Spanier JA, Howden CW, Jones MP. A systematic review of alternative therapies in the irritable bowel syndrome. Arch Intern Med 2003;163: 265–74.

# 111

## Decreased postmenopausal libido

A 62-year-old woman presents with a decreased libido. She relates that this is of no great worry to her, but she is concerned about comments her husband has recently made. She continues to be sexually active "to keep the peace" and can achieve orgasm with appropriate stimulation and time. However, she denies having sexual thoughts or desires on her own. She satisfactorily uses an over-the-counter lubricant for vaginal dryness and occasional dyspareunia. Her husband has recently retired due to ongoing health problems, and she is his primary caretaker. She tells you that their relationship is comfortable but "not particularly intimate." She states, "This isn't how I envisioned my golden years." She is healthy and takes no medications. Physical examination reveals mild genital atrophy. The most appropriate next step is

    (A) referral to a sex therapist
    (B) vaginal estrogen therapy
    (C) combined oral estrogen and testosterone therapy
\*   (D) marital and relationship counseling
    (E) treatment for depression

Hypoactive sexual desire disorder is the persistent or recurrent deficiency or absence of sexual fantasies and desire for sexual activity. It is a common complaint for women of all ages. Up to 33% of women aged 18–59 years report some degree of sexual dysfunction each year with 20% of the population reporting lack of sexual desire. The disorder is particularly common among perimenopausal and menopausal women, and with the aging trend of the U.S. population, it is sure to become even more common. It is differentiated from arousal disorders, or inability to attain or maintain sexual excitement, in that women with low desire have little inclination to partake in sexual activity.

The reasons for low desire can be varied and include physical, hormonal, mental, and relationship factors. Decreased levels of estrogen in the menopausal years can lead to genital atrophy, decreased lubrication, fragility of the vulvar skin, and dyspareunia. Fear of painful or uncomfortable sexual intercourse may dampen the patient's enthusiasm and desire for it. Circulating androgen levels do not correlate with low sexual desire or low sexual satisfaction in women. Psychologic and mental illness also can play a significant role in the development of decreased libido.

Depression, a history of sexual abuse or conflict, and other emotional disorders can all effectively lower a woman's desire for sexual activity. Recent studies, however, have shown that a woman's sexual desire is most highly correlated with her sense of well-being and happiness with her current marital or significant interpersonal relationship. For women, sexual desire takes place within the context of the relationship with her partner, and it is the quality of the relationship that determines the degree of sexual motivation. Women seek tenderness, emotional closeness, and appreciation from their partners. In situations in which anger, fear, resentment, boredom, or relationship complacency exist, the desire for sexual activity suffers. For many women, low desire may compound the issue and strain an already troubled relationship further.

The woman described has several factors that may affect her sexual desire. Topical estrogen may improve her vulvar health and ameliorate problems with lubrication and dyspareunia, and combined oral estrogen and testosterone therapy also may provide some benefit. However, the cause of her low sexual desire is manifest at an interpersonal level. Her history indicates that she has many concerns with her marital relationship, including a lack of emotional intimacy, lost expectations, and the prospect of long-term custodial care of her husband.

Serious concern exists for the possibility of depression, and consideration should be given to future treatment if it occurs. Referral to a qualified sex therapist may be a useful adjunct in this case. However, sex therapy frequently focuses on techniques and modalities for improving the sexual act or removing sexual inhibitions or habits. The key to her low sexual desire rests in the complaints that she has voiced about her relationship with her husband. Therefore, referral for marital and relationship counseling would be the most beneficial next step.

Basson R. Recent advances in women's sexual function and dysfunction. Menopause 2004;11:714–25.

Basson R. Sexual desire and arousal disorders in women. N Engl J Med 2006;354:1497–506.

Brezsnyak M, Whisman MA. Sexual desire and relationship functioning: the effects of marital satisfaction and power. J Sex Marital Ther 2004;30:199–217.

Davis SR. Circulating androgen levels and self-reported sexual function in women. JAMA 2005;294:91–6.

Hartmann U, Philippsohn S, Heiser K, Ruffer-Hesse C. Low sexual desire in midlife and older women: personality factors, psychosocial development, present sexuality. Menopause 2004;11:726–40.

Walsh KE, Berman JR. Sexual dysfunction in the older woman: an overview of the current understanding and management. Drugs Aging 2004;21:655–75.

# 112

## Positive tuberculin skin test result in pregnancy

A healthy, 25-year-old woman, gravida 1, comes to the office at 14 weeks of gestation for consultation regarding tuberculin screening results. She works in an acute care hospital on an adult medicine unit. She has cared for patients with tuberculosis during the past 12 months. Last year, her tuberculin skin test result was negative; this year, the induration measures 10 mm. Her chest X-ray is negative, and she has no symptoms of tuberculosis. You advise her that the best treatment is

* (A) isoniazid and pyridoxine hydrochloride (vitamin $B_6$) for 9 months
    (B) isoniazid for 9 months
    (C) postpartum isoniazid and pyridoxine for 9 months
    (D) postpartum isoniazid for 9 months
    (E) isoniazid, rifampin, and ethambutol

Annually, tuberculosis (TB) is responsible for 2 million deaths worldwide, and 8 million new cases occur. However, the incidence of TB has been decreasing in the United States since 1992. In 2002, for the first time in the United States, TB cases among foreign-born individuals accounted for the majority (51%) of TB cases. In most people, their *Mycobacterium tuberculosis* infection is contained by their immune system walling off the still living mycobacteria. This is latent tuberculosis infection and it causes no symptoms.

Targeted tuberculin testing is recommended for latent tuberculosis infection with intent to treat those at high risk for developing active TB. This was previously called "prevention therapy" or "chemoprophylaxis." Routine screening of all pregnant patients is not recommended. Rather, screening only high-risk and moderate-risk women is recommended.

The tuberculin skin test should be performed with an intradermal injection of 0.1 mL (5 tuberculin units) on the volar surface of the forearm. A delayed type of hypersensitivity reaction usually begins 5–6 hours after injection, peaks at 48–72 hours, and subsides over a few days. Positive reactions often persist for up to 1 week. Ideally, the skin test should be read in 48–72 hours. Previous bacille Calmette-Guérin (BCG) vaccination is not a contraindication to placement of the TB skin test. There is no reliable way to distinguish a positive tuberculin reaction caused by vaccination with BCG from a reaction caused by true TB infection. In general, the larger the reaction, the longer ago the vaccination or the greater the risk of exposure (eg, from an area of the world where TB is common, exposure to someone with TB, or family history of TB), then the more likely a reaction is caused by infectious TB.

Pregnant patients at highest risk include women with human immunodeficiency virus (HIV) infection, women who receive immunosuppressant therapy, and those who have had recent close contact with a patient with infectious pulmonary TB (Table 112-1). Women at moderate risk include patients from high-prevalence countries or

**TABLE 112-1.** Recommendations for Targeted Tuberculin Testing

| Risk Level | Target Group | PPD (in mm induration) |
|---|---|---|
| High | Contacts of patients with tuberculosis* <br> Fibrotic changes on chest X-ray† <br> Organ transplant patients† <br> Individuals on prolonged corticosteroid therapy† | 5 |
| Moderate | Recent immigrants from high-prevalence countries* <br> Injection drug users* <br> Homeless individuals* <br> Resident or employee of high-risk congregate setting* <br> Mycobacteriology laboratory employee* <br> Individuals with certain clinical conditions (eg, silicosis, diabetes mellitus, renal failure, underweight, gastrectomy, certain cancers)† | 10 |
| Low | Testing not recommended | 15 |

PPD, purified protein derivative.

*The Centers for Disease Control and Prevention recommends testing for anyone with risk for recent TB infection.

†The Centers for Disease Control and Prevention recommends testing for anyone with increased risk for progression to active disease.

Bergeron KG, Bonebrake RG, Allen C, Gray CJ. Latent tuberculosis in pregnancy: screening and treatment. Curr Womens Health Rep 2003;3:304.

regions (eg, Latin America, Asia, and Africa). Other moderate-risk groups are the homeless, illicit injection drug users, and individuals who reside or work in institutional settings with people at risk for TB. Additional moderate-risk groups for whom induration of 10 mm or more is reactive include mycobacteriology laboratory personnel, adolescents exposed to high-risk adults, and individuals with certain high-risk conditions including silicosis, diabetes mellitus, renal failure, underweight, previous gastrectomy or jejunoileal bypass, and patients with certain cancers.

Pregnant women with a positive tuberculin test result should be further evaluated with a physical examination, history, and single-view chest X-ray with abdominal shielding. Ten percent of pregnant women may have extrapulmonary disease. Acid-fast bacilli on sputum smear or *M tuberculosis* culture tests are required to establish the diagnosis of active disease. Treatment of active disease should begin as soon as the diagnosis is made because untreated TB has a mortality rate of 50%. In the case of latent TB infection, with a positive tuberculin test result but a negative X-ray, treatment also should begin immediately for women at high risk for progression (ie, women with a recent skin-test conversion, who are immunocompromised, or who have had recent contact with a patient with active TB). Ninety percent of active TB cases in the United States arise from latent TB. Patients with latent TB infection should be treated regardless of age, but older patients and those with liver disease need to be monitored more carefully. For women at lower risk for progression of disease, it is acceptable to wait for treatment of latent TB infection until after delivery.

Pregnant women and women less than 3 months postpartum who are being treated for latent TB infection should be evaluated with baseline hepatic enzyme functions, and then administered isoniazid (INH) with pyridoxine added. The pregnant woman needs a monthly clinical history to screen for symptoms of hepatitis and, when indicated, a physical examination looking for clinical signs of hepatitis while being treated.

The duration of INH therapy for latent TB infection should be 6–9 months. Directly observed daily or twice weekly doses are recommended. Pyridoxine doses may prevent peripheral neuropathy and central nervous system effects. Alternative treatments for latent disease include rifampin and pyrazinamide for 2 months or rifampin for 4 months.

A widely cited study that indicated an increase in hepatotoxicity with isoniazid in pregnancy lacked adequate statistical power. Nor was monitoring of the pregnant patients in the study close enough to conclude that the increase in hepatotoxicity with isoniazid in pregnancy was real. Pregnant patients seen for antepartum care can be easily monitored, and may be more compliant with their medications. Because postpartum compliance has been shown to be as low as 6%, obstetrician–gynecologists should emphasize the ongoing need for treatment if postpartum therapy is chosen. Breastfeeding may begin or continue with INH therapy. Because 20% of the INH dose and approximately 11% of other anti-TB medications' doses accumulate in breast milk, neonates should receive supplemental vitamin $B_6$.

Active TB in pregnancy is treated with INH, rifampin, and ethambutol, with all three drugs given for the first 2 months. Remaining therapy is given based on sensitivities of the cultured bacillus.

Bergeron KG, Bonebrake RG, Allen C, Gray CJ. Latent tuberculosis in pregnancy: screening and treatment. Curr Womens Health Rep 2003;3:303–8.

Lake MF. Tuberculosis in pregnancy. This old disease is presenting new challenges. AWHONN Lifelines 2001;5:35–40.

Ormerod P. Tuberculosis in pregnancy and the puerperium. Thorax 2001;56:494–9.

Targeted tuberculin testing and treatment of latent tuberculosis infection. American Thoracic Society; Centers for Disease Control and Prevention. Am J Respir Crit Care Med 2000;161:S221–47.

# 113

## Outpatient therapy for venous thrombosis

A 55-year-old woman is seen in the emergency department with new onset of a swollen, mottled left lower leg. She had one episode of shortness of breath that lasted 10 minutes this morning. She had a hysterectomy 7 weeks ago for uterine prolapse. Until now, her postoperative course was uncomplicated. Examination shows her pulse is 90 beats per minute, blood pressure 100/70 mm Hg, temperature 37°C (98.6°F), respirations 17 per minute and unlabored, weight 70 kg (154 lb), and height 156 cm (65 in.). Her lungs are clear. Her left lower leg is 3 cm larger than the right leg, 9 cm below the knee, and it is erythematous. Doppler ultrasonography of the left lower extremity reveals a deep vein thrombosis (DVT) in the left popliteal vein. Spiral computed tomography (CT) scan shows a small embolus in the right middle lobe of her lung. The best initial therapy is

* (A) low-molecular-weight heparin
  (B) nonsteroidal antiinflammatory drugs (NSAIDs)
  (C) warfarin
  (D) unfractionated heparin

Traditionally, patients with venous thromboembolism were admitted to the hospital, immobilized, and administered unfractionated heparin intravenously and then overlapping warfarin sodium for 5 days until the International Normalized Ratio (INR) was therapeutic for 2 days. Warfarin was continued on an outpatient basis for a minimum of 3 months. Patients were initially immobilized to decrease the frequency of embolization.

Recently, clinical studies have shown that low-molecular-weight heparin is easier to administer, and as efficacious as unfractionated heparin. Therapy with low-molecular-weight heparin may be given as an inpatient in a short-stay unit or as an outpatient with one or two daily doses. Continued care with warfarin for several months remains the recommended long-term care for DVT and pulmonary embolism.

The goals of therapy for DVT, with or without pulmonary embolization, are several:

- Arrest of thrombus growth
- Prevention of recurrence
- Prevention of embolization
- Minimization of limb swelling and postphlebitic syndrome

Low-molecular-weight heparin has been shown to be as effective as unfractionated heparin in the treatment of uncomplicated venous thromboembolism. Although inappropriate for initial use, warfarin is added for a minimum of 3 months, as with unfractionated heparin. Compared with unfractionated heparin, low-molecular-weight heparin has better bioavailability, a longer half-life, and more predictable antithrombotic effects. It prevents recurrent thrombotic events as well as unfractionated heparin does, but has a lower incidence of major bleeding.

Three low-molecular-weight therapies are available in the United States. Not enough information is available to determine if they are interchangeable. The different low-molecular-weight heparin therapies are all given at fixed doses once or twice daily based on body weight. The complete blood count, prothrombin time, and partial thromboplastic time (PTT) need to be measured at baseline. The platelet count should be monitored between days 3 and 7 in heparin-naïve patients to screen for heparin-induced thrombocytopenia. The PTT does not need to be followed serially.

Outpatient and inpatient low-molecular-weight heparin regimens have been advocated for the acute treatment of venous thromboembolism and uncomplicated pulmonary embolism. A multidisciplinary team made up of physicians, pharmacists, home health care personnel, and patient educators must be in place to coordinate the care and follow-up of outpatients. If this type of team is available, outpatient therapy has been shown to be more cost-effective than inpatient or short-stay treatment in multiple heath care systems. Low-molecular-weight heparin also is used in inpatient settings, but with less cost savings.

If a multidisciplinary team is available to coordinate outpatient therapy, patients should be hemodynamically stable, able to administer their own medications, and reside close to a hospital. Outpatient therapy should not be considered in patients with the following health care concerns:

- Two or more previous pulmonary emboli or DVTs
- Active bleeding at the time of DVT diagnosis
- More than two transfusions in a 48-hour period before DVT diagnosis
- Active peptic ulcer disease

- High risk for falls
- Patient or family history of a bleeding disorder
- Pregnancy
- Known deficiency of antithrombin 3, protein C, protein S, or activated protein C resistance
- Concomitant medical illness that necessitates hospital admission
- Cardiopulmonary instability
- Potential for medication noncompliance

Clearly, outpatient therapy should be used only in patients at low risk.

Studies have shown NSAIDs to be effective in patients with superficial thrombophlebitis. However, because this patient demonstrates evidence of DVT and pulmonary embolism, NSAIDs should not be the primary therapy.

The patient described is hemodynamically stable despite DVT and a small pulmonary embolus. Her best initial therapy is low-molecular-weight heparin whether as an inpatient or an outpatient depending on the availability of a team to manage outpatients, and then administration of subsequent warfarin therapy for a minimum of 3 months.

ASHP therapeutic position statement on the use of low-molecular-weight heparins for adult outpatient treatment of acute deep-vein thrombosis [published erratum appears in Am J Health Syst Pharm 2004;61:2243]. Am J Health Syst Pharm 2004;61:1950–5.

Boucher M, Rodger M, Johnson J, Tierney M. Shifting from inpatient to outpatient treatment of deep venous thrombosis in a tertiary care center: a cost-minimization analysis. Pharmacotherapy 2003;23:301–9.

Groce JB 3rd. Treatment of deep venous thrombosis using low-molecular-weight heparins. Am J Manag Care 2001;7 suppl:S510–5; discussion S515–23.

Merli GJ. Low molecular weight heparin in the treatment of acute deep vein thrombosis and pulmonary embolism: a paradigm change in care. J Thromb Thrombolysis 2000;9(suppl 1):S21–7.

O'Brien JA, Caro JJ. Direct medical cost of managing deep vein thrombosis according to the occurrence of complications. Pharmacoeconomics 2002;20:603–15.

# 114

## Hirsutism in patient with polycystic ovary syndrome

A 24-year-old woman presents with facial hair. She has a history of irregular menses over several years with slowly increasing facial hair during that time. Her last menstrual period was 3 months ago. She is not sexually active and not interested in seeking pregnancy. Examination is normal with the exception of mild to moderate facial hair and acne. She weighs 85.7 kg (189 lb) and is 1.6 m (64 in.) tall. Her body mass index (weight in kilograms divided by height in meters squared [$kg/m^2$]) is 32.4. Laboratory evaluation reveals a total testosterone level that is slightly elevated and normal 17$\alpha$-hydroxyprogesterone, prolactin, and thyroid-stimulating hormone (TSH) levels. A pregnancy test result is negative. The best treatment option to care for this patient is

     (A) spironolactone
     (B) norethindrone acetate
  *  (C) oral contraceptives
     (D) electrolysis and waxing
     (E) metformin

This patient has the characteristics typical of polycystic ovary syndrome (PCOS), that is, obesity, oligomenorrhea, and symptoms of hyperandrogenism (hirsutism and acne). The condition is a diagnosis of exclusion. Laboratory evaluations will rule out other etiologies, including adult onset adrenal hyperplasia, pituitary dysfunction, and adrenal or ovarian malignancy. The condition often is associated with a hyperandrogen state characterized by a low sex-hormone-binding globulin, upper limit of normal or only slightly elevated total testosterone, and elevated free testosterone.

Although the patient's main concern is facial hair, she is at risk for several reproductive, metabolic, and cardiovascular disorders. Oligoovulation–anovulation is a common cause of infertility in PCOS patients and is associated with an increased risk of endometrial cancer after prolonged exposure to unopposed estrogen. Insulin resistance is recognized to be commonly associated with PCOS; 30–40% of PCOS patients have impaired glucose tolerance or type 2 diabetes mellitus. Both insulin resistance and elevated androgens contribute to an abnormal lipid profile, which can place the patient at increased risk for cardiovascular disease. While managing her condition, this is an ideal opportunity to address issues of greater long-term health concerns and initiate lifestyle recommendations to include dietary restrictions and exercise.

Several options are available to treat the patient's hirsutism. Spironolactone dosages of at least 100 mg daily have been effective in management of hirsutism but will not treat her irregular menses. Clinical results are not seen until the drug has been used for 6–9 months. Lower doses of spironolactone will have little to no effect in managing the disorder. Periodic administration of norethindrone acetate is a derivative of 19-nortestosterone; periodic administration will induce withdrawal bleeding and reduce the risk of future endometrial hyperplasia, but will not treat her hirsutism or acne.

Low-dose oral contraceptives (ethinyl estradiol, 35 mcg or less) can effectively manage many of the symptoms of PCOS, including irregular menses and the associated risks of endometrial neoplasia, hirsutism, and acne. Oral contraceptives increase sex-hormone-binding globulin, which binds circulating androgens. Although any low-dose oral contraceptive can be used, those with less androgenic progestins, including desogestrel, norgestimate, and drospirenone, may be particularly advanta-

geous. A randomized trial of oral contraceptives and metformin found the contraceptives more effective in inducing regular menstruation, reducing free testosterone, and treating hirsutism.

Electrolysis will remove current hair but will have no effect on the underlying cause of her hirsutism. Ideally, she should receive treatment that will address the metabolic derangement that has led to the hirsutism.

Christian RC, Dumesic DA, Behrenbeck T, Oberg AL, Sheedy PF 2nd, Fitzpatrick LA. Prevalence and predictors of coronary artery calcification in women with polycystic ovary syndrome. J Clin Endocrinol Metab 2003;88:2562–8.

Ehrmann DA, Barnes RB, Rosenfield RL, Cavaghan MK, Imperial J. Prevalence of impaired glucose tolerance and diabetes in women with polycystic ovary syndrome. Diabetes Care 1999;22:141–6.

Guido M, Romualdi D, Giuliani M, Suriano R, Selvaggi L, Apa R, et al. Drospirenone for the treatment of hirsute women with polycystic ovary syndrome: a clinical, endocrinological, metabolic pilot study. J Clin Endocrinol Metab 2004;89:2817–23.

Morin-Papunen LC, Vauhkonen I, Koivunen RM, Ruokonen A, Martikainen HK, Tapanainen JS. Endocrine and metabolic effects of metformin versus ethinyl estradiol-cyproterone acetate in obese women with polycystic ovary syndrome: a randomized study. J Clin Endocrinol Metab 2000;85:3161–8.

Spritzer PM, Lisboa KO, Mattiello S, Lhullier F. Spironolactone as a single agent for long-term therapy of hirsute patients. Clin Endocrinol (Oxf) 2000;52:587–94.

# 115

## Emergency contraception

A 32-year-old married woman and her husband are using condoms for contraception. She calls your office 3 days after an episode of sexual intercourse that resulted in a condom breakage. Her last normal menstrual period began 10 days ago. She has regular menses and wishes to receive emergency contraception. Your best next step in management of this case is

      (A) prescribe estradiol
\*   (B) prescribe levonorgestrel
      (C) observation and pregnancy testing in 3 weeks
      (D) prescribe intramuscular depot medroxyprogesterone acetate
      (E) prescribe oral medroxyprogesterone acetate

Of the 3.5 million unintended pregnancies in the United States each year, approximately 40% result in birth, 13% in miscarriage, and 45–50% in abortion. It is believed that education and easy access to emergency contraception could prevent more than half of the unintended pregnancies and subsequently decrease the abortion rate.

Emergency contraception prevents pregnancy after a woman has unprotected intercourse. Four methods are available in the United States:

1. High-dose regimen of combination oral contraceptives

2. Progestin-only oral contraceptives

3. Emergency contraceptive formulation of levonorgestrel

4. Placement of a copper-containing T-shaped intrauterine device (IUD) within 5 days of the unprotected intercourse

The protective effect of emergency contraception is greatest when the oral contraceptive is prescribed within 72 hours after unprotected intercourse, but some protection is afforded when the contraceptive is used even up to 5 days after unprotected coitus. Therefore, initiation of emergency contraception is indicated for this patient.

The most commonly prescribed oral contraceptive regimen is two progestin-only 0.75-mg doses of levonorgestrel, given 12 hours apart, and this should be the emergency contraception regimen that would be recommended for the patient described. Note that similar efficacy has been demonstrated by taking both doses at the same time. This progestin-only dose of levonorgestrel is commercially available under the name Plan B. Emergency contraception also may be accomplished by taking at 12-hour intervals a combination estrogen plus progesterone oral contraceptive (Table 115-1). Compared with the combination oral contraceptives, the progestin-only

regimen causes less nausea. An antiemetic taken 60 minutes before ingesting the combination oral contraceptive may decrease nausea.

Oral regimens are highly effective and available at affordable costs. No pregnancy test is necessary before prescribing emergency contraception. No teratogenic effects have been reported from the use of emergency contraceptives, and no adverse effects on concurrent medical conditions have been noted. Effectiveness in prevention of pregnancy is estimated at 75%. The rate of unintended pregnancy is reduced from 8% to 2% after unprotected intercourse. Menses begin within 21 days in 98% of patients, and more than 50% of patients will have their menses at the expected time. Failure to note an expected menses should prompt a physician visit.

The mechanism of action of emergency contraception is primarily inhibition or delay of ovulation. Other less important functions include alteration of cervical mucus to decrease sperm penetration and capacitation and altered endometrial histology. No emergency contraceptive interrupts an established pregnancy. Because ovulatory inhibition or delay is the primary mechanism of action, patients should begin a reliable contraceptive regimen shortly after they receive emergency contraception.

Neither estradiol alone nor medroxyprogesterone acetate alone provide emergency contraception or contraceptive efficacy. Although depot medroxyprogesterone acetate is a safe, effective long-term contraceptive that may be initiated after emergency contraceptive use, it has not been studied as an emergency contraceptive regimen. Combination levonorgestrel–ethinyl estradiol is an oral contraceptive formulation and may be used for emergency contraception at higher doses (Table 115-1).

**TABLE 115-1.** Twenty-one Brands of Oral Contraceptives That Can Be Used for Emergency Contraception in the United States

| Brand | Company | Pills per Dose* | Ethinyl Estradiol per Dose (mcg) | Levonorgestrel per Dose (mg)[†] |
|---|---|---|---|---|
| Plan B[‡] | Barr | 1 white pill | 0 | 0.75 |
| Ovral | Wyeth-Ayerst | 2 white pills | 100 | 0.50 |
| Ogestrel | Watson | 2 white pills | 100 | 0.50 |
| Cryselle | Barr | 4 white pills | 120 | 0.60 |
| Levora | Watson | 4 white pills | 120 | 0.60 |
| Lo/Ovral | Wyeth-Ayerst | 4 white pills | 120 | 0.60 |
| Low-Ogestrel | Watson | 4 white pills | 120 | 0.60 |
| Levlen | Berlex | 4 light orange pills | 120 | 0.60 |
| Nordette | Wyeth-Ayerst | 4 light orange pills | 120 | 0.60 |
| Portia | Barr | 4 pink pills | 120 | 0.60 |
| Seasonale | Barr | 4 pink pills | 120 | 0.60 |
| Trivora | Watson | 4 pink pills | 120 | 0.50 |
| Tri-Levlen | Berlex | 4 yellow pills | 120 | 0.50 |
| Triphasil | Wyeth-Ayerst | 4 yellow pills | 120 | 0.50 |
| Enpresse | Barr | 4 orange pills | 120 | 0.50 |
| Alesse | Wyeth-Ayerst | 5 pink pills | 100 | 0.50 |
| Lessina | Barr | 5 pink pills | 100 | 0.50 |
| Levlite | Berlex | 5 pink pills | 100 | 0.50 |
| Lutera | Watson | 5 white pills | 100 | 0.50 |
| Aviane | Barr | 5 orange pills | 100 | 0.50 |
| Ovrette | Wyeth-Ayerst | 20 yellow pills | 0 | 0.75 |

*The treatment schedule is one dose as soon as possible after unprotected intercourse, and another dose 12 hours later. However, recent research has found that both doses of Plan B or Ovrette can be taken at the same time.

[†]The progestin in Cryselle, Lo/Ovral, Low-Ogestrel, Ogestrel, Ovral, and Ovrette is norgestrel, which contains two isomers, only one of which (levonorgestrel) is bioactive; the amount of norgestrel in each tablet is twice the amount of levonorgestrel. Levonorgestrel regimens also can be formulated by substituting double the amount of norgestrel as is indicated for levonorgestrel.

[‡]Plan B is the only dedicated product specifically marketed for emergency contraception in the United States. Preven, a combined emergency contraception pill, is no longer available on the U.S. market.

NOT-2-LATE.com: the emergency contraception website. Princeton University Office of Population Research. Princeton (NJ): Office of Population Research; 2005. Available at: http://ec.princeton.edu/ questions/dose.html. Retrieved October 13, 2005.

Emergency contraception. ACOG Practice Bulletin No. 69. American College of Obstetricians and Gynecologists. Obstet Gynecol 2005; 106:483–91.

Trussell J, Ellertson C, Stewart F, Raymond EG, Shochet T. The role of emergency contraception. Am J Obstet Gynecol 2004;190 suppl: S30–S38.

# 116

## Palpable breast lump with negative mammography test result

A 45-year-old woman found a mass on breast self-examination. You palpate a 2-cm rubbery mass in the upper outer quadrant of the left breast. She has no family history of breast cancer. A screening mammogram 1 month earlier was interpreted as normal. The next step is

        (A) repeat mammography with compression views
\*    (B) cytohistologic diagnosis
        (C) restrict caffeine
        (D) magnetic resonance imaging (MRI) of the breast
        (E) reexamination after next menstrual cycle

Breast masses occur in women of all ages. The differential diagnoses include benign tumors and cysts, ductal and lobular hyperplasia, carcinoma in situ, and invasive cancer. Cysts may occur at any age, but are more common in women in their forties and in perimenopausal women. One third of breast cancer cases occur in women younger than 50 years; therefore, history, physical examination, and clinical judgment should guide evaluation.

Mammography fails to detect approximately 10% of breast cancers, so the fact that a mass does not show up on mammography is not reassuring. In order to avoid the error of failing to further evaluate a patient with a mass, definitive diagnosis should be pursued while obtaining mammography to ascertain whether a potentially malignant lesion is multifocal or has spread. Delaying evaluation for repeat studies is not indicated.

Ultrasonography or cyst aspiration can enable the diagnosis of a simple cyst. If clear nonbloody fluid is obtained on fine-needle aspiration (FNA), the likelihood of cancer is low. The technique for FNA involves prepping the skin and stabilizing the mass with one hand. A fine-gauge needle on a syringe is introduced into the mass and moved back and forth at least 10 times while suction is maintained in the syringe. The suction should be broken before the needle is withdrawn. The aspirated material can be fixed onto a slide and evaluated. Surgical biopsy is indicated for bloody aspirate, recurrence, or solid masses. The false-negative rate of FNA is 10%. The patient should be reevaluated in 4–6 weeks to be sure the mass has not recurred.

Core needle biopsy is useful for obtaining a sufficiently large sample for histologic examination. Excisional biopsy in the operating room allows the entire lesion to be removed. Needle localization biopsy would be used to evaluate a nonpalpable lesion found on imaging, such as mammography.

The role of MRI in evaluating breast masses and for screening is not yet well defined. Any palpable, dominant mass should be fully evaluated even if fibrocystic change is suspected and the mass is tender. Attempting to treat fibrocystic change by dietary means such as eliminating caffeine should not delay diagnosis.

Hansen N, Morrow M. Breast disease. Med Clin North Am 1998;82:203–22.

Scott S, Morrow M. Breast cancer. Making the diagnosis. Surg Clin North Am 1999;79:991–1005.

Winchester DP. Evaluation and management of breast abnormalities. Cancer 1990;66 suppl:1345–7.

# 117

## Diagnosis of skin condition

A 22-year-old woman comes to your office with vulvar swelling and erythema. She states that she awoke with the condition this morning and has noted similar symptoms over the past 2 months to a lesser degree. She states that she had "rough intercourse" last night. An over-the-counter antifungal cream caused burning when applied this morning. Physical examination reveals labia minora that are diffusely edematous with an intense edema that extends to the labia majora and crural folds. The vulva is mildly tender to the touch. Her hands appear red and scaly. When questioned, she states, "I always get that in the winter, but it's worse than usual this year." Her partner has been using unlubricated condoms for contraception. The patient works as a surgical technician at a local hospital. Wet mount testing of the vagina reveals a few nonbudding yeasts. The most likely diagnosis is

  (A) eczema
* (B) latex allergy
  (C) monilial infection
  (D) local trauma
  (E) recurrent herpes

Latex allergy was first described in 1979; since then, the reported incidence of latex sensitization and allergy has been increasing steadily. Although the incidence of latex allergy in the general population is less than 1%, workers in industries that have significant exposure to latex have a much greater chance of sensitization. Currently, 12% of health care workers are either sensitized or allergic to latex. Other risk factors for latex allergy include a history of atopy and certain food allergies (eg, bananas or kiwi fruit). Patients with spina bifida and children with genitourinary malformations carry a high risk for developing the allergy.

Natural rubber latex is a product of the *Hevea brasiliensis* tree. Currently, 11 distinct proteins have been identified in latex that can contribute to sensitization and allergy. Allergic reaction from latex exposure can range from contact dermatitis to anaphylaxis. Contact exposure typically leads to erythema and irritation with swelling, pruritus, and urticaria. Depending on the duration of exposure, the reaction may be delayed. Reaction to contact exposure frequently occurs first on the hands after removing latex surgical gloves. More significant exposure can be life-threatening and may lead to generalized urticaria and laryngeal edema.

This patient's history suggests multiple risk factors for developing latex sensitization and allergy, including a history of seasonal atopy (hand eczema), her job as a surgical technician, and the use of unlubricated condoms. She does not report significant discharge or vulvar tenderness, which would be expected if she had a monilial or herpes infection. Even though the reported "rough sex" may have exacerbated the condition, her history is most consistent with a recently developed latex allergy.

Alenius H, Turjanmaa K, Palosuo T. Natural rubber latex allergy. Occup Environ Med 2002;59:419–24.

Hepner DL, Castells MC. Latex allergy: an update. Anesth Analg 2003;96:1219–29.

Margesson LJ. Contact dermatitis of the vulva. Dermatol Ther 2004;17:20–7.

Toraason M, Sussman G, Biagini R, Meade J, Beezhold D, Germolec D. Latex allergy in the workplace. Toxicol Sci 2000;58:5–14.

# 118

## Treatment of severe osteopenia

A 60-year-old woman, posthysterectomy, comes to the office to discuss results of a recent dual-energy X-ray absorptiometry (DXA) examination that showed her *T*-scores of the spine and hip to be –2.4 and –1.9, respectively. She quit smoking 8 years ago; her vasomotor symptoms are no longer bothersome. The best pharmacologic therapy for this patient is

        (A) calcitonin nasal spray
\*   (B) oral bisphosphonate therapy
        (C) oral calcium carbonate
        (D) human parathyroid hormone analog injections
        (E) estrogen therapy

Annually in the United States, osteoporosis causes some 1.5 million fractures; most of these fractures involve postmenopausal women. The most common skeletal sites for osteoporotic fractures are the spine, hip, and wrist. As the number of postmenopausal women increases, osteoporosis has the potential to cause an increasing burden of suffering, disability, and economic costs.

After attainment of peak bone mass in the mid-20s, bone loss gradually occurs until menopause, which is associated with accelerated bone loss. Bone density studies suggest that in the first 5 years postmenopause, untreated women lose 15–20% of their bone mineral density. When women have lost more than 2.5 standard deviations of their bone mass (*T*-score less than –2.5) compared with women at peak bone mass, a diagnosis of osteoporosis is made. Osteopenia, or low bone mass, refers to *T*-scores between –1.0 and –2.5. The American College of Obstetricians and Gynecologists (ACOG) recommends initiation of therapy (ie, hormone therapy, bisphosphonate, or raloxifene hydrochloride [Evista]) to prevent fractures if the *T*-score is less than –2.0, or if risk factors are present when the *T*-score is less than –1.5.

Common risk factors for osteoporosis include the following:

- Early age at menopause
- Prior fracture as an adult
- Cigarette smoking
- Weight less than 56.7 kg (125 lb)
- Poor health or frailty

It is important to be aware that age is an independent risk factor for fracture. Given the same *T*-score, a woman aged 60 years, for instance, has a substantially higher fracture risk and may benefit from fracture prevention therapy more than a woman aged 50 years.

Hormone therapy (HT) represents effective fracture prevention therapy and is particularly appropriate in women at risk for fractures who also suffer from vasomotor symptoms. However, the woman in this case no longer is bothered by vasomotor symptoms. Accordingly, bisphosphonate therapy (eg, weekly alendronate, weekly risedronate, or monthly ibandronate) offers this woman effective fracture prevention therapy without the risks associated with HT. However, it should be noted that in clinical trials of ibandronate, the drug has not been found to prevent hip fractures. Because use of the selective estrogen-receptor modulator, raloxifene, is associated with an increased risk of venous thromboembolic disease and hip fracture prevention has not been demonstrated, this agent is less preferred than bisphosphonates.

Although menopausal women should be counseled to ensure adequate intake of calcium and vitamin D, such nutritional measures by themselves are not effective in preventing fractures. Calcitonin nasal spray is not helpful in fracture prevention. Accordingly, calcitonin does not represent optimal treatment for this patient. Two years of daily subcutaneous injections of human recombinant parathyroid hormone have been found to build bone mass and prevent fractures in women with osteoporosis. Currently, use of this expensive therapy is recommended for patients who have already experienced fractures while using the fracture prevention treatments recommended by ACOG, as described.

Anderson GL, Limacher M, Assaf AR, Bassford T, Beresford SA, Black H, et al. Effects of conjugated equine estrogen in postmenopausal women with hysterectomy: the Women's Health Initiative randomized controlled trial. Women's Health Initiative Steering Committee. JAMA 2004;291:1701–12.

Body JJ, Gaich GA, Scheele WH, Kulkarni PM, Miller PD, Peretz A, et al. A randomized double-blind trial to compare the efficacy of teriparatide [recombinant human parathyroid hormone (1-34)] with alendronate in postmenopausal women with osteoporosis. J Clin Endocrinol Metab 2002;87:4528–35.

Bone HG, Hosking D, Devogelaer JP, Tucci JR, Emkey RD, Tonino RP. Ten years' experience with alendronate for osteoporosis in postmenopausal women. Alendronate Phase III Osteoporosis Treatment Study Group. N Engl J Med 2004;350:1189–99.

McClung MR, Geusens P, Miller PD, Zippel H, Bensen WG, Roux C, et al. Effect of risedronate on the risk of hip fracture in elderly women. Hip Intervention Study Group. N Engl J Med 2001;344:333–40.

Osteoporosis. American College of Obstetricians and Gynecologists. Obstet Gynecol 2004;104 suppl:66S–76S.

# 119

## Methods to increase lactation

A 28-year-old woman, gravida 1, para 1, who is 6 weeks postpartum, calls your office about her decreased lactation and a desire to continue to breastfeed her infant. The infant required surgery for hypertrophic pyloric stenosis, and breastfeeding was discontinued throughout the postoperative period. The patient wishes to resume breastfeeding but notes that her milk supply is decreased. The most appropriate next step is

* (A) frequent breastfeeding with formula supplementation
(B) metoclopramide therapy
(C) bromocriptine therapy
(D) valerian therapy
(E) one or two alcoholic beverages per day

The best method for this woman to increase her breast-feeding would be to use a mechanical breast pump and supplement breast milk with formula. Maintenance of an adequate milk supply is necessary for infant weight gain, nutrition, and satisfaction. Many factors affect maternal lactation, including medical and psychologic stressors. Periods of reduced feeding often result in a transient or permanent reduction in milk supply. Attempts to supplement breast-feeding with formula when the milk supply is reduced may result in less milk production for a 24-hour period.

Pharmacologic agents evaluated for lactation augmentation include metoclopramide and domperidone (Motilium). These are central dopamine agents, which were initially indicated for gastrointestinal disorders. The purported mechanism of action to increase lactation is inhibition of dopamine resulting in prolactin production from the pituitary gland.

A small number of poorly controlled studies have supported the use of metoclopramide to assist lactation in mothers of full-term infants. A recent, well-controlled study in mothers of preterm infants has questioned the efficacy of metoclopramide for lactation supplementation when initiated immediately postpartum. The customary duration of metoclopramide use is approximately 14 days. No studies support longer use of this agent. Metoclopramide crosses the blood–brain barrier and is secreted in significant amounts in breast milk. This is a potential concern, but no adverse outcomes in humans have been reported. This medication has been reported to effect dopamine-mediated responses in the offspring of nursing rats.

Alternative therapies consist of largely untested supplements to maternal nutrition. Herbal therapies may be oriented toward altering maternal life events such as stress reduction, rather than increasing lactation or milk production by physiologic change. Valerian is an herb that has been used as an antianxiety agent. It is not recommended for maternal consumption to enhance lactation, given the lack of scientific studies demonstrating safety or efficacy.

Traditional wisdom in many parts of the world has advocated alcohol consumption, especially beer, to enhance lactation. No studies are available on nonalcoholic beer. However, studies on lactation habits of infants whose mothers consume alcohol-containing beverages indicate a decreased quantity of breast milk consumption and shortened breastfeeding times. Therefore, alcohol-containing beverages may result in an adverse effect on breastfeeding.

Bromocriptine is a dopamine agonist that inhibits pituitary prolactin secretion. It is contraindicated in women who want to breastfeed.

da Silva OP, Knoppert DC, Angelini MM, Forret PA. Effect of domperidone on milk production in mothers of premature newborns: a randomized, double-blind, placebo-controlled trial. CMAJ 2001;164:17–21.

Koletzko B, Lehner F. Beer and breastfeeding. In: Koletzko B, Michaelson KF, Hernell O, eds. Short and long term effects of breast feeding on child health. New York (NY): Kluwer Academic/Plenum Publishers; 2000. p. 23–8.

Schanler RJ, Gartner LM, Krebs NF, Dooley S, Mass SB, editors. Breastfeeding handbook for physicians. Washington, DC: American Academy of Pediatrics and American College of Obstetricians and Gynecologists; 2006.

# 120

## *Helicobacter pylori* and peptic ulcer disease

A 50-year-old woman with dyspepsia has experienced weight loss of 10% of her usual weight over the past 3 months. She denies any melena. She has a history of *Helicobacter pylori* duodenal ulcer diagnosed without endoscopy 5 years ago. She was treated with antibiotics and a proton pump inhibitor. She has done well until the past 3 months. She placed herself on enteric-coated aspirin for mild rheumatoid arthritis approximately 6 months ago. The next step to determine the etiology of her recurrent dyspepsia is

*    (A) endoscopy with biopsy
     (B) anti-*H pylori* antibody testing
     (C) *H pylori* stool antigen testing
     (D) urea breath test
     (E) barium swallow

The 1983 discovery of *H pylori*, a cause of peptic ulcer disease, changed the management of peptic ulcer disease from symptom relief to eradication of an infectious disease. In patients with *H pylori*-positive peptic ulcer disease, the yearly relapse rates have decreased from 80% for duodenal ulcers and 60% for gastric ulcers to less than 5% for both types of ulcer after successful *H pylori* eradication. *Helicobacter pylori* is associated with low-grade gastric mucosa-associated lymphoid tissue lymphoma, gastric adenocarcinoma, type B chronic atrophic gastritis, and peptic ulcer dyspepsia. No relationship between gastroesophageal reflux disease (GERD) and *H pylori* has been found. Gastritis due to *H pylori* is associated with an increased risk of peptic ulcer disease.

An increasingly important alternative cause of peptic ulcer disease is nonsteroidal antiinflammatory drugs (NSAIDs). Patients older than 65 years are at increased risk of gastrotoxicity with NSAID use. Within 1 year of starting NSAIDs, 1–8% of elderly NSAID users are hospitalized for peptic ulcer disease complications. Approximately 20% of patients on long-term NSAID therapy develop peptic ulcer disease. Use of NSAIDs also increases the risk of bleeding and other complications in peptic ulcer disease by fourfold to sixfold. Overall, NSAID use accounts for approximately 25% of ulcers, ulcer complications, and ulcer-related mortality in the elderly. *Helicobacter pylori* and NSAIDs cause ulcers by different mechanisms and are not synergistic.

Women use NSAIDs more frequently than men and thus have a higher incidence of peptic ulcer disease caused by NSAIDs. Other risk factors for NSAID-associated gastric toxicity include alcoholism, coffee consumption, smoking, previous peptic ulcer disease (14–17-fold increased risk of peptic ulcer disease complications), prostaglandin deficiency, poor health, family history of peptic ulcer disease, and concomitant medication use.

Frequently associated drugs that increase the risk of ulcer disease include bisphosphonates, corticosteroids, antineoplastic agents, anticoagulants, and use of multiple NSAIDs. Long-term use and high dosages of NSAIDs also increase the risk of developing ulcer disease.

Diagnostic testing for patients with symptoms of nausea, vomiting, abdominal pain, dyspepsia, anorexia, pyrosis (pain that radiates substernally), melena, or hematemesis may be noninvasive or invasive. The noninvasive approach includes anti-*H pylori* antibody testing. In the absence of antibodies, an NSAID-induced ulcer is suggested. When antibodies are present, *H pylori*-induced ulcer is probable. However, in previously treated patients, the *H pylori* antibodies can persist for months to years, and therefore such testing is not used in patients previously treated for *H pylori*-associated ulcer disease. Another noninvasive test is urea breath testing. Orally ingested urea with carbon 13 or carbon 14 is hydrolyzed by the *H pylori* urease and excreted by the lungs as labeled carbon dioxide. A positive urea breath test result indicates active infection. This test is accurate to determine *H pylori* eradication posttreatment. Patients on proton pump inhibitors need to stop their medications 2 weeks before this study. Radioisotope capabilities may not always be available.

Invasive tests (eg, esophagogastroduodenoscopic evaluation of the upper gastrointestinal tract) are appropriate for patients with previously diagnosed peptic ulcer disease with recurrent symptoms, patients with long-standing GERD, or those with alarm symptoms, such as unexplained weight loss, anemia with dyspeptic symptoms, or dysphagia. Endoscopy also may be indicated in patients with acute gastrointestinal bleeding, fecal occult blood, unremitting dyspepsia, iron deficiency anemia, and abdominal pain of undetermined cause, especially if they use NSAIDs. Histology is still considered to be the criterion standard for diagnosis. However, it can be affected by antibiotic use or antisecretory medications. The rapid urea test also is performed on biopsy-obtained specimens in a tissue medium that contains urea. The urease in *H pylori* produces ammonia, which causes an increased pH and a color change. This test is 90% sensitive and 100% specific for *H pylori* infections. Recent antibiotic or proton pump inhibitor treatment may cause a false-negative test finding. Culture of mucosal biopsies is usually reserved for evaluation of patients with possible antibiotic resistance. If available, culture may be used on biopsy samples instead of the rapid urea test. *Helicobacter pylori* antigen testing on stool samples is generally reserved to check for eradication of *H pylori*

after treatment. Barium swallows are used for diagnosis of esophageal motility, not for evaluation of peptic ulcer disease.

Cappell MS, Schein JR. Diagnosis and treatment of nonsteroidal anti-inflammatory drug-associated upper gastrointestinal toxicity. Gastroenterol Clin North Am 2000;29:97–124, vi.

Cohen H. Peptic ulcer and Helicobacter pylori. Gastroenterol Clin North Am 2000;29:775–89.

Pilotto A. Helicobacter pylori-associated peptic ulcer disease in older patients: current management strategies. Drugs Aging 2001;18:487–94.

Sivri B. Trends in ulcer pharmacotherapy. Fundam Clin Pharmacol 2004;18:23–31.

Wildner-Christensen M, Touborg Lassen A, Lindebjerg J, Schaffalitzky de Muckadell OB. Diagnosis of Helicobacter pylori in bleeding peptic ulcer patients, evaluation of urea-based tests. Digestion 2002;66:9–13.

# 121
## Chronic cough caused by drug therapy

A 66-year-old woman, gravida 2, with a history of urge incontinence, comes to your office for her periodic examination. During the past year, she was admitted to the hospital with a heart attack, at which time diabetes mellitus and hypertension also were diagnosed. She underwent cardiac catheterization with stent placement and was started on lisinopril (Zestril, Prinivil), atorvastatin (Lipitor), metformin hydrochloride (Glucophage), and aspirin.

Since that time she has done well. She quit smoking and made major lifestyle changes with dietary improvements and daily exercise including aerobics. For the past 3 months, she has had worsening incontinence with a cough that she describes as dry and hacking. She is still taking extended-release tolterodine, but notes no improvement. She voids approximately every 3 hours and denies frequency or dysuria. On examination, her vital signs include a blood pressure reading of 142/82 mm Hg, pulse rate of 84 beats per minute, and temperature 37.1°C (98.8°F). Her lungs are clear to auscultation and cardiac examination findings are normal. Abdominal examination is normal without hepatomegaly. Pelvic examination reveals a normal cervix, a small anteverted uterus, a minimal cystocele, minimal hypermobility of the urethrovesical junction, and a postvoid residual volume of 15 mL. Urine is negative for nitrates and leukocyte esterase. The medication that is most likely contributing to her incontinence is

* (A) lisinopril (Prinivil, Zestril)
  (B) atorvastatin (Lipitor)
  (C) metformin hydrochloride (Glucophage)
  (D) aspirin
  (E) tolterodine tartrate (Detrol)

As the population ages, more patients present with multiple medical problems and polypharmacy. Most studies in the past have underrepresented women in clinical investigations, but sex differences in responses to medications are increasingly recognized. Current knowledge and understanding of a broad spectrum of medications is needed to provide optimal care for older women.

By history, the inciting event of the worsening incontinence in this patient is the dry cough. Although other causes of incontinence need to be considered, the new onset of the chronic cough must be recognized and identified. The three most common causes of chronic cough are asthma, gastroesophageal diseases, and rhinitis. In a chronic cough after starting to take an angiotensin-converting enzyme (ACE) inhibitor, suspicion should be high for the medicine as the cause of the cough.

Although estimates vary, ACE inhibitors have been associated with a dry cough in 20% or more of patients.

The cough is an apparent class effect that may occur with all of the ACE inhibitors, but is much less common in the newer angiotensin II receptor blockers. Many patients have a cough severe enough to require discontinuation of the medicine. Resolution of the cough may occur within days of withdrawing the ACE inhibitor or it may require weeks for complete resolution. Women, nonsmokers, and individuals of black or Asian ethnicity have been reported to be at increased risk of an ACE inhibitor–induced cough. In this patient, the recommended course of action would be to discontinue the ACE inhibitor in consultation with her primary physician. The incontinence would return to baseline with resolution of the cough if the ACE inhibitor is the cause.

Atorvastatin (Lipitor) is a hydroxy-methyl-glutaryl co-enzyme A (HMG CoA) reductase inhibitor. This statin used in dyslipidemias has few adverse reactions. Hepatic dysfunction has been reported in 0.5–3.0% of patients who use statins, but it is now unclear if statins actually cause hepatic dysfunction. Although this relationship has recently been questioned, currently the U.S. Food and Drug Administration recommends liver function testing before and 12 weeks after the initiation of a statin, then periodically thereafter. Another side effect of statins is muscle injury in 2–11% that presents as myalgias, myositis, and rarely rhabdomyolysis. Muscle injury symptoms from statins usually begin within a few weeks to months after starting the medicine then resolve following discontinuation.

Metformin hydrochloride (Glucophage), an insulin sensitizer, has gastrointestinal side effects in more than 10% of patients with nausea, vomiting, diarrhea, flatulence, abdominal discomfort, and indigestion. Metformin is associated with a rare but potentially severe lactic acidosis. Therefore, it should be discontinued in patients predisposed to hypoxia, such as congestive heart failure, respiratory failure, acute myocardial infarction, and septicemia.

The most common side effects of aspirin use are gastrointestinal and hematologic. Aspirin should be used with caution in patients with platelet and bleeding disorders. It can lead to erosive gastritis or peptic ulcer disease.

Tolterodine tartrate (Detrol) is effective for use in urge incontinence and can be used at dosages of 2–4 mg per day. With this extended-release anticholinergic agent, anticholinergic symptoms such as dry mouth are less common but present in up to 23% of patients. Tolterodine tartrate would not be contributing to the stress incontinence.

Dykewicz MS. Cough and angioedema from angiotensin-converting enzyme inhibitors: new insights into mechanisms and management. Curr Opin Allergy Clin Immunol 2004;4:267–70.

Morice AH, Kastelik JA. Cough. 1: Chronic cough in adults. Thorax 2003;58:901–7.

Morimoto T, Ghandi TK, Fiskio JM, Seger AC, So JW, Cook EF, et al. An evaluation of risk factors for adverse drug events associated with angiotensin-converting enzyme inhibitors. J Eval Clin Pract 2004; 10:499–509.

Schwartz JB. Gender-specific implications for cardiovascular medication use in the elderly optimizing therapy for older women. Cardiol Rev 2003;11:275–98.

# 122

## Use of intrauterine device

A 22-year-old woman, para 2, with children ages 2 years and 1 year, requests contraception. She and her husband of 4 years do not want more children. A deep vein thrombosis (DVT) was diagnosed while she was taking oral contraceptives at age 17 years and received heparin prophylaxis during both pregnancies. She conceived her last child while using condoms, and is currently using condoms intermittently. Her menses occur every 28–30 days but are becoming increasingly heavier and longer. She was told she cannot donate blood because of mild anemia. She has had difficulty losing weight since she was a teenager, and she currently weighs 95.3 kg (210 lb) and is 1.6 m (63 in.) tall. Her body mass index (weight in kilograms divided by height in meters squared [kg/m$^2$]) is 37.2. Her examination findings, including pelvic examination, are otherwise normal. You tell her that the most appropriate contraceptive for her would be

(A) depot medroxyprogesterone acetate injections
(B) tubal sterilization
(C) contraceptive vaginal ring
* (D) levonorgestrel-containing intrauterine device (IUD)
(E) combination oral contraceptives with 20 mcg ethinyl estradiol

Although this patient states at this time that she does not desire future childbearing, at her young age she is at risk for regret if she has permanent sterilization. In the U.S. Collaborative Review of Sterilization (CREST), a prospective cohort study that enrolled more than 10,000 women and followed for up to 14 years, the cumulative probability of regret was 20% for women aged 30 years and younger. Any form of tubal occlusion, hysteroscopic or laparoscopic, would not be an ideal choice for this patient. Because of her history of DVT, she is not a candidate for any method of estrogen-containing contraceptives including very low-dose combination oral contraceptives, the transdermal contraceptive patch, or the contraceptive vaginal ring. When given every 3 months, depot medroxyprogesterone acetate is highly effective but is associated with weight gain, an issue for this patient.

This patient is an ideal candidate for an IUD. She is multiparous in a monogamous relationship for several years and is not considering childbearing in the near future, if ever. Two IUDs are currently available in the United States: the levonorgestrel IUD and the copper-containing IUD. Both are highly effective and have been shown to have similar efficacy rates to sterilization procedures. An additional benefit of the levonorgestrel IUD is that it greatly reduces uterine blood loss. The local release

of levonorgestrel into the endometrium creates an atrophic decidualized endometrium even though ovulation is still occurring in most patients. One year after insertion, there is an 80% reduction in blood loss, and approximately 20% of patients are amenorrheic. If the patient chooses to have more children, there is immediate return of fertility on removal. The device is currently approved for 5 years of contraceptive use. The currently approved copper-containing IUD is effective for 10 years but is not an ideal choice in this patient because of its association with increased uterine bleeding and cramping.

Andersson K, Odlind V, Rybo G. Levonorgestrel-releasing and copper-releasing (Nova T) IUDs during five years of use: a randomized comparative trial. Contraception 1994;49:56–72.

Hillis SD, Marchbanks PA, Tylor LR, Peterson HB. Poststerilization regret: findings from the United States Collaborative Review of Sterilization. Obstet Gynecol 1999;93:889–95.

Hurskainen R, Teperi J, Rissanen P, Aalto AM, Grenman S, Kivela A, et al. Clinical outcomes and costs with the levonorgestrel-releasing intrauterine system or hysterectomy for treatment of menorrhagia: randomized trial. JAMA 2004;291:1456–63.

Intrauterine device. ACOG Practice Bulletin No. 59. American College of Obstetricians and Gynecologists. Obstet Gynecol 2005;105:223–32.

Milsom I, Andersson K, Andersch B, Rybo G. A comparison of flurbiprofen, tranexamic acid, and a levonorgestrel-releasing intrauterine contraceptive device in the treatment of idiopathic menorrhagia. Am J Obstet Gynecol 1991;164:879–83.

# 123

## Role of diet in lowering blood pressure

A 60-year-old woman comes to your office for a periodic health maintenance visit. She has a blood pressure of 150/95 mm Hg, weight 72.6 kg (160 lb), and height 1.52 m (60 in.). Her body mass index (weight in kilograms divided by height in meters squared [kg/m$^2$]) is 31.3. Along with weight reduction, the best next dietary management step to help reduce her blood pressure is to decrease consumption of

(A) potassium
(B) calcium
(C) fish oil
* (D) sodium
(E) magnesium

An initial step to reduce the risk of cardiovascular disease should be simple dietary and lifestyle modifications that affect blood pressure. A variety of dietary modifications have been demonstrated to be beneficial in the treatment of hypertension, but the single modification most likely to be helpful in blood pressure reduction is sodium restriction. Limiting sodium has been associated with mean decreases in systolic and diastolic blood pressures by 4.1 mm Hg and 2.5 mm Hg, respectively. A 1,600-mg sodium Dietary Approaches to Stop Hypertension (DASH) eating plan has effects similar to single-drug antihypertensive therapy.

All hypertensive patients should be encouraged to maintain high rather than reduced potassium intake. Potassium supplementation has been shown to decrease systolic and diastolic blood pressures by a mean of 3.3 mm Hg and 2.1 mm Hg, respectively. Maintenance of adequate potassium balance may be important in hypertensive patients independent of the possible increase in the risk of sudden death associated with hypokalemia. Potassium supplements may be indicated, both for blood pressure control and vascular disease prevention, in patients who ingest a high-sodium, low-potassium diet. This combination is particularly common in blacks who, compared to whites, have a higher incidence of hypertension and are at greater risk for hypertensive cardiovascular complications.

Both dietary and nondietary calcium supplements have a minimal effect on blood pressure. This effect is too small to recommend the use of these supplements to treat hypertension. Calcium supplements, as opposed to dietary calcium, also may slightly increase the risk of kidney stones in susceptible individuals.

Although magnesium supplementation has been shown to cause vasodilation, it has not been proven to be a clinically effective antihypertensive agent. Mild hypomagnesemia is a common electrolyte abnormality, particularly in elderly individuals who may have increased urinary magnesium losses because of diuretic therapy or interstitial renal disease. Whether this abnormality should be treated or prevented with prophylactic magnesium administration is unclear.

High-dose fish oil (50 mL containing 15 g of n-3 polyunsaturated fatty acids, such as eicosapentaenoic acid), not low-dose fish oil or safflower oil, produced an average decline in systolic and diastolic blood pressures of 6.5 mm Hg and 4.4 mm Hg, respectively. This response was associated with a fall in the levels of the vasoconstrictor thromboxane A2. For hypertensive patients, increased consumption of fish in combination with weight loss may have additive effects on blood pressure reduction and a variety of protective cardiovascular effects. A separate issue is whether fish intake has a beneficial effect on cardiovascular disease in general. Data suggest that fish intake may be associated with a reduced risk of fatal myocardial infarction, sudden death, and total mortality.

Recent research has focused on patients identified as having prehypertension. The Trials of Hypertension Prevention phase II studied a group who had systolic and diastolic blood pressures less than 140 mm Hg and 83–89 mm Hg, respectively, and who were 110–165% of ideal body weight. The patients were randomized to usual care, sodium restriction, weight reduction, or both. Compared with usual care, combined therapy of sodium restriction and weight reduction resulted in the greatest decrease in blood pressure.

Viewed together, these observations suggest that diet plays an important role in many susceptible patients in the genesis of hypertension. Weight reduction and salt restriction may both lower the blood pressure and have an additive effect when used in conjunction with antihypertensive medications. A diet rich in fruits and vegetables and low-fat dairy products is beneficial. One additional important lifestyle modification is cessation of smoking. Although smoking itself does not appear to cause persistent hypertension, it markedly increases the cardiovascular risk in hypertensive patients. If these strategies are not successful, then pharmacologic intervention is indicated.

Chobanian AV, Bakris GL, Black HR, Cushman WC, Green LA, Izzo JL Jr, et al. The seventh report of the Joint National Committee on Prevention, Detection, Evaluation, and Treatment of High Blood Pressure: the JNC 7 report. National Heart, Lung, and Blood Institute Joint National Committee on Prevention, Detection, Evaluation, and Treatment of High Blood Pressure; National High Blood Pressure Education Program Coordinating Committee [published erratum appears in JAMA 2003;290:197]. JAMA 2003;289:2560–72.

Effects of weight loss and sodium reduction intervention on blood pressure and hypertension incidence in overweight people with high–normal blood pressure. The Trials of Hypertension Prevention, phase II.

The Trials of Hypertension Prevention Collaborative Research Group. Arch Intern Med 1997;157:657–67.

Geleijnse JM, Kok FJ, Grobbee DE. Blood pressure response to changes in sodium and potassium intake: a metaregression analysis of randomised trials. J Hum Hypertens 2003;17:471–80.

He FJ, MacGregor GA. Fortnightly review: beneficial effects of potassium. BMJ 2001;323:497–501.

Knapp HR, FitzGerald GA. The antihypertensive effects of fish oil. A controlled study of polyunsaturated fatty acid supplements in essential hypertension. N Engl J Med 1989;320:1037–43.

Kotchen TA, McCarron DA. Dietary electrolytes and blood pressure: a statement for healthcare professionals from the American Heart Association Nutrition Committee. Circulation 1998;98:613–7.

Sacks FM, Svetkey LP, Vollmer WM, Appel LJ, Bray GA, Harsha D, et al. Effects on blood pressure of reduced dietary sodium and the Dietary Approaches to Stop Hypertension (DASH) diet. DASH—Sodium Collaborative Research Group. N Engl J Med 2001;344:3–10.

# 124
## Informed consent

A 42-year-old school principal was considering a hysterectomy for uterine leiomyoma. Her physician advised her that this procedure is the definitive treatment for her symptoms of menorrhagia. She was counseled and given written information on the possibility of injury to other abdominal organs. During the surgery, a ureteral transection occurred, and the patient successfully pursued a lawsuit based on inadequate informed consent. The element missing from her preoperative discussion was

     (A) assessment of competence
\*   (B) discussion of alternatives
     (C) discussion of benefits
     (D) discussion of risks
     (E) discussion of physician's professional liability history

The basis of the doctrine of informed consent is that any competent individual has the right to determine what shall be done to her body. The informed consent process is applicable to all surgical procedures and some medical treatments whether in the hospital or in the office. It should be understood as a process and not simply the signing of a consent form, which does not address all the issues involved in the care of the patient and which she may not understand fully. For proper informed consent, the physician must explain to the patient the risks and benefits of the proposed procedure, as well as the health implications if she refuses therapy.

Assessment of competence is part of assessing the patient's ability to give consent. All risks that a reasonable person would expect to be made aware of must be discussed. The alternative therapies also must be presented to the patient. In the case presented, there was no discussion of the alternatives, including expectant management, medical treatment, or uterine artery embolization, any of which might have avoided ureteral injury. Informed consent discussions should use language a patient can understand. It often helps to have the patient repeat back to you her understanding of the situation in her own words. In addition, documentation in the chart of the discussion, perhaps with the patient's signature, is just as important as the standard consent form.

In the case under discussion, even though risks and benefits were discussed, this was not adequate consent, because alternative treatments were not discussed with the patient. The physician's professional liability history is not part of the informed consent process.

American College of Obstetricians and Gynecologists. Informed consent. In: Ethics in obstetrics and gynecology. 2nd ed. Washington, DC: ACOG; 2004. p. 9–17.

Finkelstein D, Smith MK, Faden R. Informed consent and medical ethics. Arch Ophthalmol 1993;111:324–6.

Gold JA. Informed consent. Arch Ophthalmol 1993;111:321–3.

Informed refusal. ACOG Committee Opinion No. 306. American College of Obstetricians and Gynecologists. Obstet Gynecol 2004; 104:1465–6.

# 125

## Domestic violence

A 33-year-old woman comes to your office for evaluation of headaches and panic attacks. She reports that she lives with her husband and is home all day with her three small children. She says that there is a great deal of tension with her husband and that they have many arguments. She describes him as very jealous and controlling, limiting her contact with friends and family. Last night he threw her against the wall when he accused her of looking at someone else when they were out. She states that she remains with her husband because he has a job that provides health insurance and he is her only source of income. She says she does not want to leave him. She believes that he would never hurt the children and she will be all right. This patient's stage of behavior can be described best as

* (A) precontemplation
  (B) contemplation
  (C) preparation
  (D) action
  (E) relapse

Approximately 31% of women experience domestic violence at some stage of their life, and 68% of incidents result in physical injury, more than any other violent crime. Only approximately 30% of women seek help after the first or second attack. Up to 25% of all female emergency department visits are related to domestic violence. In one study, one third of the women who attended a general practice had experienced physical violence from a male partner, and most incidents were not identified by the general practitioner. Women who have been pregnant in the past year are at high risk for physical violence, double the risk of nonpregnant women. Because the risk during pregnancy is so high, screening for domestic violence is a critical component of prenatal care that should be carried out in each trimester.

Studies show that less than 10% of primary care providers screen for domestic violence. Reported barriers to screening are frustration with the patient's denial, fear of opening "Pandora's box," and the overwhelming scope of the problem. One study demonstrated that more than 75% of women believe their providers should ask about domestic violence. For providers who are concerned about offending their patients with a domestic violence screen, the following statement can be useful: "I would like to ask you a few questions about the possibility of physical, sexual, or emotional trauma, because we know these things are common and affect women's health."

In a stage-based approach to behavior change, the goal is not to fix the problem, but rather to partner with the patient and offer her options that may help shift her perspective. This woman is in the precontemplative stage. She is not considering change because she has a partner on whom she depends. She does not recognize her husband's behavior as abusive nor does she appreciate the risks involved in staying in the relationship. She appears to be resistant, reluctant, or resigned, or she is rationalizing. At this stage, the patient is not ready for concrete action, but by inquiring about domestic violence, the physician redefines the woman's reality as being in an abusive relationship and increases her awareness of alternatives.

In the contemplative stage, the patient is ambivalent about change. She recognizes the abusive relationship as a problem and has an increased awareness of the advantages and disadvantages of change. The patient will demonstrate an increased willingness to consider taking action, even though she is not yet ready to do so.

In the preparation stage, the patient's ambivalence toward change is lifting. The patient begins to prepare for change, to explore options, and to make plans.

In the action stage, the patient is ready to stop the abuse by separating from her abuser. At this point, the patient will follow through on referrals to a shelter for battered women, counseling, and legal help. It often takes several attempts for a woman to finally sever ties with her abuser, and relapse is frequent.

Physicians are less likely to be overwhelmed if they adopt a stage-based approach to understanding the problem of domestic violence. There will be less frustration on the physician's part when there is recognition of the progressive nature of the cycle of change. Individual physicians cannot be the sole solution to their patients' domestic violence problems. However, they can and should be able to recognize the problem and to act as a conduit for assistance, including referral to domestic vio-

lence support workers, state and local departments of social services, and legal services.

Campbell JC. Health consequences of intimate partner violence. Lancet 2002;359:1331–6.

Chrestman KR, Prins A, Koss MP. Enhancement of primary care treatment for women trauma survivors. NC-PTSD Clin Q 1996;6(4):83–6.

Wathen CN, MacMillan HL. Interventions for violence against women: scientific review. JAMA 2003;289:589–600.

Zink T, Elder N, Jacobson J, Klostermann B. Medical management of intimate partner violence considering the stages of change: precontemplation and contemplation. Ann Fam Med 2004;2:231–9.

# 126

## Indications for hepatitis B vaccine

A 35-year-old primigravid woman is enrolled in medical technology courses. She is 6 weeks pregnant. Her hepatitis B surface antibody (HBsAb) and hepatitis B surface antigen (HBsAg) test results are negative. She has never received vaccination for hepatitis B. She is due to start clinical training in the laboratory today. You advise her that the ideal time for her to receive hepatitis B vaccine would be

* (A) immediately
  (B) in the second trimester
  (C) in the third trimester
  (D) postpartum

Hepatitis B virus (HBV) is a DNA virus, which causes acute and chronic liver infections. One third of the world's population has serologic evidence of past infection. In the United States, approximately 5,000 deaths occur annually from hepatocellular carcinoma and cirrhosis as a result of chronic hepatitis B infection. Transmission is most often from sexual exposure or intravenous drug use in the United States. Occupational exposure and perinatal transmission are less common, but still occur. Before HBV vaccine was available, 15–30% of U.S. health care workers with frequent exposure to blood and body fluids had serologic evidence of hepatitis B. The incidence of new infections yearly in health care personnel without vaccine was 1%. Before universal precautions and hepatitis B vaccine were introduced, 6–8% of new infections occurred in health care personnel. Now new infections in health care workers are less than 1%.

Employees in occupations associated with increased risk of blood and body fluid exposure include health care personnel, individuals who work in laboratories with blood or tissue sample exposures, staff of institutions for the developmentally disabled, morticians, public safety employees (ie, police, emergency medical service providers, firefighters), and commercial sex workers. Individ-

uals in these high-risk occupations may be screened for immunity with anti-HBs and, if negative, offered vaccine. The Occupational Safety and Health Administration requires that HBV immunization be offered to personnel at risk of exposure to blood and body fluids at no cost to the employee and prohibits employers from requiring serologic testing before vaccination.

A number of medical conditions and lifestyles place patients at higher risk of HBV infection:

- Individuals with a history of sexually transmitted diseases
- Household contacts of HBV-infected individuals
- Hemodialysis patients
- Intravenous drug users
- Immigrants from endemic countries
- Men who have sex with men
- Sexual partners of HBV-infected individuals
- Individuals who have had more than one sexual partner in the previous 6 months

All of these at-risk individuals should be offered vaccination if they have not already been immunized.

Perinatal infection occurs only when the mother is HBsAg positive. Infectivity to the infant is higher when the mother is also hepatitis e antigen (HBeAg) positive (90% if the mother is HBeAg positive and 10% if the mother is HBeAg negative). Most vertical transmission occurs at birth. Vaccination of infants and administration of hepatitis B immune globulin (HBIG) at birth prevents approximately 97% of infections. Up to 90% of infants of mothers who contract hepatitis B in the last trimester of pregnancy develop chronic hepatitis unless they receive prophylaxis at birth. Breastfeeding is compatible with HBsAg-positive mothers. All mothers should be screened for HBsAg during pregnancy.

The HBV vaccine is made from noninfectious particles of HBsAg obtained from recombinant technology. Recombivax and Engerix-B are the vaccines currently available. There is no infectivity to the patient or her fetus. These are not live attenuated vaccines and are not derived from plasma. The vaccine is safe in pregnancy. Adults receive three intramuscular (upper arm) doses of vaccine at 0, 1, and 6 months. Contraindications to vaccination are previous anaphylactic reactions to the vaccine or to yeast.

The protocol for hepatitis B prophylaxis for percutaneous or mucosal exposure depends on knowledge of the source HBsAg status or the source risk for having acute or chronic hepatitis B. Treatment is not modified for the pregnant patient with exposure because both hepatitis B vaccine and immune globulin are safe in pregnancy.

This patient with risk of occupational exposure to hepatitis B should begin the HBV vaccine series immediately. The vaccine is safe in all trimesters of pregnancy, and the benefits of preventing maternal and neonatal infection if the mother is exposed are great. Both maternal and neonatal acute and chronic disease may be avoided. If the pregnant patient is exposed to hepatitis B before completion of her series of three HBV vaccinations and seroconversion, she also may receive the HBIG.

Gartner LM, Morton J, Lawrence RA, Naylor AJ, O'Hare D, Schanler RJ, et al. Breastfeeding and the use of human milk. American Academy of Pediatrics Section on Breastfeeding. Pediatrics 2005;115:496–506.

Lin KW, Kirchner JT. Hepatitis B. Am Fam Phys 2004;69:75–82.

Tillett J. The use of vaccines in pregnancy. J Perinat Neonat Nurs 2004; 18:216–29.

Zimmerman RK, Ahwesh ER. Adult vaccination, part 2: vaccines for persons at high risk. Teaching Immunization for Medical Education (TIME) Project. J Fam Pract 2000;49(9 suppl):S51–S63; quiz S64.

# 127

## Atypical gastroesophageal reflux disease

A 35-year-old active woman with mild adult-onset asthma presents with chest pain that has grown worse over the past several months. Her pain occurs in the middle of her chest, lasts for a few hours, and sometimes occurs at night. She occasionally coughs at night as well as during the day, but she denies fever, chills, or sputum production. She has tried antacids with significant improvement. She has had minimal improvement with her albuterol metered-dose inhaler and notes that her asthma has seemed worse during this time. On physical examination, the patient has only a few scattered wheezes. The most appropriate diagnostic step is

 (A) endoscopy
 (B) stress thallium cardiac evaluation
 (C) chest X-ray
 (D) trial of long-acting bronchodilator
* (E) trial of proton pump inhibitor

Chronic reflux of acid into the esophagus may be associated with significant complications of erosive esophagitis, stricture, and Barrett esophagus. Whether or not the patient presents with classic gastroesophageal reflux symptoms, such as heartburn or any extraesophageal symptoms, early diagnosis and intervention are imperative to prevent complications.

The evaluation of symptoms should be the primary method for diagnosing gastroesophageal reflux disease (GERD) because, for a large proportion of patients, the disorder will not be diagnosed by endoscopy. Endoscopy can be falsely negative in 50–66% of patients with clinically significant reflux. Nonetheless, endoscopy is important to identify cancer or alternative diagnoses and, therefore, it is indicated in a patient with alarm symptoms, such as weight loss or dysphagia, or in a patient older than 50 years with new symptoms.

Heartburn, the burning feeling rising from the stomach or lower chest toward the neck, is the hallmark symptom of GERD. The clustering of symptoms during the postprandial period and their prompt relief by antacids point to GERD as the correct diagnosis. Despite these classic symptoms, a substantial proportion of patients with GERD exhibit a broad spectrum of less classic, extraesophageal symptoms. Extraesophageal symptoms include manifestations related to the pulmonary system, noncardiac chest pain, and ear, nose, and throat problems (Boxes 127-1 and 127-2). An awareness of these associated signs and symptoms is critical in the identification and diagnosis of GERD.

This patient with asthma presents with new onset chest pain that is intermittent, occurs sometimes at night, and is relieved with antacids. Epidemiologic studies have shown a significant association of GERD and asthma. In patients with asthma, the prevalence of symptoms of GERD ranges from 65% to 72%. In some patients, both asthma and GERD are present and unrelated; in others, both diseases are present with one exacerbating the other. Exacerbation of asthma because of GERD may occur from esophageal acid-induced bronchoconstriction, neural enhancement of bronchial reactivity, or microaspiration. It has been demonstrated that GERD may cause or exacerbate asthma. Studies have shown symptom improvement with proton pump inhibitor therapy. The constellation of symptoms should prompt the clinician to suspect GERD as an exacerbating factor.

Traditional approaches for treatment of reflux disease have begun with changes in lifestyle and diet with eventual progression to medications in a step-wise fashion. For diagnostic and therapeutic reasons, many experts now recommend an initial trial with a proton pump inhibitor, and this should be the initial therapy of choice for the patient described. To determine if asthma is related to reflux, a 3-month trial with a proton pump inhibitor twice daily is recommended.

Cardiac testing (eg, a stress thallium examination) is necessary when coronary artery disease is suspected. In this fairly young patient, the pain is not anginal in character and is not associated with activity. Although a chest X-ray is a diagnostic option, pneumonia would be less likely with this type of chest pain and with no history of fever or sputum production. Congestive heart failure would be unlikely without additional symptoms of fatigue, shortness of breath, or peripheral edema.

Long-acting bronchodilators can be used to improve asthmatic control for up to 12 hours. However, this patient does not get relief from a bronchodilator such as albuterol; therefore, a longer-acting medication would not be likely to provide any improvement because her worsened symptoms are triggered by reflux.

---

**BOX 127-1**

### Extraesophageal Manifestations of Gastroesophageal Reflux Disease

Pulmonary symptoms
- Asthma (nonseasonal, nonallergic)
- Chronic bronchitis
- Aspiration pneumonia
- Bronchiectasis
- Pulmonary fibrosis
- Chronic obstructive pulmonary disease
- Pneumonia

Ear, nose, and throat symptoms
- Chronic cough
- Laryngitis
- Hoarseness
- Globus
- Pharyngitis
- Sinusitis
- Vocal cord granuloma
- Laryngeal carcinoma (possible)

Other symptoms
- Noncardiac chest pain
- Dental erosion
- Sleep apnea

---

Reprinted from American Journal of Medicine, Vol. 117(suppl 5A), Nord HJ, "Extraesophageal symptoms: what role for the proton pump inhibitors?" pages 56S–62S, Copyright © 2004, with permission from Excerpta Medica Inc.)

---

**BOX 127-2**

### Clinical Clues to Gastroesophageal Reflux-Related Asthma

Asthma symptoms manifesting in adulthood
No family history of asthma
Diagnosis of reflux disease that precedes onset or diagnosis of asthma
Asthma worsening with eating, exercise, or supine posture
Nocturnal respiratory symptoms
Pharmacologic agents such as theophylline or $\beta_2$-agonists have no effect on or worsen asthma
Difficult-to-control asthma symptoms requiring systemic corticosteroids
Absence of an allergic component to asthma symptoms

---

Reprinted from American Journal of Medicine, Vol. 117(suppl 5A), Nord HJ, "Extraesophageal symptoms: what role for the proton pump inhibitors?" pages 56S–62S, Copyright © 2004, with permission from Excerpta Medica Inc.)

An evidence-based appraisal of reflux disease management—the Genval Workshop Report. Gut 1999;44(suppl 2):S1–16.

Dent J. Definitions of reflux disease and its separation from dyspepsia. Gut 2002;50(suppl 4):iv17–20; discussion iv21–2.

Nord HJ. Extraesophageal symptoms: what role for the proton pump inhibitors? Am J Med 2004;117(Suppl 5A):56S–62S.

# 128

## Alcohol and drug screening

A 28-year-old woman comes to your office for her first prenatal visit at 6 weeks of gestation. She states that she and her fiancé "like to party a lot." You ask her if she has been drinking or taking drugs more than she has meant to in the past year and she hesitatingly says she has. She reports that she needs to cut down on her drinking, especially now that she is pregnant. You ask her what she knows about the risks of alcohol exposure to her developing fetus. You offer her additional information that includes the recommendation for abstinence during pregnancy. She responds that curtailing her drinking will not be a problem and indicates that she does not consume that much alcohol. The most appropriate screening tool for this patient is the

   (A) T-ACE questionnaire
   (B) CAGE questionnaire
 *  (C) TWEAK questionnaire
   (D) Conjoint Screening Test
   (E) Alcohol Use Disorders Identification Test (AUDIT)

It is well documented that maternal prenatal alcohol use is a leading cause of birth defects and developmental disabilities. The Centers for Disease Control and Prevention (CDC) estimate that 1 in 1,000 U.S. babies are born with fetal alcohol syndrome. Studies demonstrate that even low levels of prenatal alcohol exposure can affect the developing fetus negatively. Because no safe level has been identified, the U.S. Surgeon General recommends abstinence from preconception through completion of pregnancy.

The CDC's 2002 Behavioral Risk Factor Surveillance System (BRFSS) results indicate that half of all reproductive-aged women are drinkers and 21% are binge drinkers. Studies report that 10–20% of women admit to drinking alcohol during pregnancy, and that 19% consume alcohol in the first trimester. These findings led the U.S. Preventive Services Task Force (USPSTF) to recommend that all adults and pregnant women have primary care screening for alcohol and drug use as an essential component of preventive and preconception care.

Several reliable and valid screening tools are available for primary caregivers to assess alcohol and drug misuse. The best method is one that is easy and is used on a regular basis. In the initial interview of the patient described, two questions required by the Conjoint Screening Test were included:

• In the past year, have you ever drunk or used drugs more than you meant to?

• In the past year, have you felt you wanted or needed to cut down on your drinking or drug use?

A positive response to these two questions detects substance abuse with nearly 80% specificity and sensitivity.

The Conjoint Screening Test is an excellent tool to determine which patients would benefit from further screening. Because this patient has already answered these two questions affirmatively, she requires more comprehensive screening. More extensive queries will help the physician decide the appropriate level of intervention.

Several screening tools have been developed to assess alcohol and drug use: the CAGE, AUDIT, TWEAK, and T-ACE questionnaires (Boxes 128-1–4, respectively). However, the screening tools that have been validated for use in women are the TWEAK, T-ACE, and AUDIT questionnaires. The TWEAK questionnaire was developed specifically for use in pregnancy and has been shown to

---

**BOX 128-1**

**Substance Abuse Questionnaire: CAGE**

**C**  Have you ever felt you ought to **C**ut down on your drinking?

**A**  Have people **A**nnoyed you by criticizing your drinking?

**G**  Have you ever felt bad or **G**uilty about your drinking?

**E**  Have you ever had a drink first thing in the morning to steady your nerves or get rid of a hangover (**E**ye opener)?

Two or more affirmative responses are indicative of alcoholism; however, even one positive response calls for further investigation.

Ewing JA. Detecting alcoholism: the CAGE questionnaire. JAMA 1984;252:1907. Copyright 1984, American Medical Association

## BOX 128-2

### Substance Abuse Questionnaire: AUDIT

1. How often do you have a drink containing alcohol?
   - (0) Never
   - (1) Monthly or less
   - (2) 2–4 times per month
   - (3) 2 to 3 times per week
   - (4) 4 or more times per week

2. How many drinks containing alcohol do you have on a typical day when you are drinking?
   - (0) 1 or 2
   - (1) 3 or 4
   - (2) 5 or 6
   - (3) 7 to 9
   - (4) 10 or more

3. How often do you have six or more drinks on one occasion?
   - (0) Never
   - (1) Less than monthly
   - (2) Monthly
   - (3) Weekly
   - (4) Daily or almost daily

4. How often during the past year have you found that you were not able to stop drinking once you started?
   - (0) Never
   - (1) Less than monthly
   - (2) Monthly
   - (3) Weekly
   - (4) Daily or almost daily

5. How often during the past year have you failed to do what was normally expected from you because of drinking?
   - (0) Never
   - (1) Less than monthly
   - (2) Monthly
   - (3) Weekly
   - (4) Daily or almost daily

6. How often during the past year have you needed a first drink in the morning to get yourself going after a heavy drinking session?
   - (0) Never
   - (1) Less than monthly
   - (2) Monthly
   - (3) Weekly
   - (4) Daily or almost daily

7. How often during the past year have you had a feeling of guilt or remorse after drinking?
   - (0) Never
   - (1) Less than monthly
   - (2) Monthly
   - (3) Weekly
   - (4) Daily or almost daily

8. How often during the past year have you been unable to remember what happened the night before because you had been drinking?
   - (0) Never
   - (1) Less than monthly
   - (2) Monthly
   - (3) Weekly
   - (4) Daily or almost daily

9. Have you or someone else been injured as a result of your drinking?
   - (0) No
   - (2) Yes, but not in the past year
   - (4) Yes, during the past year

10. Has a relative or friend, or a doctor or other health care worker been concerned about your drinking or suggested you cut down?
   - (0) No
   - (2) Yes, but not in the past year
   - (4) Yes, during the past year

The minimum score (for nondrinkers) on the AUDIT is 0 and the maximum possible score is 40. A score of 8 or more indicates a strong likelihood of hazardous or harmful alcohol consumption. (Available online at http://www.niaaa.nih.gov/publications/insaudit.htm.)

Reprinted with permission from World Health Organization. AUDIT, the Alcohol Use Disorders Identification Test: guidelines for use in primary health care. 2nd ed. Geneva: WHO; 2000.

be the most reliable and valid screening tool in identifying harmful drinking in pregnant women. It is the questionnaire that would be most appropriate for the woman under discussion.

The TWEAK questionnaire is superior to the T-ACE questionnaire because it incorporates a question about blackouts, which serve as a marker of severity. Both the

TWEAK and T-ACE questionnaires have a tolerance question that is important for circumventing the denial that can be provoked by more direct questions. Because pregnant women have been told that drinking is unsafe for their baby, they may downplay the amount of their drinking. Asking, "How many drinks does it take to make you feel high?" (T-ACE) or "How many drinks can you

BOX 128-3

**Substance Abuse Questionnaire: TWEAK**

| | |
|---|---|
| **T** | **T**olerance: How many drinks can you hold? If five or more drinks—score 2 points |
| **W** | Have close friends or relatives **W**orried or complained about your drinking in the past year? If "Yes"—score 2 points |
| **E** | **E**ye Opener: Do you sometimes take a drink in the morning when you get up? If "Yes"—score 1 point |
| **A** | **A**mnesia: Has a friend or family member every told you about things you said or did while you were drinking that you could not remember? If "Yes"—score 1 point |
| **K (C)** | Do you sometimes feel the need to **C**ut down on your drinking? If "Yes"—score 1 point. |

The TWEAK is used to screen for pregnant at-risk drinking defined here as the consumption of 1 ounce or more of alcohol per day while pregnant. A total score of 2 or more points indicates a positive screen for pregnancy risk drinking.

Reprinted with permission from Chan AW, Pristach EA, Welte JW, Russell M. Use of the TWEAK test in screening for alcoholism/heavy drinking in three populations. Alcohol Clin Exp Res 1993;17:1188–92.

BOX 128-4

**Substance Abuse Questionnaire: T-ACE**

| | |
|---|---|
| **T** | **T**olerance: How many drinks does it take to make you feel high? More than two drinks is a positive response—score 2 points |
| **A** | Have people **A**nnoyed you by criticizing your drinking? If "Yes"—score 1 point. |
| **C** | Have you ever felt you ought to **C**ut down on your drinking? If "Yes"—score 1 point. |
| **E** | **E**ye opener: Have you ever had a drink first thing in the morning to steady your nerves or get rid of a hangover? If "Yes"—score 1 point. |

A total score of 2 or more points indicates a positive screen for pregnancy risk drinking.

Reprinted from Am J Obstet Gynecol, Vol 160, Sokol RJ, Martier SS, Ager JW. The T-ACE questions: practical prenatal detection of risk drinking. p. 863-8; discussion 868–70, 1989, with permission from Elsevier.

hold?" (TWEAK) is more sensitive for detecting risky drinking than asking, "Have you ever felt you ought to cut down on your drinking?" (CAGE).

Although the CAGE questionnaire is the most popular tool to screen for alcohol misuse in primary care settings, it has been demonstrated to be less effective in identifying drinking problems among women. The CAGE questionnaire also is less sensitive for early problem drinking or heavy drinking than the AUDIT questionnaire. Because the AUDIT questionnaire screens for quantity, frequency, and binge drinking behaviors, it offers high sensitivity for harmful or hazardous drinking. However, it has the disadvantage of being longer and therefore less convenient for daily use.

The obstetrician–gynecologist has an opportunity to create a respectful environment for women to have an open dialogue about substance use. Supportive inquiry

opens the door to referral and treatment. Physicians should assume that, although many women do not welcome a pregnancy and over one half of pregnancies are unplanned, all women want a healthy baby. The goal of Healthy People 2000 was to increase the obstetrics screening rate from 34% in 1987 to 75% in 2000. This goal was not met. Routine screening for alcohol and drug consumption among women of childbearing age should be a standard component of provider practice. Obstetric providers should screen at the initiation of prenatal care and continue to screen throughout the pregnancy if a substance abuse issue is identified.

Bradley KA, Boyd-Wickizer J, Powell SH, Burman ML. Alcohol screening questionnaires in women: a critical review. JAMA 1998; 280:166–71.

Brown RL, Leonard T, Saunders LA, Papasouliotis O. A two-item conjoint screen for alcohol and other drug problems. J Am Board Fam Pract 2001;14:95–106.

Screening and behavioral counseling interventions in primary care to reduce alcohol misuse: recommendation statement. U.S. Preventive Services Task Force. Ann Intern Med 2004;140:554–6.

Taylor P, Zaichkin J, Baily D, editors. Substance abuse during pregnancy: guidelines for screening. Revised ed. Olympia (WA): Washington State Department of Health; 2002.

# 129

## Appropriate therapy for dysmenorrhea

A 34-year-old nulliparous woman consults you in regard to worsening secondary dysmenorrhea that she has experienced for the past 8 months. Her pain begins approximately 4 days before the onset of menses and peaks with her second day of flow. Initially, the pain resolved at completion of her menses but in the past few months it has persisted at a lower level well into the next cycle. She describes the pain as midline cramping with some rectal pain and a sense of constipation during menses. She would like to maintain fertility. Oral contraceptives were initiated 4 months ago on advice from her primary care provider with little relief of symptoms. Her history is negative for abnormal cervical cytology, sexually transmitted diseases, or gynecologic procedures. Her medical history is significant for severe asthma for which she is on several regular medications. Pelvic examination reveals no detectable masses and a normal size retroverted uterus. There is mild posterior tenderness on rectovaginal examination but no nodularity. The most appropriate next step is

      (A) laparoscopy
      (B) medroxyprogesterone acetate
      (C) hysterectomy with adnexectomy
*    (D) gonadotropin-releasing hormone (GnRH) therapy
      (E) danazol (Danocrine) therapy

Dysmenorrhea is defined as abnormal pain with menses. An important component of the differential diagnosis of secondary dysmenorrhea is endometriosis. Endometriosis is defined as endometrial glands and stroma present outside the endometrial cavity. These glands and stroma continue to respond to cyclic menstrual hormones and result in inflammation, adhesion formation, and an influx of hemosiderin laden macrophages. The condition is associated with secondary dysmenorrhea, pelvic pain, and infertility.

Endometriosis occurs in 7–10% of women in the general population. Its etiology is debated in the literature. Prevailing theories include retrograde menstruation, hematogenous or lymphatic spread, coelomic metaplasia, and genetic origin. The condition is more common in women with menorrhagia, any type of cervical or vaginal outflow obstruction, and early menarche. Because the condition is estrogen-dependent, patients with decreased estrogen (eg, athletes, individuals with eating disorders, and tobacco smokers) have a lower rate of the condition. Endometriosis is characterized by secondary dysmenorrhea that starts before menses in the late luteal phase, peaks with onset of menses, and then dissipates in the follicular phase. Some women with endometriosis report deep dyspareunia during menses, sacral back pain, and perimenstrual diarrhea or tenesmus. An association between the degree or location of endometriosis and the degree of a patient's pain has not been documented. Many women with endometriosis, even severe cases, are asymptomatic while some women with less evident disease experience great pain. It is known, however, that deeply infiltrating endometriosis is more likely to be associated with pain.

The only way to confirm the presence of endometriosis is by histologic confirmation. This is typically accomplished by laparoscopy and biopsy. Experience with visualizing endometriosis improves the accuracy of laparoscopic diagnosis because the disease has many symptoms. However, visual confirmation alone is inadequate because it is quite common to find endometriosis histologically on biopsy sample of normal-appearing peritoneum.

Because the symptoms of endometriosis include secondary dysmenorrhea and the disease is a hormonally responsive condition, initial empiric therapy is identical to that of simple dysmenorrhea. The options include oral contraceptives, nonsteroidal antiinflammatory agents (NSAIDs), and progestins. The hormonal medications suppress the estrogen-predominant hormonal cycle and can reduce the size of endometriosis lesions. In particular, women with mild endometriosis are excellent candidates for these initial therapies. When effective, oral contraceptives and medroxyprogesterone acetate typically demonstrate relief within 3 months. When they fail, second-line therapies include danazol (Danocrine), depot medroxyprogesterone acetate (Depo-Provera), and GnRH agonists. Each has a fairly high efficacy for reducing symptoms. Danazol has been shown to be equal to GnRH agonists for relief of symptoms; however, it has a significantly higher side effect profile and is usually poorly tolerated by patients. Depot medroxyprogesterone acetate has a similar efficacy to medroxyprogesterone acetate and carries with it a significant side effect profile including weight gain and a tendency to exacerbate depression. All hormonal therapies for endometriosis impact a patient's fertility while she is taking them because all affect the ovulatory cycle.

Another option in patients who fail first-line therapy is laparoscopy. The advantage of laparoscopy is that it can function as a diagnostic and therapeutic maneuver. Disadvantages include the fact that laparoscopy can fail to make the diagnosis in cases where the appearance of disease is atypical and that effective therapy depends on the surgeon's skill. The effectiveness of medical vs surgical therapy for symptom relief in patients who wish to maintain long-term fertility is the subject of debate. It is known that surgical intervention for endometriosis results in significant reduction of symptoms in the first 6 months postoperatively. Approximately 44% of patients, however, will have recurrent symptoms within a year. Two thirds will have recurrence within 2 years. The recurrence rate of symptoms that require retreatment is 53% in the first 5 years after discontinuation of GnRH agonist therapy. No long-term data are available on symptom relief after discontinuation of oral contraceptives, medroxyprogesterone acetate, or danazol. However, treatment with oral contraceptives, danazol, or progestins after either surgical or GnRH agonist therapy has been shown to reduce recurrent symptoms in the short term.

A major component of effective surgical intervention is the expertise of the surgeon in recognizing endometriosis and eradicating all lesions. In recent years, research has examined whether empiric medical therapy without definitive surgical diagnosis and treatment is an efficacious and cost-effective option. Arguments against the use of surgery for endometriosis include the known imprecision of surgical diagnosis and risks of surgery and anesthesia. If effective, empiric therapy is a good option for endometriosis because the consequences of an inaccurate diagnosis are minimal. The therapies for dysmenorrhea are essentially the same as for endometriosis so that, at the very least, the symptom is being addressed. It is important in considering empiric therapy to rule out other causes of pelvic pain such as gastrointestinal and urologic disorders and sexually transmitted diseases.

One well-designed prospective randomized controlled trial demonstrated that after an appropriate evaluation to rule out other causes and failure of first-line oral contraceptives and NSAIDs, empiric therapy with GnRH agonists was effective. This treatment method achieved clinically and statistically significant reduction in symptoms including dysmenorrhea and pelvic tenderness. If the patient failed to respond to the initial therapy of oral contraceptives and NSAIDs, subsequent laparoscopy revealed the presence of endometriosis 87% of the time. Adhesions and cul-de-sac obliteration were present in an additional 9% of patients, which brought the total number of patients likely to have endometriosis to 96%. Thus, GnRH agonists may be successfully used as a diagnostic and therapeutic agent in patients who fail first-line therapy for endometriosis with NSAIDs and oral contraceptives. This method identified the patients with endometriosis without initial surgical diagnosis. Although a cost-effectiveness study to compare these methods has not been done, it is believed that 3 months of GnRH agonist therapy is less costly than laparoscopy.

The patient described has a history suspicious for endometriosis. In addition, she has uterosacral tenderness, which is strongly associated with this diagnosis. Her physical examination otherwise is consistent with mild endometriosis. She wishes to maintain fertility and has a medical history that puts her at a higher risk of complications with surgery (ie, her history of asthma). This patient is thus an excellent candidate for GnRH agonist therapy with a high likelihood of symptomatic relief.

Hysterectomy with adnexectomy is the definitive therapy for endometriosis. It should be, however, the last line of therapy, because it requires the most intervention. In addition, this patient wishes to maintain fertility and this option would leave her incapable of having a child of her own.

American College of Obstetricians and Gynecologists. Medical management of endometriosis. ACOG Practice Bulletin No. 11. Washington, DC: ACOG; 1999.

Bulletti C, Flamigni C, Polli V, Giacomucci E, Albonetti A, Negrini V, et al. The efficacy of drugs in the management of endometriosis. J Am Assoc Gynecol Laparosc 1996;3:495–501.

Sutton CJ, Ewen SP, Whitelaw N, Haines P. Prospective, randomized, double-blind, controlled trial of laser laparoscopy in the treatment of pelvic pain associated with minimal, mild, and moderate endometriosis. Fertil Steril 1994;62:696–700.

Sutton CJ, Pooley AS, Ewen SP, Haines P. Follow-up report on a randomized controlled trial of laser laparoscopy in the treatment of pelvic pain associated with minimal to moderate endometriosis. Fertil Steril 1997;68:1070–4.

# 130

## Cervical length screening

A 32-year-old woman, gravida 2, para 1, sees you for her first obstetric visit. She is currently 8 weeks pregnant with unsure dates and healthy. Her prior pregnancy was uncomplicated and delivered vaginally at term. She has no history of sexually transmitted diseases, abnormal cytology, or gynecologic procedures. Her examination is normal. Transvaginal ultrasonography reveals a singleton gestation with crown–rump length consistent with 8 weeks of gestation. The ultrasound technician, noting a subjectively short cervical length, measures it. This reveals a cervical length of 2.5 cm without funneling. Given the ultrasound finding, the best workup would be

      (A) ultrasonographic measurement of cervical length at 11–12 weeks of gestation
      (B) ultrasonographic measurement of cervical length at 12–14 weeks of gestation
  *  (C) ultrasonographic measurement of cervical length at 16–20 weeks of gestation
      (D) cerclage at 16–17 weeks of gestation
      (E) no further workup

*Cervical insufficiency* or *incompetence* is defined as the inability of the uterine cervix to retain a pregnancy to term. The diagnosis of cervical insufficiency has been based historically on the presence of painless cervical dilation. This symptom combined with the history of cervical trauma is highly suggestive of the diagnosis. Assessment of risk as well as screening for this and other etiologies of preterm birth is not well described because of incomplete and often conflicting data in the literature.

Various studies have been performed to attempt to delineate an appropriate screening test for cervical insufficiency. Transvaginal ultrasonographic measurement of the cervix has been investigated because it is objective, repeatable, and widely available. Such measurement of the cervix during pregnancy in normal women has revealed a wide range of normal lengths for the cervix during the first 20 weeks of gestation. It is thought that some of the difficulty in measuring the cervix at this early gestational age relates to the difficulty differentiating between the cervix and the lower uterine segment myometrium through the mid-second trimester. Thus, ultrasonographic measurements of cervical length before 16–20 weeks of gestation are not considered very precise or accurate. One study demonstrated a mean cervical length of 4 cm between 14 and 28 weeks of gestation in normal pregnancies. This average decreased after 30 weeks to between 2.5 and 3 cm. These lengths have been confirmed in other studies. It has been demonstrated that there is a correlation between cervical shortening and preterm delivery when serial ultrasonograms of the cervical length are obtained between 24 and 28 weeks of gestation.

Evidence of cervical shortening (effacement) and funneling (wedge-shaped opening at the internal os) can be measured by transvaginal ultrasonography. To elicit these changes, transfundal pressure techniques such as coughing have been used. Despite this, serial measurement of cervical length in low-risk women (ie, women without a history of early pregnancy loss) has shown low sensitivity and positive predictive value, and thus, its use in screening is limited in the low-risk group. The American College of Obstetricians and Gynecologists has recommended against the use of ultrasonography as a screening tool for cervical insufficiency in low-risk women from a lack of supporting evidence. Further unnecessary screening will only raise the patient's concerns.

Despite the lack of evidence of its effectiveness, assessment of the cervical length is often a routine component of an early ultrasound examination to confirm dating or to complete an obstetric anatomy survey. Evidence exists to support screening at 16–20 weeks of gestation for women who have a history of early pregnancy loss. If an abnormal cervical length is incidentally demonstrated in the low-risk patient before 16–20 weeks of gestation, it is recommended that the examination be repeated during that time frame given the common difficulty of distinguishing the lower uterine segment from the cervix. In cases where a short cervical length is demonstrated at or beyond 20 weeks of gestation in a low-risk patient, a workup should be initiated for preterm labor or fetal abnormalities. Cervical length measurement has been shown to be a significant prognostic indicator for preterm delivery in women with threatened preterm labor. In addition, a short cervical length (2.5 cm or less) with funneling has been shown to be a significant risk factor for even earlier preterm delivery and serious neonatal morbidity.

In this patient, the ultrasonographic finding of a cervical length of 2.5 cm is abnormal in the first trimester.

However, given that the pregnancy is very early and there is the known difficulty of distinguishing cervix from lower uterine segment at this time, it is recommended that the measurement be repeated at 16–20 weeks of gestation when the measurement is more accurate. Follow-up ultrasonographic measurement before the time frame when reliable measurement can be achieved is not useful.

In this patient, without any history to support the diagnosis of cervical insufficiency, a planned cerclage would be considered unnecessary. The risk–benefit ratio would not support such a level of intervention.

Botsis D, Papagianni V, Vitoratos N, Makrakis E, Aravantinos L, Creatsas G. Prediction of preterm delivery by sonographic estimation of cervical length. Biol Neonate 2005;88:42–5.

Cervical insufficiency. ACOG Practice Bulletin No. 48. American College of Obstetricians and Gynecologists. Obstet Gynecol 2003; 102:1091–9.

Iams JD, Johnson FF, Sonek J, Sachs L, Gebauer C, Samuels P. Cervical competence as a continuum: a study of ultrasonographic cervical length and obstetric performance. Am J Obstet Gynecol 1995;172:1097–1103; discussion 1104–6.

Iams JD, Goldenberg RL, Meis PJ, Mercer BM, Moawad A, Das A, et al. The length of the cervix and the risk of spontaneous premature delivery. National Institute of Child Health and Human Development Maternal Fetal Medicine Unit Network. N Engl J Med 1996;334: 567–72.

Romero R, Espinoza J, Erez O, Hassan S. The role of cervical cerclage in obstetric practice: can the patient who could benefit from this procedure be identified? [Editorial.] Am J Obstet Gynecol 2006;194:1–9.

Rust OA, Atlas RO, Kimmel S, Roberts WE, Hess LW. Does the presence of a funnel increase the risk of adverse perinatal outcome in a patient with a short cervix? Am J Obstet Gynecol 2005;192:1060–6.

# 131

## Management of prehypertension

A healthy 50-year-old woman comes to the office for a periodic health maintenance visit. Her blood pressure is 135/85 mm Hg. The patient has had blood pressure readings in a similar range on two other occasions in the past 6 months. The most important recommendation would be

* (A) lifestyle changes to decrease blood pressure
(B) pharmacologic therapy with one drug
(C) recheck blood pressure in 1 year
(D) renal spiral computerized tomography
(E) echocardiography for ventricular hypertrophy

The ultimate public health goal of treatment for hypertension is the reduction of cardiovascular and renal morbidity and mortality. The treatment of hypertension is the most common reason for office visits of nonpregnant adults to physicians in the United States and for use of prescription drugs. The number of patients with hypertension is likely to grow as the population ages, because either systolic hypertension or combined systolic and diastolic hypertension occurs in more than one half of individuals older than 65 years. An increased incidence of obesity also will increase the number of hypertensive individuals. Despite the prevalence of hypertension and its associated complications, control of the disease is far from adequate. Only 34% of individuals with hypertension have their blood pressure under control, defined as a level below 140/90 mm Hg. This failure reflects the inherent problem of maintaining long-term therapy for a usually asymptomatic condition, particularly when the therapy may interfere with the patient's quality of life and when its immediate benefits may not be obvious to the

patient. Thus, hypertension will likely remain the most common risk factor for heart attack and stroke.

Patients with prehypertension (systolic blood pressure 120–139 mm Hg or diastolic blood pressure 80–89 mm Hg) are treated with nonpharmacologic therapies such as weight reduction, sodium restriction, and avoidance of excess alcohol ingestion. They also should have their blood pressure measured every 12 months, because they are at significant risk for developing hypertension. The higher the blood pressure, the higher the risk. Individuals with prehypertension have a greater risk of cardiovascular events over time than do individuals with normal blood pressure. However, there is no need for further investigation, such as renal spiral computerized tomography or echocardiography for ventricular hypertrophy, in otherwise healthy individuals with prehypertension.

If lifestyle modification does not effectively lower the blood pressure of a patient with prehypertension to the target range, antihypertensive medication should be initiated if there exists a compelling indication such as diabetes mellitus or renal disease. In the absence of an indication for any other specific drug, the Antihypertensive and Lipid-Lowering Treatment to Prevent Heart Attack Trial (ALLHAT) suggested that a low-dose thiazide diuretic should be the preferred initial therapy.

Lowering the blood pressure is especially beneficial in some patients who have blood pressures near but not in the hypertensive range, primarily with concomitant conditions (eg, diabetes or chronic renal failure). The best evidence for a causal role of increasing blood pressure in cardiovascular complications is an improvement in outcome with antihypertensive therapy. Treatment studies have demonstrated the efficacy of lowering both diastolic and systolic pressures in patients with hypertension. Early treatment of hypertension is particularly important in patients with diabetes both to prevent cardiovascular disease and to minimize progression of renal disease and diabetic retinopathy. Treatment of even mild hypertension is important in patients with chronic renal failure to protect against both progressive renal failure and cardiovascular disease, which is markedly increased with even moderate chronic renal disease.

Chobanian AV, Bakris GL, Black HR, Cushman WC, Green LA, Izzo JL Jr, et al. The seventh report of the Joint National Committee on Prevention, Detection, Evaluation, and Treatment of High Blood Pressure: the JNC 7 report. National Heart, Lung, and Blood Institute Joint National Committee on Prevention, Detection, Evaluation, and Treatment of High Blood Pressure; National High Blood Pressure Education Program Coordinating Committee [published erratum appears in JAMA 2003;290:197]. JAMA 2003;289:2560–72.

Diuretic versus alpha-blocker as first-step antihypertensive therapy: final results from the Antihypertensive and Lipid-Lowering Treatment to Prevent Heart Attack Trial (ALLHAT). Antihypertensive and Lipid-Lowering Treatment to Prevent Heart Attack Trial Collaborative Research Group. Hypertension 2003;42:239–46.

# 132

## Parvovirus exposure during pregnancy

A 34-year-old woman at 19 weeks of gestation informs you that she has just been exposed to a child infected with fifth disease while at work in a child care center. Measuring titers for parvovirus B19 immunoglobulin (Ig) G and IgM found no parvovirus infection. The next step in her care is

    (A) serial obstetric ultrasonographic examinations
\*   (B) repeat the IgG titer measurement in 3–4 weeks
    (C) percutaneous umbilical blood sampling
    (D) amniocentesis for parvovirus culture of amniotic fluid

Fifth disease, also known as erythema infectiosum, is caused by parvovirus B19. The infection is transmitted by the respiratory route. Most clinically apparent infections are in school-aged children. Many adults have evidence of prior infection. Infection of pregnant women can lead to transplacental transmission of parvovirus. Clinicians should be aware of the testing and follow-up required after exposure of their pregnant patients to parvovirus B19.

In children, parvovirus B19 infection causes a characteristic rash, with erythematous facial flushing consistent with a "slapped cheek" appearance. Adults with parvovirus B19 infection have a characteristic reticular rash on the trunk along with peripheral arthropathy. Approximately one third of adults infected with parvovirus B19 are asymptomatic. Patients with an underlying hemoglobinopathy may develop a transient aplastic crisis.

Infected individuals usually are infectious for 5–10 days after exposure and before the onset of the rash. Once the rash is present, the individual is no longer infectious.

A positive immunoglobulin (Ig) M titer result provides serologic evidence of infection within 1 month. A positive IgG titer result indicates prior infection and immunity, particularly in the absence of IgM antibodies. More than 60% of adults and adolescents are seropositive for IgG. The risk of transmission from a household member infected with parvovirus B19 is 50%. In child care centers or schools, the risk of transmission may vary from 20% to 50%.

Fetal risks from maternal parvovirus B19 infection include hydrops fetalis, spontaneous abortion, and stillbirth. Transplacental transmission occurs in 33% of cases; however, the rate of fetal loss among newly infected pregnant women ranges from 2% to 9%. The most severe fetal effects occur in pregnant women infected before 20 weeks of gestation. Most fetal effects are seen within 8 weeks of infection. Teratogenic effects have not been reported in association with parvovirus B19 infection.

Maternal infection can be diagnosed by examining both IgG and IgM titers. The presence of IgM parvovirus-specific antibodies is diagnostic of primary infection. If measurement of the IgG titers is positive in the absence of IgM antibodies, previous infection has occurred and the fetus is not at risk for adverse perinatal outcome. Parvovirus B19 also can be diagnosed by the finding of characteristic nuclear inclusions within erythroblasts.

Pregnant women exposed to parvovirus B19 should have IgG titers measured to determine if immunity to infection is present. If immunity is present, no further workup is required. If the IgG titers are negative, they should be repeated in 3–4 weeks to determine if seroconversion has occurred. In the absence of seroconversion, no further maternal or fetal testing is required. In the event of seroconversion, ultrasonographic monitoring of the fetus for anemia or hydrops should be performed for 10 weeks postexposure. Development of hydrops fetalis indicates the need for percutaneous umbilical blood sampling. A fetal complete blood count plus testing for parvovirus DNA should be performed on the sample, with

transfusion of red cells as needed. Polymerase chain reaction (PCR) testing has been used on fetal samples to document infection with parvovirus B19 with high sensitivity, although data are limited.

The patient described had negative IgG and IgM antibody titer results. Percutaneous umbilical blood sampling or amniocentesis is not indicated, because there is no documented maternal infection and these tests carry significant risks to the fetus. Similarly, serial ultrasonographic evaluation of the fetus is not recommended in the absence of maternal seroconversion.

Al-Khan A, Caligiuri A, Apuzzio J. Parvovirus B-19 infection during pregnancy. Infect Dis Obstet Gynecol 2003;11:175–9.

American College of Obstetricians and Gynecologists. Perinatal viral and parasitic infections. ACOG Practice Bulletin 20. Washington, DC: ACOG; 2000.

Koch WC. Parvovirus B19. In: Behrman RE, Kliegman RM, Jenson HB, editors. Nelson textbook of pediatrics. 17th ed. Philadelphia (PA): WB Saunders; 2004. p. 1048–51.

# 133

## Contraception in epilepsy

To prevent focal and generalized seizures, a 32-year-old woman takes carbamazepine (Epitol, Tegretol) and lamotrigine (Lamictal). She previously used depot medroxyprogesterone acetate contraceptive injections, but discontinued the injections because of weight concerns. The best contraceptive choice for this patient is

(A) a combination oral contraceptive
(B) vaginal contraceptive ring
(C) a progestin-only oral contraceptive
* (D) intrauterine device (IUD)
(E) transdermal contraceptive patch

For women with seizure disorders, the frequency of seizures may increase during pregnancy. Furthermore, many anticonvulsants are teratogens. Accordingly, effective contraception is important for women who take anticonvulsant medications and who do not wish to conceive. In many cases, women take anticonvulsant medications for indications other than seizure disorders (eg, bipolar disease, migraine prophylaxis, and chronic pain). Therefore, the contraceptive considerations relevant to this case extend beyond the population of patients with seizure disorders. Carbamazepine, similar to the anticonvulsants, phenytoin sodium (Dilantin), felbamate (Felbatol), and topiramate (Topamax), is known to induce hepatic enzymes that can decrease serum concentrations of the estrogen or progestin component of oral contracep-

tives. Therefore, in theory, the lower the dose of the oral contraceptive, the higher the failure rate in the setting of concomitant use of enzyme-inducing medications. Although no data support this recommendation, some experts prescribe oral contraceptives formulated with 50 mcg of ethinyl estradiol for women who use enzyme inducers. Although few data have examined the pharmacokinetic impact of concomitant enzyme-inducing drug use in women who use the contraceptive patch or vaginal ring, it is prudent to assume that considerations are similar to those for oral contraceptives. Because the dose of progestin-only oral contraceptives is low, and ovulation often occurs during use, progestin-only oral contraceptives may not provide effective contraception in women who use hepatic enzyme inducers.

Injectable depot medroxyprogesterone acetate has intrinsic anticonvulsant qualities, and pregnancies have not been reported in women who use this effective contraceptive. Accordingly, some experts consider depot medroxyprogesterone acetate to be the hormonal contraceptive of choice in women with seizure disorders. Unfortunately, no published pharmacokinetic data address the impact that concomitant enzyme inducers have in women who take depot medroxyprogesterone acetate.

Because the effectiveness of the T-copper IUD should not be impacted by concomitant liver enzyme-inducing medications and this IUD offers users annual (and 10-year) failure rates as low as surgical sterilization, it would represent a sensible contraceptive choice for the woman

in this case. No data assess the contraceptive efficacy of the levonorgestrel-releasing IUD in women who use iver enzyme inducers, although any effect on efficacy is likely to be low given the low systemic absorption of the progestin.

Crawford P. Interactions between antiepileptic drugs and hormonal contraception. CNS Drugs 2002;16:263–72.

Intrauterine device. ACOG Practice Bulletin No. 59. American College of Obstetricians and Gynecologists. Obstet Gynecol 2005;105:223–32.

Kaunitz AM. Injectable long-acting contraception. Clin Obstet Gynecol 2001;44:73–91.

Use of hormonal contraception in women with coexisting medical conditions. ACOG Practice Bulletin No. 73. American College of Obstetricians and Gynecologists. Obstet Gynecol 2006;107:1453–72.

# 134
## Blood pressure in type 2 diabetes mellitus

A 66-year-old woman with type 2 diabetes mellitus is observed to have systolic and diastolic blood pressures of 139 mm Hg and 89 mm Hg, respectively, during her periodic health maintenance examination. Previous interventions have included weight loss, exercise, and low-dose diuretic therapy. Her glycemic control is good with hemoglobin $A_{1C}$ in the normal range. The best approach to minimize progression of renal disease and diabetic retinopathy is to add therapy with

   (A) insulin
   (B) metformin hydrochloride (Glucophage)
\*  (C) angiotensin-converting enzyme (ACE) inhibitor
   (D) high-dose diuretic
   (E) glyburide

In patients with diabetes mellitus, hypertension is associated with the progression of diabetic renal disease and retinopathy. Around 39% of patients with newly diagnosed diabetes already are hypertensive; the patient's blood pressure typically begins to rise within the normal range approximately 3 years after the onset of microalbuminuria. Ultimately, the incidence of hypertension is approximately 15–25% in all patients with microalbuminuria and 75–85% in patients with overt diabetic nephropathy.

All patients with diabetes mellitus should have their blood pressure lowered to below 130 mm Hg systolic and 80 mm Hg diastolic. Intensive drug therapy with appropriate drugs has been shown to be protective. A lower-than-usual blood pressure may be required to protect maximally against cardiovascular disease and progressive diabetic nephropathy. The results of the Hypertension Optimal Treatment Trial suggest that a lower target diastolic pressure has a cardioprotective effect in individuals with diabetes and that 80 mm Hg rather than 85 mm Hg

should be the ideal target diastolic pressure in these patients. The goal for patients with concurrent renal insufficiency is a reduction in blood pressure to less than 130/80 mm Hg. However, evidence suggests that an even lower systolic pressure may be more effective in slowing progressive renal disease in patients with a protein excretion of greater than 1 g per day.

Among patients with type 2 diabetes mellitus, the benefits of tight blood pressure control may be as great as or greater than the benefit of strict glycemic control. The UK Prospective Diabetes Study Group showed that tight blood pressure control in patients with hypertension and type 2 diabetes mellitus achieves a clinically important reduction in the risk of deaths related to diabetes mellitus and its complications, progression of diabetic retinopathy, and deterioration in visual acuity. This randomized controlled trial compared tight control of blood pressure using the ACE inhibitor, captopril (Capoten, Capozide), or the β-blocker, atenolol (Tenoretic, Tenormin).

Intensive drug therapy is unequivocally protective, so the benefits of antihypertensive drugs quickly outweigh the adverse effects. Initial therapy should include non-pharmacologic methods (eg, weight reduction, exercise, sodium restriction, and avoidance of smoking and excess alcohol ingestion). However, all patients with diabetes mellitus who have blood pressures higher than 130 mm Hg systolic and 80 mm Hg diastolic are considered to be at such high risk of cardiovascular complications that they also should be immediately begun on antihypertensive drug therapy. Intensified multifactorial intervention in patients with type 2 diabetes mellitus and microalbuminuria slows progression to nephropathy and progression of retinopathy and autonomic neuropathy. Although there are concerns about masking hypoglycemic symptoms and possible exacerbation of peripheral vascular disease, β-blockers are effective therapy for hypertension in patients with diabetes.

Metabolic complications and a possible increase in cardiovascular risk have been a major concern with high doses of diuretics in patients with diabetes mellitus. However, as shown by data from the Antihypertensive and Lipid-Lowering Treatment to Prevent Heart Attack Trial (ALLHAT) and other studies, the increase in blood glucose is usually quite small with low-dose therapy (eg, 12.5–25 mg of hydrochlorothiazide or chlorthalidone per day). Low-dose thiazide therapy also can minimize the decrease in plasma potassium concentration and the increase in triglyceride and uric acid concentrations induced by 50 mg of hydrochlorothiazide (or its equivalent) in hypertensive patients with type 2 diabetes mellitus.

Chobanian AV, Bakris GL, Black HR, Cushman WC, Green LA, Izzo JL Jr, et al. The seventh report of the Joint National Committee on Prevention, Detection, Evaluation, and Treatment of High Blood Pressure: the JNC 7 report. National Heart, Lung, and Blood Institute Joint National Committee on Prevention, Detection, Evaluation, and Treatment of High Blood Pressure; National High Blood Pressure Education Program Coordinating Committee [published erratum appears in JAMA 2003;290:197]. JAMA 2003;289:2560–72.

Hansson L, Zanchetti A, Carruthers SG, Dahlof B, Elmfeldt D, Julius S, et al. Effects of intensive blood-pressure lowering and low-dose aspirin in patients with hypertension: principal results of the Hypertension Optimal Treatment (HOT) randomised trial. HOT Study Group. Lancet 1998;351:1755–62.

Major outcomes in high-risk hypertensive patients randomized to angiotensin-converting enzyme inhibitor or calcium channel blocker vs diuretic: The Antihypertensive and Lipid-Lowering Treatment to Prevent Heart Attack Trial (ALLHAT). ALLHAT Officers and Coordinators for the ALLHAT Collaborative Research Group. The Antihypertensive and Lipid-Lowering Treatment to Prevent Heart Attack Trial [published errata appear in JAMA 2003;289:178; JAMA 2004;291:2196]. JAMA 2002;288:2981–97.

Mogensen CE. Combined high blood pressure and glucose in type 2 diabetes: double jeopardy. British trial shows clear effects of treatment, especially blood pressure reduction. BMJ 1998;317:693–4.

Tight blood pressure control and risk of macrovascular and microvascular complications in type 2 diabetes: UKPDS 38. UK Prospective Diabetes Study Group [published erratum appears in BMJ 1999;318:29]. BMJ 1998;317:703–13.

Vijan S, Hayward RA. Treatment of hypertension in type 2 diabetes mellitus: blood pressure goals, choice of agents, and setting priorities in diabetes care. Ann Intern Med 2003;138:593–602.

# 135

## Gastrointestinal illness

A 31-year-old woman has a 3-year history of heartburn that occurs several times a month and she treats it with antacids. She describes her heartburn as a burning sensation rising from her stomach that occurs after she has eaten and sometimes manifests itself at night waking her up. She is concerned because cancer was recently diagnosed in an uncle. She denies pain with swallowing, weight loss, or gastrointestinal bleeding. The best management strategy is to

    (A) continue antacids and add lifestyle changes
    (B) order a barium swallow
    (C) obtain a gastrointestinal consultation for endoscopy
    (D) start an $H_2$-receptor antagonist
\*     (E) start a proton pump inhibitor

The separation of dyspepsia and gastroesophageal reflux is critical, but not always simple. Dyspepsia has a variety of definitions, but is most commonly defined as chronic or recurrent pain or discomfort centered in the upper abdomen or epigastrium. Most patients in the primary care setting have uninvestigated dyspepsia. Many of these patients may have an underlying structural cause, such as peptic ulcer disease or reflux esophagitis, but a substantial number of these patients will have "functional dyspepsia" in which there is no definite structural or biochemical explanation for their symptoms. A key element of effective care of symptomatic patients is the identification and exclusion of those patients who have gastroesophageal reflux disease (GERD).

Gastroesophageal reflux disease is estimated to affect 4–7% of the population, although only a small percentage will seek medical attention. It is defined as being present in all individuals who exhibit physical complications from reflux (ie, esophageal erosions or ulcerations, stricture, and Barrett's syndrome) or in those who experience clinically significant impairment in quality of life because of reflux-related symptoms. This definition tries to distinguish individuals whose symptoms are troublesome enough to define reflux as a disease from the many individuals in the general population who experience clinically insignificant reflux-induced symptoms. The pattern of symptoms in GERD usually is distinctive with the predominant symptom being heartburn. Heartburn is best defined as a burning feeling rising from the stomach or lower chest toward the neck. The diagnosis is further secured if symptoms are positional (ie, increased when supine and when stooping), occur postprandially and at night, or are transiently relieved with antacids.

Patients with typical or mild symptoms compatible with GERD can be treated empirically, without further evaluation. The traditional approach to treatment has been to initiate treatment with lifestyle changes (including weight loss, smoking cessation, no food before bedtime, and elevation of the head of the bed) and antacids, then to increase the intensity of therapy until there is an adequate response. The logic of this approach has been questioned given the superior and prompt response of GERD to a 2–4-week course of a proton pump inhibitor such as omeprazole (Prilosec). Other therapies are much less effective; their use is less likely to provide prompt relief of symptoms, confirmation of the diagnosis, and reassurance for the patient. Therefore, in the primary care setting with no alarm symptoms (eg, weight loss, dysphagia, or new symptoms in a patient older than 50 years), a patient with typical reflux symptoms can be treated without an additional workup. Minimization of drug cost would seem to be the only logical reason for not using a proton pump inhibitor as the initial therapy for reflux.

No consensus exists on long-term management strategies for the treatment of GERD. The options of withdrawal of initial successful therapy, its continuation unchanged, step down therapy, or even antireflux surgery are all appropriate depending on individual patient characteristics.

Referral or gastrointestinal consultation is always an option. Endoscopy can be useful in the initial phase of management for both diagnosis and severity assessment, but less than one half of patients with troublesome reflux symptoms have definitive esophagitis by endoscopy. Endoscopy is clearly indicated when alarm symptoms are present that suggest the presence or coexistence of serious problems such as chronic peptic ulcer disease, esophageal or gastric cancer, esophageal stricture, or bleeding secondary to esophagitis.

An evidence-based appraisal of reflux disease management—the Genval Workshop Report. Gut 1999;44(suppl 2):S1–16.

Dent J. Definitions of reflux disease and its separation from dyspepsia. Gut 2002;50(suppl 4):iv17–20, discussion iv21–2.

Dent J. Management of reflux disease. Gut 2002;50(suppl 4):iv67–71.

Talley NJ. Dyspepsia: management guidelines for the millennium. Gut 2002;50(Suppl 4):iv72–8, discussion iv79.

# 136

## Home evaluation of asthma in the pregnant patient

A 32-year-old woman with a history of asthma is seen at 22 weeks of gestation. She tells you that for the past 7–10 days, her breathing has been tighter than usual. She uses her β-sympathomimetic inhaler approximately four times a day. Her breathing has improved somewhat with the use of the inhaler but the effect does not last. She has experienced more coughing, especially at night, and has difficulty climbing the 14 steps to the second floor without feeling shortness of breath. She denies any fever or sputum production. On examination, she does not appear distressed. Her respiratory rate is 26 breaths a minute; blood pressure, 130/80 mm Hg; and pulse rate, 104 beats per minute. She is mentally alert and oriented, speaks in complete sentences, and her lips are pink in color. Pulmonary examination demonstrates loud wheezing with inspiration and expiration. She is not using her accessory muscles for respiration. A peak expiratory flow rate in the office is 250 L/min. The symptom or sign that correlates best with the severity of her asthma is

        (A) nocturnal coughing
        (B) respiratory rate
        (C) tachycardia
        (D) loud wheezing
\*     (E) peak expiratory flow rate

Asthma has been estimated to affect at least 4–7% of pregnant women. The incidence of asthma is increasing in all population groups in the United States. Asthma appears to affect pregnancy outcome with increased rates of preeclampsia, preterm birth, fetal growth restriction, and perinatal mortality. A correlation exists between the severity of asthma and outcomes. Patients with more persistent symptoms of asthma suggestive of inadequate control have been found to be at higher risk of fetal growth restriction. Such observations suggest that it is the disease and not the treatment that increases adverse pregnancy outcomes. Poor asthma control may cause acute or chronic maternal hypoxia, potentially treatable with therapy. The U.S. National Institutes of Health sponsored a multicenter study that showed similar perinatal outcomes in patients with mild and moderate to severe asthma and in controls. This was likely related to incorporation of objective assessment of asthma severity with appropriate aggressive management.

Asthma has been noted to improve, worsen, or maintain the same clinical course in pregnancy. Anecdotal observations suggest that more severe asthma has a tendency to worsen whereas milder disease tends to maintain its course or lessen.

Asthma currently is recognized as a chronic inflammatory disease punctuated by acute, intermittent exacerbations. As part of the effective management of asthma, triggers that induce exacerbations should be identified and avoided where possible. Such avoidable triggers include the following:

- Allergens (eg, pet dander, house mites, mold, pollen)
- Irritants (eg, tobacco smoke)
- Occupational exposures (eg, grain dust)
- Food additives (eg, sulfites)
- Weather (eg, cold air)

Objective measures of maternal lung function provide the most reliable method for evaluating severity of asthma in pregnancy. Such methods include pulmonary function testing by an office spirometer to measure forced expiratory volume in 1 second ($FEV_1$). In lieu of $FEV_1$, which is an office-based measure not designed for home use, the peak expiratory flow rate (PEFR) correlates well, is inexpensive, and can be used by patients to monitor their own lung function. The PEFR remains fairly constant throughout pregnancy with an average of 430–450 L per minute. For the patient under discussion, home evaluation of her

PEFR provides the best measure of the severity of her asthma.

Nocturnal cough is useful in the diagnosis of asthma, and its appearance in the setting of asthma may indicate worsening control. Other etiologies include allergic reaction and gastroesophageal reflux; both may contribute to asthma symptoms. Persistent use of a β-sympathomimetic inhaler generally indicates inadequate control and suggests the need to evaluate severity objectively and to modify the treatment regimen. Physical findings such as tachycardia, wheezing, use of accessory muscles (eg, sternocleidomastoid), tachypnea, tachycardia, and a pulsus paradoxicus of greater than 10 mm occur with an acute exacerbation but are generally insensitive signs of severity of airflow obstruction.

The goal of treatment is to attain pulmonary function as near normal as possible. Antiinflammatory treatment includes steroids (either oral or inhaled or both) and cromolyn sodium. The National Asthma Education Program has published guidelines for the management of asthma in pregnancy (see Appendices C and D). In general, for mild asthma ($FEV_1$ or PEFR greater than 80% of baseline), intermittent use of a β-sympathomimetic inhaler will suffice. Use of cromolyn for prophylaxis is recommended when exposure to a trigger (eg, cold air) is expected. With increasing severity, increasing persistence of symptoms, and decreasing $FEV_1$ or PEFR, the physician may choose to add antiinflammatory agents including cromolyn, inhaled steroids, and oral steroids.

Bracken MB, Triche EW, Belanger K, Saftlas A, Beckett WS, Leaderer BP. Asthma symptoms, severity, and drug therapy: a prospective study of effects on 2205 pregnancies. Obstet Gynecol 2003;102:739–52.

Dombrowski MP, Schatz M, Wise R, Momirova V, Landon M, Mabie W, et al. Asthma during pregnancy. National Institute of Child Health and Human Development Maternal–Fetal Medicine Units Network and the National Heart, Lung, and Blood Institute. Obstet Gynecol 2004;103:5–12.

Dombrowski MP, Schatz M, Wise R, Thom EA, Landon M, Mabie W, et al. Randomized trial of inhaled beclomethasone dipropionate versus theophylline for moderate asthma during pregnancy. National Institute of Child Health and Human Development Maternal–Fetal Medicine Units Network and the National Heart, Lung, and Blood Institute. Am J Obstet Gynecol 2004;190:737–44.

Kallen B, Rydhstroem H, Aberg A. Asthma during pregnancy—a population based study. Eur J Epidemiol 2000;16:167–71.

Management of asthma during pregnancy. Report of the working group on asthma and pregnancy. NIH Publication No. 93-3279. September 1993. Bethesda (MD): National Institutes of Health, 1993.

NAEPP expert panel report. Managing asthma during pregnancy: recommendations for pharmacologic treatment—2004 update. National Heart, Lung, and Blood Institute; National Asthma Education and Prevention Program Asthma and Pregnancy Working Group [published erratum appears in J Allergy Clin Immunol 2005;115:477]. J Allergy Clin Immunol 2005;115:34–46.

Namazy JA, Schatz M. Pregnancy and asthma: recent developments. Curr Opin Pulm Med 2005;11:56–60.

Schatz M, Dombrowski MP, Wise R, Momirova V, Landon M, Mabie W, et al. Spirometry is related to perinatal outcomes in pregnant women with asthma. Am J Obstet Gynecol 2006;194:120–6.

# 137

## Coronary heart disease in women

A 48-year-old woman, gravida 2, para 2, comes to your office for her period health maintenance examination. She is concerned because coronary artery disease was diagnosed in her mother at age 59 years requiring bypass surgery. The patient's earlier fasting laboratory readings revealed a high-density lipoprotein (HDL) cholesterol level of 45 mg/dL, triglycerides level of 189 mg/dL, and fasting blood sugar level of 105 mg/dL. On examination, she is noted to have a blood pressure of 125/84 mm Hg, weight 81.7 kg (180 lb), and height 1.57 m (62 in.). Her body mass index (weight in kilograms divided by height in meters squared [kg/m$^2$]) is 32.9. A possible diagnosis of metabolic syndrome can be confirmed by

  (A) body mass index
* (B) waist circumference
  (C) low-density lipoprotein (LDL) cholesterol
  (D) total cholesterol
  (E) high-sensitivity C-reactive protein

Obesity is a major health problem in the United States and is increasing in prevalence. Data from the Third National Health and Nutrition Examination Survey (NHANES III) indicate that while the mean height for women (aged 20–74 years) increased less than 2.54 cm (1 in.) over the past 4 decades, mean body weight has risen from 63.7 kg to 74.0 kg, representing a 10.3-kg (16.2%) increase. The increase in obesity in the United States is commonly attributed to the ready availability of high-calorie food (fast food) and sedentary lifestyle. The number one health consequence of obesity is atherosclerotic cardiovascular disease (ASCVD), a substantial portion of which is mediated by type 2 diabetes mellitus.

Obesity is defined as an excess of body fat. A measure of body fat is the body mass index (BMI). Table 137-1 shows a chart for calculation of BMI. A body mass index of 25–29 is called overweight, and BMI of 30 or higher is defined as obesity. Clinically, the best way to estimate obesity is to measure waist circumference. An excess of abdominal fat is most closely associated with risk for ASCVD. In the United States, abdominal obesity is defined as a waist circumference in men of 102 cm or more and in women of 88 cm or more. Truncal fat is more strongly related to risk of ASCVD than is gluteofemoral fat.

A constellation of metabolic risk factors for heart disease have been defined as the metabolic syndrome (Appendix B). The National Cholesterol Education Program Adult Treatment Panel III has proposed a simple scheme for its routine diagnosis. When three of the five risk factors listed in Appendix B for metabolic syndrome are found in the patient, the diagnosis is confirmed. The advantage of measuring waist circumference is that an excess of abdominal fat is correlated more closely with the presence of metabolic risk factors than total body fat. Individuals meeting the criteria for metabolic syndrome have at least a twofold increase in risk for ASCVD and a fivefold increase in risk for type 2 diabetes mellitus. Patients typically have an atherogenic dyslipidemia characterized by increasing triglycerides, increasing small LDL particles, and low HDL cholesterol.

The patient presented has two risk factors for metabolic syndrome: elevated triglycerides and low HDL cholesterol. If her waist circumference is greater than 88 cm (35 in.), she meets the criteria for metabolic syndrome. Elevation of high-sensitivity C-reactive protein is emerging as another marker for heart disease in women, but is not included in the diagnosis of metabolic syndrome.

**TABLE 137-1.** Body Mass Index Calculation, Chart, and Categories

The body mass index (BMI) is an indirect measure of body fat and is used to determine obesity. The BMI is calculated as weight in kilograms (kg) divided by the square of height in meters (m²).

$$\mathrm{BMI} = \frac{\text{weight (kg)}}{\text{height squared (m}^2\text{)}}$$

Using a BMI chart is an easy and rapid way of identifying the BMI for all adult patients.

### Body Mass Index Table

| BMI | Normal | | | | | | Overweight | | | | | Obese | | | | | | | | | | Extreme Obesity | | | | | | | | | | | | | | |
|---|---|---|---|---|---|---|---|---|---|---|---|---|---|---|---|---|---|---|---|---|---|---|---|---|---|---|---|---|---|---|---|---|---|---|---|---|
| | 19 | 20 | 21 | 22 | 23 | 24 | 25 | 26 | 27 | 28 | 29 | 30 | 31 | 32 | 33 | 34 | 35 | 36 | 37 | 38 | 39 | 40 | 41 | 42 | 43 | 44 | 45 | 46 | 47 | 48 | 49 | 50 | 51 | 52 | 53 | 54 |
| Height (inches) | | | | | | | | | | | | | | | | Body Weight (pounds) | | | | | | | | | | | | | | | | | | | | |
| 58 | 91 | 96 | 100 | 105 | 110 | 115 | 119 | 124 | 129 | 134 | 138 | 143 | 148 | 153 | 158 | 162 | 167 | 172 | 177 | 181 | 186 | 191 | 196 | 201 | 205 | 210 | 215 | 220 | 224 | 229 | 234 | 239 | 244 | 248 | 253 | 258 |
| 59 | 94 | 99 | 104 | 109 | 114 | 119 | 124 | 128 | 133 | 138 | 143 | 148 | 153 | 158 | 163 | 168 | 173 | 178 | 183 | 188 | 193 | 198 | 203 | 208 | 212 | 217 | 222 | 227 | 232 | 237 | 242 | 247 | 252 | 257 | 262 | 267 |
| 60 | 97 | 102 | 107 | 112 | 118 | 123 | 128 | 133 | 138 | 143 | 148 | 153 | 158 | 163 | 168 | 174 | 179 | 184 | 189 | 194 | 199 | 204 | 209 | 215 | 220 | 225 | 230 | 235 | 240 | 245 | 250 | 255 | 261 | 266 | 271 | 276 |
| 61 | 100 | 106 | 111 | 116 | 122 | 127 | 132 | 137 | 143 | 148 | 153 | 158 | 164 | 169 | 174 | 180 | 185 | 190 | 195 | 201 | 206 | 211 | 217 | 222 | 227 | 232 | 238 | 243 | 248 | 254 | 259 | 264 | 269 | 275 | 280 | 285 |
| 62 | 104 | 109 | 115 | 120 | 126 | 131 | 136 | 142 | 147 | 153 | 158 | 164 | 169 | 175 | 180 | 186 | 191 | 196 | 202 | 207 | 213 | 218 | 224 | 229 | 235 | 240 | 246 | 251 | 256 | 262 | 267 | 273 | 278 | 284 | 289 | 295 |
| 63 | 107 | 113 | 118 | 124 | 130 | 135 | 141 | 146 | 152 | 158 | 163 | 169 | 175 | 180 | 186 | 191 | 197 | 203 | 208 | 214 | 220 | 225 | 231 | 237 | 242 | 248 | 254 | 259 | 265 | 270 | 278 | 282 | 287 | 293 | 299 | 304 |
| 64 | 110 | 116 | 122 | 128 | 134 | 140 | 145 | 151 | 157 | 163 | 169 | 174 | 180 | 186 | 192 | 197 | 204 | 209 | 215 | 221 | 227 | 232 | 238 | 244 | 250 | 256 | 262 | 267 | 273 | 279 | 285 | 291 | 296 | 302 | 308 | 314 |
| 65 | 114 | 120 | 126 | 132 | 138 | 144 | 150 | 156 | 162 | 168 | 174 | 180 | 186 | 192 | 198 | 204 | 210 | 216 | 222 | 228 | 234 | 240 | 246 | 252 | 258 | 264 | 270 | 276 | 282 | 288 | 294 | 300 | 306 | 312 | 318 | 324 |
| 66 | 118 | 124 | 130 | 136 | 142 | 148 | 155 | 161 | 167 | 173 | 179 | 186 | 192 | 198 | 204 | 210 | 216 | 223 | 229 | 235 | 241 | 247 | 253 | 260 | 266 | 272 | 278 | 284 | 291 | 297 | 303 | 309 | 315 | 322 | 328 | 334 |
| 67 | 121 | 127 | 134 | 140 | 146 | 153 | 159 | 166 | 172 | 178 | 185 | 191 | 198 | 204 | 211 | 217 | 223 | 230 | 236 | 242 | 249 | 255 | 261 | 268 | 274 | 280 | 287 | 293 | 299 | 306 | 312 | 319 | 325 | 331 | 338 | 344 |
| 68 | 125 | 131 | 138 | 144 | 151 | 158 | 164 | 171 | 177 | 184 | 190 | 197 | 203 | 210 | 216 | 223 | 230 | 236 | 243 | 249 | 256 | 262 | 269 | 276 | 282 | 289 | 295 | 302 | 308 | 315 | 322 | 328 | 335 | 341 | 348 | 354 |
| 69 | 128 | 135 | 142 | 149 | 155 | 162 | 169 | 176 | 182 | 189 | 196 | 203 | 209 | 216 | 223 | 230 | 236 | 243 | 250 | 257 | 263 | 270 | 277 | 284 | 291 | 297 | 304 | 311 | 318 | 324 | 331 | 338 | 345 | 351 | 358 | 365 |
| 70 | 132 | 139 | 146 | 153 | 160 | 167 | 174 | 181 | 188 | 195 | 202 | 209 | 216 | 222 | 229 | 236 | 243 | 250 | 257 | 264 | 271 | 278 | 285 | 292 | 299 | 306 | 313 | 320 | 327 | 334 | 341 | 348 | 355 | 362 | 369 | 376 |
| 71 | 136 | 143 | 150 | 157 | 165 | 172 | 179 | 186 | 193 | 200 | 208 | 215 | 222 | 229 | 236 | 243 | 250 | 257 | 265 | 272 | 279 | 286 | 293 | 301 | 308 | 315 | 322 | 329 | 338 | 343 | 351 | 358 | 365 | 372 | 379 | 386 |
| 72 | 140 | 147 | 154 | 162 | 169 | 177 | 184 | 191 | 199 | 206 | 213 | 221 | 228 | 235 | 242 | 250 | 258 | 265 | 272 | 279 | 287 | 294 | 302 | 309 | 316 | 324 | 331 | 338 | 346 | 353 | 361 | 368 | 375 | 383 | 390 | 397 |
| 73 | 144 | 151 | 159 | 166 | 174 | 182 | 189 | 197 | 204 | 212 | 219 | 227 | 235 | 242 | 250 | 257 | 265 | 272 | 280 | 288 | 295 | 302 | 310 | 318 | 325 | 333 | 340 | 348 | 355 | 363 | 371 | 378 | 386 | 393 | 401 | 408 |
| 74 | 148 | 155 | 163 | 171 | 179 | 186 | 194 | 202 | 210 | 218 | 225 | 233 | 241 | 249 | 256 | 264 | 272 | 280 | 287 | 295 | 303 | 311 | 319 | 326 | 334 | 342 | 350 | 358 | 365 | 373 | 381 | 389 | 396 | 404 | 412 | 420 |
| 75 | 152 | 160 | 168 | 176 | 184 | 192 | 200 | 208 | 216 | 224 | 232 | 240 | 248 | 256 | 264 | 272 | 279 | 287 | 295 | 303 | 311 | 319 | 327 | 335 | 343 | 351 | 359 | 367 | 375 | 383 | 391 | 399 | 407 | 415 | 423 | 431 |
| 76 | 156 | 164 | 172 | 180 | 189 | 197 | 205 | 213 | 221 | 230 | 238 | 246 | 254 | 263 | 271 | 279 | 287 | 295 | 304 | 312 | 320 | 328 | 336 | 344 | 353 | 361 | 369 | 377 | 385 | 394 | 402 | 410 | 418 | 426 | 435 | 443 |

| Weight Category | BMI |
|---|---|
| Underweight | Less than 18.5 |
| Normal weight | 18.5–24.9 |
| Overweight | 25–29.9 |
| Obesity (Class I) | 30–34.9 |
| Obesity (Class II) | 35–39.9 |
| Extreme obesity (Class III) | 40 or more |

The practical guide: identification, evaluation, and treatment of overweight and obesity in adults. National Heart, Lung, and Blood Institute and North American Association for the Study of Obesity. Bethesda (MD): National Institutes of Health; 2000.

Clinical guidelines on the identification, evaluation, and treatment of overweight and obesity in adults—the evidence report [published erratum appears in Obes Res 1998;6:464]. National Institutes of Health. Obes Res 1998;6(Suppl 2):51S–209S.

Detection, evaluation, and treatment of high blood cholesterol in adults (Third Adult Treatment Panel, ATP III): National Cholesterol Education Program, National Heart, Lung, and Blood Institute, National Institutes of Health. NIH Publication No. 02-5215, 2002. Bethesda (MD): National Institutes of Health, 2002.

Grundy SM, Hansen B, Smith SC Jr, Cleeman JI, Kahn RA. Clinical management of metabolic syndrome: report of the American Heart Association/National Heart, Lung, and Blood Institute/American Diabetes Association conference on scientific issues related to management. American Heart Association; National Heart, Lung, and Blood Institute; American Diabetes Association. Circulation 2004;109:551–6.

Ogden CL, Fryar CD, Carroll MD, Flegal KM. Mean body weight, height, and body mass index, United States 1960–2002. Advance Data from Vital and Health Statistics, No. 347. National Center for Health Statistics, Centers for Disease Control and Prevention, 2004.

# 138

## Simple adnexal cyst in postmenopausal women

A 65-year-old menopausal woman is referred for evaluation of a 2.3-cm simple cyst on her right ovary visualized by transvaginal ultrasonography. The cyst was initially noted on ultrasound examination of the abdomen performed for evaluation of gallbladder disease. The rest of the pelvic structures were reported as ultrasonographically normal. Her CA 125 level was normal. She denies pelvic pain. The next step in management should be

       (A) exploratory laparotomy with adnexectomy
       (B) laparoscopic bilateral salpingo-oophorectomy
\*   (C) repeat transvaginal ultrasonography in 2–3 months
       (D) magnetic resonance imaging (MRI) of the pelvis
       (E) pelvic examination in 1 year

Before the widespread availability of high-resolution pelvic imaging, the presence of an adnexal mass in a postmenopausal patient indicated the need for surgical exploration to exclude ovarian malignancy. Increasingly, ultrasonography is being used to evaluate postmenopausal bleeding, which has led to frequent incidental detection of asymptomatic simple ovarian cysts. Presumably, the postmenopausal ovary should not contain functional masses. Simple ovarian cysts are defined as unilocular anechoic structures with thin walls.

Recently, data have been published on the natural history and appropriate management of postmenopausal ovarian simple cystic masses. Three studies in the past decade have documented that the risk of malignancy in postmenopausal women with simple ovarian cysts is extremely low. One series from Kentucky examined 2,763 women with unilocular ovarian cysts up to 10 cm in diameter. Spontaneous resolution within 1 year was seen in 69% of cases; 7% of cases did not change in appearance. Of those cysts that stayed the same or progressed to a complex mass, none were found to be malignant at subsequent surgery. In a series of 215 menopausal women from Spain, the investigators found that 74% of simple cysts resolved within 2 years. A stage 1A ovarian squamous carcinoma was found in a patient with a 3-cm simple cyst and elevated CA 125 level.

The question of how long these masses can be followed safely has been addressed by a study from the United Kingdom. Women with persistent unilocular ovarian cysts less than 5 cm were followed annually with ultrasonography and CA 125 for 5 years. The investigators found that 76% of women in this series did not have any change in ovarian cyst diameter over the follow-up period nor did their CA 125 levels increase. Of the rest of the women in whom the cysts increased in size or CA 125 level increased, two cases (2%) were found to have stage

1B serous cystadenocarcinoma. Both of these women also had elevated CA 125 levels.

Based on the results of these studies, it appears safe to follow asymptomatic postmenopausal women with simple ovarian cystic masses less than 5 cm in diameter with serial ultrasonographic examination. Surgical exploration is indicated if the cyst increases in diameter or develops septations or wall abnormalities, or an increase in CA 125 is noted. More than 50% of unilocular ovarian cysts in postmenopausal women resolve spontaneously, sparing many from surgical intervention or further evaluation.

Color Doppler ultrasonography has been used as an adjunct to the gray scale B-mode images in the evaluation of adnexal masses. Quantitative Doppler indices and flow parameters do not provide sufficient discriminatory value alone to distinguish between benign and malignant masses. The information obtained from color Doppler may be useful in combination with gray scale imaging for diagnosing ovarian malignancy.

Magnetic resonance imaging may be useful in evaluation of adnexal masses because of the ability to identify different tissue types and because of the excellent soft tissue contrast. Many of the benign ovarian tumors, such as teratomas, endometriomas, and ovarian fibromas, have characteristic or specific MRI features. Despite the advantages of MRI, pelvic ultrasonography is still recommended as the primary method for evaluation of the adnexal mass. The cost of MRI is several times that of ultrasonography. In addition, MRI cannot definitively exclude malignancy and eliminate the need for follow-up imaging or surgical evaluation. For the ultrasonographically indeterminate pelvic mass, MRI can provide a noninvasive method to characterize the origin and nature of such lesions in up to 98% of cases. In the patient described, the simple ovarian cyst was clearly visualized by ultrasonography. No significant additional information regarding the mass would be added by MRI. If the mass was not well defined or if the ovaries were not visualized by ultrasonography, MRI would be an excellent option.

In this patient, ultrasonographic follow-up is indicated instead of surgery because many simple cysts will resolve and virtually all are benign. If follow-up imaging reveals a complex change in the cyst or enlargement, surgery would be indicated. Surgical management of the adnexal mass is undergoing evolution from laparotomy to laparoscopic approaches. Although laparotomy remains an acceptable approach to the suspicious adnexal mass, laparoscopic removal and even staging appear not to compromise prognosis or survival.

Castillo G, Alcazar JL, Jurado M. Natural history of sonographically detected simple unilocular adnexal cysts in asymptomatic postmenopausal women. Gynecol Oncol 2004;92:965–9.

Chi DS, Abu-Rustum NR, Sonoda Y, Ivy J, Rhee E, Moore K, et al. The safety and efficacy of laparoscopic surgical staging of apparent stage I ovarian and fallopian tube cancers. Am J Obstet Gynecol 2005;192:1614–9.

Modesitt SC, Pavlik EJ, Ueland FR, DePriest PD, Kryscio RJ, van Nagell JR Jr. Risk of malignancy in unilocular ovarian cystic tumors less than 10 centimeters in diameter. Obstet Gynecol 2003;102:594–9.

Nardo LG, Kroon ND, Reginald PW. Persistent unilocular ovarian cysts in a general population of postmenopausal women: is there a place for expectant management? Obstet Gynecol 2003;102:589–93.

Oyelese Y, Kueck AS, Barter JF, Zalud I. Asymptomatic postmenopausal simple ovarian cyst. Obstet Gynecol Surv 2002;57:803–9.

# 139

## Suppressive herpes simplex virus therapy

A 33-year-old woman presents with a confirmed history of three episodes of genital herpes simplex virus (HSV-2) in the past year. The treatment that would be most effective in preventing transmission to her unaffected sexual partner is

* (A) continuous daily oral valacyclovir hydrochloride (Valtrex)
  (B) valacyclovir during the viral prodrome
  (C) valacyclovir while genital herpes lesions are present
  (D) topical acyclovir (Zovirax)
  (E) herpes vaccine

Genital herpes is a common and highly contagious sexually transmitted disease. Although most cases are due to HSV-2, approximately 25% are caused by herpes simplex virus 1 (HSV-1). In the United States, 22% of adults have been exposed to HSV-2, and 1.6 million new cases are estimated to occur yearly. Viral shedding can occur without symptoms or signs of active lesions. Decreasing asymptomatic viral shedding is the chief goal in prevention strategies for HSV-2. Many patients are unaware of the risk of transmission to an unaffected partner in the absence of symptoms. Clinicians can help prevent further spread of the disease by counseling infected women about appropriate prevention methods.

Establishment of the diagnosis of genital herpes should be confirmed with laboratory testing. A significant proportion of women with clinically diagnosed herpes will not have the infection. Further, the vesicular lesions commonly described are actually present only in a minority of women with the infection. Laboratory testing is not required for every episode. One positive test is sufficient to establish the diagnosis of genital HSV infection. The most commonly used test and among the most accurate is viral culture. Although highly specific, culture may not detect up to 25% of infections. The older the lesions cultured, the less likely that the virus will be isolated by culture.

Polymerase chain reaction (PCR) testing is up to four times more sensitive than viral culture. The advantages of the increased sensitivity, ease of obtaining samples, and the stability of the sample may lead to PCR replacing viral culture in the future.

Type-specific antibody testing is available. Of the marketed tests, only those that detect glycoprotein G-2 for HSV-2 and glycoprotein G-1 for herpes simplex virus 1 (HSV-1) are truly type specific. This testing has the disadvantage of not detecting newly acquired infections or of discriminating between infection sites. It may be useful for establishing the diagnosis when culture proves negative or lesions are not present.

Recurrence is common in women who are infected with HSV-2, with an average of four episodes in the first year of infection. By contrast, HSV-1 infections are far less likely to recur, with an average of once a year. Frequent recurrences may be managed with daily suppressive therapy with antiviral drugs such as acyclovir, valacyclovir, or famciclovir. Daily suppression with antivirals will prevent 80% of recurrences in HSV-infected women.

Episodic therapy with these agents also may be used to manage recurrent HSV episodes. Use of episodic therapy decreases the duration of symptoms and viral shedding. Effectiveness of such therapy is maximized when it is started at the beginning of prodromal symptoms and continued until the lesions are healed.

Another benefit of daily suppression demonstrated for daily valacyclovir is prevention of transmission of HSV to an unaffected sexual partner. Unaffected sexual partners were 48% less likely to acquire HSV-2 infection when their affected partner was given daily valacyclovir therapy. Asymptomatic viral shedding is decreased by use of daily valacyclovir as well. Prevention of transmission of HSV-1 has not been studied for this regimen.

In couples with one partner with known HSV infection, type-specific serology may be obtained from both. For couples with discordant HSV serotypes, prevention methods should be discussed. Condoms and dental dams can be used; they decrease but do not eliminate the risk of transmission. Failure of barrier methods to prevent HSV transmission is likely secondary to skin-to-skin contact or condom failure.

Topical acyclovir is indicated for treatment of recurrent herpes labialis (cold sores). It is not effective for genital herpes.

A vaccine for genital herpes is under development. Initial studies indicate that the vaccine has efficacy only in women, and efficacy also seems to be limited by serologic status. There is some efficacy for women who are serologically negative for both HSV-1 and HSV-2, but not for those seropositive for HSV-1 and seronegative for HSV-2.

Corey L, Wald A, Patel R, Sacks SL, Tyring SK, Warren T, et al. Once-daily valacyclovir to reduce the risk of transmission of genital herpes. Valacyclovir HSV Transmission Study Group. N Engl J Med 2004; 350:11–20.

Gynecologic herpes simplex virus infections. ACOG Practice Bulletin No. 57. American College of Obstetricians and Gynecologists. Obstet Gynecol 2004;104: 1111–8.

Sexually transmitted diseases treatment guidelines, 2006. Centers for Disease Control and Prevention [published erratum appears in MMWR Recomm Rep 2006;55(36):997]. MMWR Recomm Rep 2006;55 (RR-11):1–94.

Stanberry LR, Spruance SL, Cunningham AL, Bernstein DI, Mindel A, Sacks S, et al. Glycoprotein-D-adjuvant vaccine to prevent genital herpes. GlaxoSmithKline Herpes Vaccine Study Group. N Engl J Med 2002;347:1652–61.

# 140

## Office testing for fetal fibronectin

A 32-year-old woman, gravida 3, comes to your office for a prenatal visit at 28 weeks of gestation. Her first pregnancy ended in a first-trimester spontaneous miscarriage at 10 weeks of gestation. Her second pregnancy, 3 years ago, delivered preterm at 28 weeks, preceded by spontaneous preterm labor. She now reports that in the past 7–10 days she has experienced increased lower abdominal cramping feelings. These episodes occur typically more often with activity and during the afternoon of her workday. However, contractions occur also on weekends when she is not working. She notes that some of the contractions are painful. The maximum frequency is approximately 7–10 cramping feelings in an hour. She is not currently experiencing contractions. The fetus is active. Vaginal discharge has not changed. She is concerned about the risk of preterm labor. The best laboratory test to evaluate her risk of preterm birth is

      (A) serum corticotropin-releasing hormone (CRH)
      (B) vaginal wet mount
      (C) cervical interleukin-6 (IL-6)
\*   (D) cervical fetal fibronectin
      (E) serum alpha-fetoprotein

Preterm birth, which accounted for 11–12% of all births in 1999, is the second leading cause of neonatal mortality. Most preterm births are the result of preterm labor. The ability to predict which populations are at increased risk of preterm labor and preterm birth has improved, although effective interventions to prevent preterm birth have not been identified.

Risk factors for preterm birth can be categorized as follows:

- Demographic factors, eg, prior obstetric history, including prior preterm birth
- Current pregnancy complications, eg, bleeding
- Maternal nutritional status
- Maternal psychosocial factors
- Infections, eg, bacterial vaginosis and periodontal disease
- Biophysical factors, eg, cervical length and uterine contractions
- Elevated fetal fibronectin

One of the strongest risk factors is a prior preterm birth, increasing the relative risk by 6-fold to 22-fold or an absolute risk of approximately 15–22%. The earlier in gestation the prior preterm birth, the higher the risk of recurrence.

In patients with uterine contractions, measuring elevated cervical fetal fibronectin (ie, fetal fibronectin level greater than 50 ng/mL) is the test that best predicts the risk of preterm birth (likelihood ratio = 5.42 with a positive test result, 95% confidence interval [CI] 4.36–6.74). The positive predictive value of a positive fetal fibro-

nectin test result remains low (range 13–30%). Currently, with the exception of possibly administering corticosteroids to stimulate fetal lung maturation, it is unclear what other therapy to offer in the event of a positive fetal fibronectin test result. Treatment with antibiotics (eg, metronidazole and erythromycin), with the presumption that elevated fetal fibronectin levels may be sequelae of subclinical infection, has not demonstrably reduced the incidence of preterm birth.

Because the diagnosis of preterm labor can be difficult and up to 30% of patients with preterm labor resolve spontaneously, the greater value of fetal fibronectin, when negative (less than 50 ng/mL), may be the avoidance of unnecessary treatment in women with uterine contractions. A negative value has been associated with a likelihood ratio of 0.25 (reduction of risk by 75%), and with a negative predictive value as high as 95–99% for preterm birth in the subsequent 7–14 days. Thus, a negative fetal fibronectin test result would permit close observation as alternative management and provide reassurance to this patient. Measurement of cervical–vaginal fetal fibronectin is the most useful laboratory test for patients at risk for preterm birth.

The National Institute of Child Health and Human Development Maternal–Fetal Medicine Units Network Preterm Prediction Study prospectively assessed approximately 3,000 pregnancies and evaluated biochemical markers that may predict preterm birth. Within the study, nested controlled studies evaluated the association of serum corticotropin-releasing hormone (CRH) and alpha-fetoprotein. Only alpha-fetoprotein was significantly elevated at 24 weeks of gestation in patients who ultimately experienced preterm birth at less than 35 weeks of gestation compared with term births (odds ratio = 3.51, 95% CI 1.84–6.71). Other studies have documented that unexplained elevated maternal serum alpha-fetoprotein in the second trimester, evaluated as part of the biochemical screening for fetal aneuploidy and neural tube anomalies, have been correlated with increased risks of adverse outcomes, including preterm birth, fetal death, preeclampsia, and placental abruption. Unexplained elevations of alpha-fetoprotein may imply an abnormal placentation. Corticotropin-releasing hormone is secreted by the fetal hypothalamus, placenta, and decidua. It is hypothesized that maternal levels reflect placental secretion. Normal metabolism demonstrates an increasing level in the second half of pregnancy, which peaks in labor and decreases postpartum. Both of these tests were used primarily to screen populations at risk of preterm birth.

Cervical interleukin-6 (IL-6) is an inflammatory cytokine that increases local prostanoid production, which in turn may stimulate uterine contractions. Cervical IL-6 levels correlated with preterm birth in one study that prospectively assessed cervical samples every 3–4 weeks. In contrast, these levels were not found to be an independent risk factor for preterm birth by the Preterm Prediction Study. In amniotic fluid of pregnancies with uterine contractions, IL-6 is highly correlated with preterm birth. Whether cervical IL-6 or the risk of amniocentesis and assessment of amniotic fluid IL-6 are of value in the evaluation of patients with uterine contractions remains unclear.

Presence of bacterial vaginosis when detected on the vaginal wet mount, in an asymptomatic pregnancy, complicated by a prior preterm birth, is modestly linked to an increased risk of recurrent preterm birth. Bacterial vaginosis is identified in approximately 20% of pregnancies, and more often in black women than in white women. However, antibiotic treatment has not been associated with a reduction in risk. In a large randomized trial involving 1,953 pregnancies, bacterial vaginosis resolved in 78% of women treated with two doses of 2 g of metronidazole and spontaneously in 38% in the placebo group. However, no difference was identified in preterm delivery rates before 32 weeks between the treated and placebo group.

Carey JC, Klebanoff MA, Hauth JC, Hillier SL, Thom EA, Ernest JM, et al. Metronidazole to prevent preterm delivery in pregnant women with asymptomatic bacterial vaginosis. National Institute of Child Health and Human Development Network of Maternal–Fetal Medicine Units. N Engl J Med 2000;342:534–40.

Goepfert AR, Goldenberg RL, Andrews WW, Hauth JC, Mercer B, Iams J, et al. The Preterm Prediction Study: association between cervical interleukin 6 concentration and spontaneous preterm birth. National Institute of Child Health and Human Development Maternal–Fetal Medicine Units Network. Am J Obstet Gynecol 2001;184:483–8.

Goldenberg RL, Iams JD, Mercer BM, Meis P, Moawad A, Das A, et al. What we have learned about the predictors of preterm birth. National Institute of Child Health and Human Development Network of Maternal–Fetal Medicine Units. Semin Perinatol 2003;27:185–93.

Honest H, Bachmann LM, Gupta JK, Kleijnen J, Khan KS. Accuracy of cervicovaginal fetal fibronectin test in predicting risk of spontaneous preterm birth: systematic review. BMJ 2002;325:301–4.

Moawad AH, Goldenberg RL, Mercer B, Meis PJ, Iams JD, Das A, et al. The Preterm Prediction Study: the value of serum alkaline phosphatase, alpha-fetoprotein, plasma corticotropin-releasing hormone, and other serum markers for the prediction of spontaneous preterm birth. Am J Obstet Gynecol 2002;186:990–6.

# 141

## Collection procedures

You meet with a new collections agency representative hired by your office administrator. The representative details the process the agency uses to collect outstanding debts on your behalf from patients with delinquent accounts. The representative says that the agency starts with a letter on the agency's official letterhead sent to the patient's home address to demand payment and detail the process. Then the agency follows up with a telephone call to the patient, in the evening, typically after dinner. The calls continue on a daily basis for a week. The phone calls are then escalated to include calls to the patient's workplace with messages left with the supervisor, regarding the amount owed to the collections agency. If, after 14 days, the account remains outstanding, then a second letter is sent to the patient to demand payment with the threat of reporting the patient to a credit bureau. Calls and letters are sent to inform the patient of a potential lawsuit if the fees are not paid. Of the processes detailed above, the one that is in violation of the Federal Fair Debt Collections Practices Act is

     (A) use of official letterhead
     (B) telephone call before 9:00 pm
  *  (C) telephone call to the supervisor with message
     (D) report to a credit bureau

Laws regarding collection of debt, including medical care fees, exist at the federal and state level. At the federal level, debt collection is addressed by the Fair Debt Collection Practices Act, passed in 1996 as part of the Consumer Credit Protection Act (15 U.S.C. 1601 et seq.) under Title VIII. At the state level, regulations may exist that further modify the federal act.

The Fair Debt Collections Practices Act contains specific language that outlines fair practices. The act has several sections and can be retrieved in its entirety on the Federal Trade Commission web site. The web site lists examples that constitute fair and unfair practices. In terms of communications between the debt collector and debtor, the act details that a debt collector may contact the debtor by mail, telephone, fax, or telegram but not by postcard. By telephone, the debt collector may not call during inconvenient times such as before 8:00 AM and after 9:00 PM, unless authorized by the debtor. Harassing or annoying calls may not be made.

Regarding the patient's debt, the debt collector is allowed to contact the patient (debtor), the debtor's attorney or a consumer reporting agency, creditor, creditor's attorney, and debt collector's attorney. The collector is forbidden to contact the patient's workplace if it is known that the employer forbids such communications. Unless specifically authorized by the debtor, the collector is forbidden to communicate with a third party, such as leaving messages about the debt at the patient's place of work.

Letters on the agency letterhead are legitimate, but debt collectors may not indicate that papers being sent are legal when they are not, nor indicate the converse, that is, indicate that the papers sent are not legal when they are. Debt collectors may take actions such as a lawsuit, but may not state that such an action will occur when such action cannot legally occur or when the agency has no intention to take such action. As noted, state laws may modify further the Fair Debt Collections Practices Act.

Federal Trade Commission. Fair debt collection. FTC facts for consumers. June 2005. Available at: http://www.ftc.gov/os/statutes/fdcpa/fdcpact.htm. Retrieved June 22, 2005.

The fair debt collection practices act. Public Law 104-208, 110 Stat. 3009 (Sept. 30, 1996). Consumers Credit Protection Act (15 U.S.C. 1601 et seq.) Title VIII Debt Collection Practices.

# 142

## Contraception use by adolescents

A 16-year-old adolescent comes in with her mother and requests oral contraceptives. Her last menstrual period was last week and occurred at the appropriate time. She initiated sexual activity 8 months ago and has had two sexual partners who, she says, have always used condoms. Her current sexual partner is 20 years old. On examination, there are a few small verrucous lesions on the labia majora. You prescribe oral contraceptives and discuss safe sex with her. You instruct her that condoms used correctly and consistently are most efficacious in decreasing the transmission of

    (A) gonorrhea
    (B) herpes simplex virus type 2 (HSV-2)
\*   (C) human immunodeficiency virus (HIV)
    (D) chlamydia
    (E) human papillomavirus (HPV)

Of the more than 18.9 million new cases of sexually transmitted diseases (STDs) in the United States each year, an estimated 9.1 million occur in adolescents and young adults. The Centers for Disease Control and Prevention reports that girls and boys aged 10–19 years are at higher risk than adults for contracting STDs. This is largely due to an adolescent's likelihood of eventually having multiple sexual partners and higher-risk partners and the immaturity of the cervical tissue in young women. Among adolescents and young adults aged 15–24 years, HPV has the highest STD incidence, with an estimated 4.6 million new cases per year. Moreover, HPV has long-term implications for women and is particularly common among sexually active adolescents. In one study of sexually active teens, 90% were found to have HPV on the cervix. The body's immune system will eventually clear this virus in most individuals who are infected, but approximately 10% of patients will carry it on the genital skin for many years— possibly a lifetime. A 2003 study reported that all confirmed cervical cancer cases are associated with high-risk HPV DNA. Women at highest risk for cervical cancer are those who become sexually active in the mid-adolescent years and have a tendency toward multiple sexual partners.

This patient presents the opportunity to offer counseling on what contraception can and cannot do, which is vital in enabling this teen to make informed decisions. Condoms, used consistently and correctly, provide an estimated 85% reduction in the risk of acquiring HIV infection. The actual degree of protection is highly variable (range of 35–94%), because consistent and correct condom use is not the norm. Because of the impressive reduction in HIV acquisition with use of condoms, sexually active adolescents must understand the importance of their consistent and correct use.

Although prevention of HIV acquisition with condom use has been documented, there appears to be lesser protection from other STDs. Protection from viral STDs such as HPV and HSV is compromised because these STDs infect skin in the genital area not covered by condoms. It would appear that condoms would be quite effective in preventing gonorrhea and chlamydia, but studies reveal mixed results. In a large study of more than 3,000 adolescents infected with chlamydia, the rate of reinfection was no different in those who stated they used condoms consistently vs those who used condoms inconsistently.

An expert panel convened by the National Institutes of Health (NIH) to review the medical literature showed that although condoms, used correctly and consistently, do greatly reduce the risk of HIV, they do not significantly reduce the risk of other STDs. The World Health Organization has noted, however, that even though condoms are not 100% effective, even partial protection can reduce the spread of STDs within populations.

Another concern with this patient is the older age of her sexual partner. Each state has laws governing the age at which individuals are legally capable of consenting to sexual activity. This age of consent varies by state, ranging from 14 to 18 years. Adolescent girls with considerably older partners are more likely than their peers to have sex, which increases their risk of pregnancy and STDs. Several studies have shown that adolescents who have older partners have an increased risk of STD infection.

Ford K, Lepkowski JM. Characteristics of sexual partners and STD infection among American adolescents. Int J STD AIDS 2004;15: 260–5.

Holmes KK, Levine R, Weaver M. Effectiveness of condoms in preventing sexually transmitted infections. Bull World Health Organ 2004;82:454–61.

Kaestle CE, Morisky DE, Wiley DJ. Sexual intercourse and the age difference between adolescent females and their romantic partners. Perspect Sex Reprod Health 2002;34:304–9.

Jacobson DL, Womack SD, Peralta L, Zenilman JM, Feroli K, Maehr J, et al. Concordance of human papillomavirus in the cervix and urine among inner city adolescents. Pediatr Infect Dis J 2000;19:722–8.

National Institutes of Health, Workshop summary: scientific evidence on condom effectiveness for sexually transmitted disease (STD) prevention, July 20, 2001. National Institute of Allergy and Infectious Diseases web site. Available at http://www.niaid.nih.gov/dmid/stds/condomreport.pdf. Retrieved June 20, 2005.

Weinstock H, Berman S, Cates W Jr. Sexually transmitted diseases among American youth: incidence and prevalence estimates, 2000. Perspect Sex Reprod Health. 2004;36(1):6–10.

Weller S, Davis K. Condom effectiveness in reducing heterosexual HIV transmission. The Cochrane Database of Systematic Reviews 2002, Issue 1. Art. No.: CD003255. DOI: 10.1002/14651858.CD003255.

# 143

## Allergies to heparin

A 32-year-old primigravid woman comes to the office for prenatal care at 17 weeks of gestation. She reports a medical history of a pulmonary embolus 3 years ago following prolonged bed rest after a motor vehicle accident. Test results for thrombophilia are negative. Her provider started subcutaneous unfractionated heparin therapy early in pregnancy. After 1 month, she reports slightly raised, red, itchy patches on her abdomen. After discontinuation of the current heparin injections, the next best step in management is

        (A) compression stockings
        (B) baby aspirin
\*    (C) no further anticoagulation
        (D) warfarin therapy

Hypersensitivity allergic reactions to unfractionated heparin, low-molecular-weight heparin, and synthetic heparinoids are seen in increasing numbers. These reactions often occur in pregnant women.

The diagnosis of a heparin allergy is made according to the patient's clinical complaints and visual evaluation of the skin. The findings of ecchymoses or skin discoloration may prompt an order for platelet counts and partial thromboplastin time (PTT) testing. Thrombocytopenia is the most common adverse reaction to heparin therapy and resolves after discontinuation.

The pathophysiology of heparin hypersensitivity and allergic reactions is incompletely understood. Portions of the heparin molecule may act as haptens by binding to dermal or subcutaneous structural proteins. All heparin and heparin alternatives have structural differences, but many have nearly identical functional groups that result in similar chemical and pharmacologic activities. Therefore the similarities that result in adequate anticoagulation properties also may lead to the resultant allergic reactions.

Findings of clinical skin lesions associated with heparin use may prompt referrals for skin biopsy or allergy testing if the diagnosis is uncertain. Skin biopsies of any scaly infiltrated plaques may reveal an increased number of CD3 and CD4 lymphocytes, plasma cells, eosinophils, mast cells, and vascular proliferation.

The best therapy for this patient is discontinuation of the current unfractionated heparin. Because she has a nonrecurring cause for a thromboembolic event and a negative thrombophilia test result, no further anticoagulation therapy is required.

The use of the oral anticoagulant, warfarin sodium (Coumadin), may be considered during the second and early third trimester of pregnancy. However, because of the teratogenic risks in the first trimester of pregnancy and the difficulty of reversing this drug's effect, it is rarely used. Discontinuation of warfarin before delivery is necessary. Nonpharmacologic methods of clot prevention intraoperatively and postoperatively may be instituted (ie, compression devices or foot pumps) but are not indicated in this patient.

In the future, therapeutic options for patients with heparin allergies may include use of synthetic heparinoids. Examples are fondaparinux, a synthetic pentasaccharide, or the semi-synthetic lepirudin (Refludan), a recombinant hirudin.

Jappe U, Juschka U, Kuner N, Hausen BM, Krohn K. Fondaparinux: a suitable alternative in cases of delayed-type allergy to heparins and semisynthetic heparinoids? A study of 7 cases. Contact Dermatitis 2004;51:67–72.

Kim J, Smith KJ, Toner C, Skelton H. Delayed cutaneous reactions to heparin in antiphospholipid syndrome during pregnancy. Int J Dermatola 2004;43:252–60.

Wutschert R, Piletta P, Bounameaux H. Adverse skin reactions to low molecular weight heparins: frequency, management and prevention. Drug Saf 1999;20:515–25.

# 144

## Treatment for depression in adolescents

A 17-year-old adolescent girl had an uneventful pregnancy and gave birth 3 weeks ago. During her hospital admission, she reported no recent contact with the father of the baby. Her family lives out of state, but her mother will visit for 1 month to assist with child care. For the past week, she reports difficulty sleeping, recurrent headaches, and nightmares. Family history is positive for depression in her mother and sister. In addition to cognitive behavioral therapy and referral for family counseling, the best treatment for this patient is

      (A) exercise and sleep
      (B) thyroid testing
      (C) tricyclic antidepressant (TCA)
\*    (D) selective serotonin reuptake inhibitors (SSRI) therapy

Postpartum depression may develop in 10–15% of women of all ages. Development of this disorder may severely compromise the ability of mothers to care for themselves and their newborns. Onset varies greatly, from 1–12 months postpartum. Up to 50% of cases may be undetected and therefore are untreated. Incidence is increased in women with a history of depressive mood disorders and in women with a positive family history of depression. Other risk factors for postpartum depression include a history of stressful life events, a poor social support system, and bipolar disease.

Depression has been estimated to affect up to 8% of adolescents. Incidence increases throughout adolescence; 20% of depressed adolescents have at least one episode of major depression by age 18 years. Suicide is the third leading cause of death in girls and boys aged 10–19 years. In determining the best management for the depressed postpartum adolescent, the practitioner should consider present and past psychiatric symptoms, present or past substance abuse, history of self-harmful behaviors or suicide attempts, medical history, and family history of psychiatric disease. Consideration also should be given to the personal concerns of the adolescent.

The overall etiologies of depression can be grouped into biologic, psychologic, and social categories. Physical examination and laboratory testing should focus on detection of medical disorders that may be associated with depression (Box 144-1). In place of verbalized complaints of depression, adolescents may express a variety of somatic symptoms such as headache, abdominal pain, musculoskeletal pain, and issues around gender identification.

The American Academy of Child and Adolescent Psychiatry recommends a treatment approach using several modalities for the treatment of children and adolescents with depressive disorders. At the present time, there is a lack of complete understanding of the benefits of different treatment modalities in depressed adolescents. However, pharmacotherapy may be strongly considered when there is a positive family history for mood disorders or a personal or family history of positive response to antidepressant medications. Medication also may be beneficial in adolescents who show neurovegetative signs and poor or limited response to psychotherapy alone.

Although psychopharmacologic treatment of depression in adolescents has become increasingly common in recent years, such treatment has been the subject of some controversy. Studies in children and adolescents have been done in regard to the use of fluoxetine and other SSRIs, such as paroxetine hydrochloride (Paxil), sertraline (Zoloft), citalopram (Celexa), and venlafaxine hydrochloride (Effexor). Although some statistical evidence exists that SSRIs are efficacious in the treatment of depressed adolescents, with response rates of 36–70%, clear clinical efficacy often is lacking and results are contradictory. The studies had high placebo response rates and minimal clinical differences between medication and placebo groups. Despite such mixed results, SSRIs have emerged as the psychopharmacologic treatment of choice for depressed adolescents.

The U.S. Food and Drug Administration (FDA) has issued a black box warning regarding increased risk of suicidal behavior in children and adolescents treated with antidepressant medications. The FDA developed a *Medication Guide for Families* that recommends close monitoring with one visit a week for the first 4 weeks, one visit every 2 weeks for the next 4 weeks, and a follow-up after 12 weeks of antidepressant use. Intermittent visits also are recommended if problems or questions arise. Practitioners must fully inform their patients and families of possible side effects. They should closely follow the patients for signs of suicidal behavior and worsening clinical symptoms.

---

**BOX 144-1**

**Medical and Psychiatric Conditions Associated With Depressive Symptomatology**

Psychiatric disorders with depressive features
- Major depressive disorder
- Dysthymia
- Adjustment disorder with depressed mood
- Adjustment disorder with mixed anxiety and depression
- Attention deficit and hyperactivity disorder
- Oppositional defiant disorder
- Conduct disorder
- Substance abuse disorders
- Anorexia nervosa
- Bulimia nervosa

General medical conditions with depressive features
- Hypothyroidism or hyperthyroidism
- Diabetes mellitus
- Anemia
- Mononucleosis
- Chronic fatigue syndrome
- Central nervous system disorder
- Multiple sclerosis
- Stroke

Substance abuse
- Marijuana
- Alcohol
- Barbiturates
- Heroin

---

Lack of sleep may exacerbate symptoms of low mood, and regular exercise may combat depressive symptoms by physiologic endorphin release. Amitriptyline therapy has been studied in adults with depressive disorders, but no data on postpartum adolescent patients are available. It may be considered an adjunctive measure in patients with sleeplessness. The best choice for this patient is SSRI therapy. Given the severity of her symptoms, neither thyroid testing nor the recommendation of exercise and sleep would be appropriate.

Birmaher B, Ryan ND, Williamson DE, Brent DA, Kaufman J, Dahl RE, et al. Childhood and adolescent depression: a review of the past 10 years. Part I. J Am Acad Child Adolesc Psychiatry 1996;35:1427–39.

Brent DA, Kolko DJ, Birmaher B, Baugher M, Bridge J, Roth C, et al. Predictors of treatment efficacy in a clinical trial of three psychosocial treatments for adolescent depression. J Am Acad Child Adolesc Psychiatry 1998;37:906–14.

Executive summary; preliminary report of the task force on SSRIs and the suicidal behavioral in youth. American College of Neuro-psychopharmacology. Available at: http://www.acnp.org/exec_summary point. Retrieved April 19, 2005.

Wagner KD, Ambrosini P, Rynn M, Wohlberg C, Yang R, Greenbaum MS, et al. Efficacy of sertraline in the treatment of children and adolescents with major depressive disorder: two randomized controlled trials. Sertraline Pediatric Depression Study Group. JAMA 2003;290: 1033–41.

Zito JM, Safer DJ, DosReis S, Gardner JF, Soeken K, Boles M, et al. Rising prevalence of antidepressants among US youths. Pediatrics 2002;109:721–7.

# 145
## Interstitial cystitis

A 49-year-old woman presents to your office for the evaluation of lower abdominal pain. She has experienced the pain for several years, and the pain seems to worsen if she allows her bladder to become full. The pain nearly completely resolves following voiding. At its worst, the patient finds herself voiding at least every hour. She notes that curiously, the consumption of tomato-based foods as well as drinking orange juice will exacerbate the situation. She also complains of pain with sexual intercourse. She smokes a pack of cigarettes per day. Prior physicians have treated her with antibiotics, but the patient has noted no improvement. A review of her records reveals two sterile urine cultures while she was symptomatic, and urinalyses noted no white blood cells and 2–3 red blood cells per high-power field. Your examination is unremarkable except for tenderness to palpation of the anterior vaginal wall. The most appropriate test to arrive at a diagnosis would be

      (A) an excretory urogram
      (B) a urine sample for cytology
      (C) a potassium sensitivity test
*   (D) a cystoscopy in the office under local anesthesia
      (E) a cystoscopy under general anesthesia with bladder hydrodistention

This patient presented with symptoms suggestive of interstitial cystitis, a painful bladder syndrome characterized by urinary frequency, urgency, and suprapubic discomfort. Bladder pain is exacerbated by filling, and alleviated to a degree by voiding. In many patients, the ingestion of particular foods and beverages is associated with a flare-up in symptoms. The problem also may worsen before menses and commonly is associated with dyspareunia. Because its etiology is unclear, interstitial cystitis remains a diagnosis of exclusion. There are no pathognomonic features. Although attempts have been made to define a diagnostic tool to identify the disorder, they have been characterized by shortcomings.

This patient presents with characteristic symptoms of interstitial cystitis: lower abdominal pain worsened with bladder filling, urinary frequency, and pain with sexual intercourse. Therefore, the workup of this entity consists of ruling out other causes that mimic its symptoms. An excretory urogram affords little information about the bladder lining and is of no assistance in completing the workup of interstitial cystitis.

The potassium sensitivity test was developed to provoke the symptoms of bladder pain due to interstitial cystitis as an adjunct in the workup of pelvic pain of unknown etiology. Its rationale revolved about the theory that interstitial cystitis might be caused by increased permeability of the bladder epithelium to certain ions in the urine, which penetrated a malfunctioning glycosaminoglycan coating to depolarize sensory nerve endings. A volume of 45-mL solution containing 0.4 M potassium is slowly instilled intravesically for 5 minutes and the response compared to the effect when the same volume of sterile water is used. Pain and urgency are measured on an 11-point scale, with an increase of 2 points or greater representing a positive test result. However, studies have shown that the probability of having interstitial cystitis when the test result is positive is only 66%, and that when negative, 46% of patients might still have interstitial cystitis.

Cystoscopy under anesthesia, performed in an operating room setting, is probably unnecessary when seeking the diagnosis of interstitial cystitis. There is no pathognomonic histologic finding on biopsy. A biopsy might be in order if carcinoma in situ is suspected. Earlier literature suggested that maximal distention of the bladder was necessary for complete evaluation of a patient for interstitial cystitis. Only this maneuver would produce the small petechial hemorrhages within the bladder known as glomerulations that are believed to be characteristic of interstitial cystitis. This degree of distention could be achieved only under anesthesia. However, this finding has subsequently been shown to be a nonspecific observation. In a prospective study, 20 asymptomatic women due to have a bilateral tubal ligation under general anesthesia consented to undergo the hydrodistention maneuver routinely used to diagnose interstitial cystitis. Photographs of the bladder mucosa were taken before and after maximal bladder filling and were shown to urologists unaware of the patients' lack of symptoms. On the basis of the photographs alone, 45% of these normal women would have been diagnosed with interstitial cystitis.

Bladder cancer should be considered in the diagnosis of irritative voiding symptoms, particularly in a patient older than 40 years who is a smoker. However, urine cytologies have a high false-negative rate when used for the detection of low-grade tumors. Cystoscopy best evaluates this possibility and can be done easily under topical anesthesia in an office setting. Filling of the bladder with small volumes of fluid during cystoscopy also can reproduce the patient's symptoms, assisting with the diagnosis. If the cystoscopy is negative and bladder cancer is excluded, the most likely diagnosis for this patient is interstitial cystitis.

Chambers GK, Fenster HN, Cripps S, Jens M, Taylor D. An assessment of the use of intravesical potassium in the diagnosis of interstitial cystitis. J Urol 1999;162:699–701.

Duldulao KE, Diokno AC, Mitchell B. Value of urinary cytology in women presenting with urge incontinence and/or irritative voiding symptoms. J Urol 1997;157:113–6.

Parsons CL, Greenberger M, Gabal L, Bidair M, Barme G. The role of urinary potassium in the pathogenesis and diagnosis of interstitial cystitis. J Urol 1998;159:1862–6; discussion 1866–7.

Waxman JA, Sulak PJ, Kuehl TJ. Cystoscopic findings consistent with interstitial cystitis in normal women undergoing tubal ligation. J Urol 1998;160:1663–7.

# 146

## Delivery method for a patient infected with human immunodeficiency virus

A 22-year-old woman with human immunodeficiency virus (HIV) infection, gravida 2, para 1, comes to the office at 36 weeks of gestation (determined by last menstrual period and second-trimester ultrasonography) to discuss mode of delivery. She has been taking antiretroviral therapy throughout the pregnancy; her most recent viral load was 1,300 copies per milliliter. The most appropriate labor and delivery management for this patient is

      (A) spontaneous labor and vaginal birth
      (B) induction of labor at 38 weeks
\*    (C) planned cesarean delivery at 38 weeks
      (D) induction of labor at 39 weeks
      (E) planned cesarean delivery at 39 weeks

Transmission of HIV from infected mothers to their fetus is a major concern. Evidence suggests that without intervention that includes antiretrovirals, 25% of infants born to HIV-infected women will become infected. Moreover, while they are breastfeeding, an additional 12–14% of women will become infected. Prevention of vertical transmission of HIV is a major health care goal in the United States and throughout the world. It has been found that treatment of the mother with zidovudine during pregnancy and labor and of the neonate for the first 6 weeks of life reduces the transmission rate from 25% to 8%.

How the fetus becomes infected is uncertain. It could occur transplacentally during pregnancy or labor, or it could occur by exposure to maternal blood and cervicovaginal secretions during labor and delivery. It is known that the rate of vertical transmission is proportional to the maternal viral load, because the vertical transmission rate is low (around 2%) when the maternal viral load is less than 1,000 copies per milliliter.

A significant relationship appears to exist between mode of delivery and vertical transmission risk. Several studies have found that planned cesarean delivery reduces the transmission when compared with unplanned cesarean delivery or vaginal birth. This finding persisted whether or not the mother took zidovudine during her pregnancy. Data do not show a reduction in transmission if the cesarean delivery is performed after the onset of labor or membrane rupture. These results suggest that the additional risk of a scheduled cesarean delivery is outweighed by the benefit it imparts to the fetus. When the mother received zidovudine during pregnancy and then had a planned cesarean delivery, the risk of transmission dropped to 2%, the same as the risk for a mother with a low viral load (less than 1,000 copies per milliliter).

Neonates of women with viral loads greater than 1,000 copies per milliliter are most likely to benefit from planned cesarean delivery. Thus, at this time, the American College of Obstetricians and Gynecologists and the Centers for Disease Control and Prevention recommend that mothers with HIV infection receive antenatal antiretroviral therapy and have a planned cesarean delivery at 38 completed weeks of gestation. Given the possibility of vertical transmission during labor, it is recommended that the delivery be performed at 38 weeks in order to allow for fetal lung maturity and not risk the patient going into labor before the delivery can be performed. Data are inadequate to support planned cesarean delivery in situations where the maternal viral load is less than 1,000 copies per milliliter.

Amniocentesis for fetal lung maturity in HIV-infected women should be avoided because it is unclear whether and to what degree this intervention affects the risk of transmission. Therefore, clinical determination of dating should be used.

Recently, the patient described had a viral load above 1,000 copies per milliliter. Because she has received zidovudine therapy, she has a risk of transmission of 8% at delivery. If she has a planned cesarean delivery at 38 weeks of gestation, before rupture of membranes or labor, data suggest that her transmission rate will drop to 2%.

American College of Obstetricians and Gynecologists. Scheduled cesarean delivery and the prevention of vertical transmission of HIV infection. ACOG Committee Opinion 234. Washington, DC: ACOG; 2000.

Elective cesarean section versus vaginal delivery in prevention of vertical HIV-I transmission: a randomised clinical trial. The European Mode of Delivery Collaboration [published erratum appears in Lancet 1999;353:1714]. Lancet 1999;353:1035–9.

The mode of delivery and the risk of vertical transmission of human immunodeficiency virus type I—a meta-analysis of 15 prospective cohort studies. The International Perinatal HIV Group. N Engl J Med 1999;340:977–87.

Mofenson LM, Lambert JS, Stiehm ER, Bethel J, Meyer WA 3rd, Whitehouse J, et al. Risk factors for perinatal transmission of human immunodeficiency virus type I in women treated with zidovudine. Pediatric AIDS Clinical Trials Group Study 185 Team. N Engl J Med 1999;341:385–93.

Sexually transmitted diseases treatment guidelines, 2006. Centers for Disease Control and Prevention [published erratum appears in MMWR Recomm Rep 2006;55(36):997]. MMWR Recomm Rep 2006;55 (RR-11):1–94.

# 147

## Health Insurance Portability and Accountability Act

You are preparing to inform a patient of the results of her amniocentesis. However, before you can inform her that the karyotype of her fetus is consistent with trisomy 18, her husband calls to request that you provide him with the results first. He is concerned that his wife will harm herself or the fetus if she receives bad news. Your immediate response to the husband's request should be to

      (A) disclose the diagnosis
\*    (B) refuse to disclose the diagnosis
      (C) obtain a release of liability from the husband
      (D) obtain legal consultation

The Health Insurance Portability and Accountability Act (HIPAA) became law in August 1996. The Act has several provisions that protect the privacy and security of health information, and it sets standards for unique identifiers and electronic health-related claim transactions. The privacy rule became effective on April 14, 2003, and affects nearly all practicing health care providers in the United States. The rule covers disclosure of any personal health information. Penalties for violation of HIPAA include civil fines or imprisonment.

Included in the designation of personal health information are all medical records and other individually identifiable health information in any form, whether communicated electronically, on paper, or orally. The disclosure of personal health information must include only the minimum necessary to complete the task or satisfy the request. The exceptions to the minimum necessary standard include disclosure to other health care providers for treatment, disclosures to the patient herself, disclosures required by law, and disclosures required by HIPAA. To meet the minimum necessary disclosure standard, physicians should take the following steps:

- Designate individuals in their office responsible for maintaining policies related to access to patient information.
- Identify which employees in the office need access to only personal health information.
- Make a reasonable effort to limit access to personal health information to individuals not authorized to access it.

Disclosure of personal health information may be made only with the patient's informed and written authorization with a few exceptions. The exceptions include disclosure to a health plan, provider, or clearinghouse only for purposes of health care treatment, payment, and operations. Patients also must be provided detailed written information on privacy rights and how their information will be used.

In the scenario described, the patient's husband is requesting personal health information. Disclosure requires the patient's authorization despite the husband's apparent concern for her well-being. A release of liability from the husband would not be useful because the personal health information does not concern him directly. It is not the husband's personal health information that is at issue. Although legal consultation may be helpful in some complex situations in regard to HIPAA, this is a case where the patient's privacy rights are clearly protected by the law. Perhaps the best approach to this scenario would be to acknowledge the husband's concerns and to offer to meet jointly with him and the patient to discuss the test results.

Code of Federal Regulations, Title 45, Subtitle A, Part 164: Chapter 502, Uses and disclosures of protected health information: general rules; Chapter 506, Uses and Disclosures to carry out treatment, payment or health care operations; and Chapter 508, Uses and disclosures for which an authorization is required. Available at: http://www.access.gpo.gov/nara/cfr/waisidx_02/45cfr164_02.html. Retrieved September 7, 2005.

HIPAA in practice—minimum necessary standard. HIPAA in practice: February 27, 2003. Washington, DC: American College of Obstetricians and Gynecologists; 2003.

Protecting the privacy of patients' health information, summary of the final regulation. Department of Health and Human Services (HHS) Fact Sheet. US Department of Health and Human Services, December 20, 2000. Available at: http://aspe.hhs.gov/admnsimp/final/pvcfact1.htm. Retrieved September 7, 2005.

# 148

## Surgery for uterine leiomyomata

A 40-year-old premenopausal woman comes to your office and describes regular menstrual cycles that have lengthened from 4 to 10 days with up to 5 days of heavy bleeding. Over the past 2 years, she has noticed slowly increasing abdominal girth with difficulty buttoning her pants. She also has increased urinary frequency and a sense of fullness. A previous examination by another provider 2 years ago revealed an enlarged uterus, which the patient was told was likely caused by leiomyomata. On examination today a large, globular abdominopelvic mass approximately 18 weeks of gestation size is palpated, consistent with a fibroid uterus. There are no adnexal masses palpable. Ultrasonographic evaluation confirms multiple uterine leiomyomata, the largest of which is anterior, intramural, and measures 5 cm. Three other scattered, intramural leiomyomata measure 2, 2.5, and 3 cm. The ovaries bilaterally are within normal limits, and the endometrial stripe is symmetric and measures 8 mm on cycle day 22. She has no further desire for childbearing and would like management of all of her symptoms. The best procedure for this patient is

   (A) laparoscopic myomectomy
   (B) hysteroscopic myomectomy with endometrial ablation
   (C) abdominal myomectomy
 * (D) abdominal hysterectomy
   (E) uterine artery embolization

Uterine leiomyomata are the most common solid pelvic tumor in women. Leiomyomata are estimated to occur in up to 80% of women although they are clinically apparent in only 25–50%. Despite the fact that most women with leiomyomata are asymptomatic, leiomyomata are nonetheless the most frequently cited indication for hysterectomy. The type and degree of symptoms with which a patient may present depend on their number, size, and location within the uterine wall.

Leiomyomata can be subserosal, intramural, or submucosal. Subserosal leiomyomata more commonly present with pressure symptoms whereas submucosal leiomyomata are more likely to cause abnormal bleeding. Intramural leiomyomata, if large, can result in both types of symptoms. The most common symptoms that women with leiomyomata report are bleeding and pelvic pain or pressure. In some instances, leiomyomata will compress surrounding organs, which can affect bowel or bladder function. A bleeding aberration typically presents as menorrhagia with increase in flow or duration of menses often leading to anemia and has significant effects on quality of life.

Although medical treatments for leiomyomata are available, the need for long-term therapy and the frequent side effects of such medications make surgical intervention more popular. In this age of minimally invasive procedures, a number of surgical alternatives to hysterectomy for the treatment of leiomyomata have emerged, each with its own efficacy, benefits, and potential problems.

The only surgical intervention that is definitive and thus guarantees no recurrence is hysterectomy. All other surgical interventions may allow for the growth of preexisting leiomyomata that were too small to treat initially. Hysterectomy, however, is also the only surgical intervention that prevents any further childbearing. The desire to have or not to have children as well as the efficacy of a given procedure for the type of tumor a patient exhibits must be taken into consideration when determining the best surgical approach.

Myomectomy removes only the visible, accessible leiomyomata leaving the remaining uterus in place. This is an option for patients who wish to maintain fertility. Traditionally this procedure was performed by laparotomy for all subserosal and intramural leiomyomata. The literature shows a reoperation rate (ie, requiring a hysterectomy or repeat myomectomy after abdominal myomectomy) of 18% after 10 years. Hysteroscopic myomectomy can be performed for small submucosal leiomyomata. More recently, laparoscopic myomectomy has emerged as an option. This procedure has the advantage of a smaller incision than laparotomy and thus faster recovery and better cosmetic results. The downside, however, is that it can only be performed for leiomyomata small enough to be visualized and safely removed through the endoscope. Thus, it is not appropriate for large uteri or deep intramural leiomyomata not well seen through the scope. In recent years, endoscopic morcellators have allowed for larger leiomyomata to be removed via this route; however, these instruments require significant expertise and leave a larger uterine incision, which is more technically difficult to repair endoscopically. Because of these issues, most recommend that leiomyomata larger than 5–8 cm, leiomyomata that are multiple in nature, or deep intramural leiomyomata be removed via laparotomy. In addition, recurrence rates after laparoscopic myomectomy are higher than laparotomy with a rate of 33% at 27 months. While fertility and future childbearing are an option after these procedures, many would recommend a cesarean delivery after a myomectomy for large or deeply intramural leiomyomata due to increased risk of uterine rupture.

Hysteroscopic myomectomy is best for small submucosal leiomyomata and symptomatic bleeding. Success rates are good for patients who are candidates for this procedure with a reoperation rate of 16% at 9 years. Large or intramural–subserosal leiomyomata cannot be removed this way, in part because they cannot be adequately visualized through the hysteroscope but also because bleeding and other surgical complications are higher in that case. Adding an endometrial ablation to the hysteroscopic myomectomy can improve relief of bleeding even in cases of remaining intramural leiomyomata. This addi-

tional procedure adds little risk to the overall intervention and lowers the reoperation rate to 8% after 6 years. Hysteroscopic procedures add the risk of media intravasation, possible water intoxication, and hyponatremia.

Uterine artery embolization is a radiologic procedure that has been used more often in recent years. This procedure involves partial blockage of the uterine arteries and thus decreased blood supply to the uterine myometrium and its leiomyomata. The procedure is considered minimally invasive because there are no abdominal incisions and the patients typically recover quickly. Most patients do experience a decrease in bleeding and reduction in tumor volume (mean reduction approximately 40%) and pressure symptoms after an embolization. However, in patients whose primary leiomyoma-related symptom is pain, the evidence suggests better efficacy with hysterectomy when compared to embolization. Uterine artery embolization is not without risk. Cases of infection, hemorrhage, ileus, and uterine necrosis that require emergent surgery and cause death have all been reported. In addition, this procedure, which was initially promoted as an outpatient procedure, now in most cases involves at least an overnight hospital stay for pain management and monitoring. Although it is technically a uterine-sparing procedure, long-term effects on the uterine wall and the eventual effect on fertility and pregnancy are unknown and considered to be high risk.

The patient described has multiple leiomyomata, all of which are intramural, and at least one is considered large (5 cm). She has no further childbearing desires and wants therapy for all of her symptoms. The only option listed that offers this is hysterectomy. Abdominal myomectomy would be an option as well; however, given that she likely has at least 10 years until menopause, her chance of recurrence and thus need for reoperation before that time is nearly 20%. Similarly, laparoscopic myomectomy would be difficult in this patient with multiple intramural leiomyomata and would leave her with an even higher recurrence risk. Hysteroscopic myomectomy with or without endometrial ablation would be suboptimal in this patient given that her leiomyomata are intramural and would not be adequately visualized for removal.

Uterine artery embolization would offer the patient some relief with up to 40% reduction in uterine volume. Additionally, data show she could expect a reduction in her heavy menstrual flow. There would still be a risk of recurrence, however, as well as incomplete symptomatic relief.

Hormonal therapies for leiomyomata are generally temporizing measures in patients who wish to maintain childbearing or who have contraindications to surgery. Each has a distinct set of side effects and risks and none offer permanent relief with virtually 100% recurrence after discontinuation. There are promising data on the use of the levonorgestrel-releasing intrauterine device (IUD) in patients with leiomyomata and abnormal bleeding. Though not appropriate for the patient in this case, this IUD is safe and shows long-term efficacy for reducing bleeding.

Acien P, Quereda F. Abdominal myomectomy: results of a simple operative technique. Fertil Steril 1996;65:41–51.

American College of Obstetricians and Gynecologists. Surgical alternatives to hysterectomy in the management of leiomyomas. ACOG Practice Bulletin 16. Washington, DC: ACOG; 2000.

Khaund A, Moss JG, McMillan N, Lumsden MA. Evaluation of the effect of uterine artery embolisation on menstrual blood loss and uterine volume. BJOG 2004;111:700–5.

Rosa e Silva JC, de Sa Rosa e Silva AC, dos Reis FJ, Manetta LA, Ferriani RA, Nogueira AA. Use of a levonorgestrel-releasing intrauterine device for the symptomatic treatment of uterine myomas. J Reprod Med 2005;50:613–17.

Spies JB, Cooper JM, Worthington-Kirsch R, Lipman JC, Mills BB, Benenati JF. Outcome of uterine embolization and hysterectomy for leiomyomas: results of a multicenter study. Am J Obstet Gynecol 2004;191:22–31.

# 149–152
## Pessary fitting and choice

Match the patient (149–152) with the type of pessary (A–E) best suited to the patient's case scenario.

(A) Incontinence ring
(B) Lever (Smith-Hodge)
(C) Gehrung
(D) Gellhorn
(E) Cube

C　**149.** A 50-year-old woman with a large rectocele who is not sexually active.

D　**150.** A 62-year-old woman with stage 3 anterior segment prolapse.

E　**151.** An 80-year-old nursing home resident with uterine procidentia and a large enterocele unable to retain a ring pessary.

B　**152.** A 25-year-old pregnant woman at 20 weeks of gestation with cervical prolapse.

Mechanical support for the pelvic organs may be provided by pessaries. They may be used to treat prolapse, incontinence, or cervical insufficiency, although there are limited data supporting their use. The types of pessaries currently in common use include the ring or donut, incontinence ring, lever (Smith-Hodge or Risser), Gehrung, Gellhorn, cube, and ball. Most pessaries are now made of silicone, which lasts longer with less risk of odor and latex allergies. Each pessary is suited to a particular indication (Tables 149–152-1 and 149–152-2). For example, only the Gehrung and cube pessaries are suitable for rectoceles. Cube pessaries work for almost all types of prolapse, but are difficult to remove and frequently induce ulceration. For anterior segment prolapse, ring or Gellhorn pessaries are good first choices. The lever-type pessaries have been used for retroverted uteri or incompetent cervix.

Pessaries are fitted and placed in the vagina in much the same way that a contraceptive diaphragm is (Fig. 149–152-1). The genital hiatus, vaginal depth, perineal body, and type of prolapse are assessed during examination. The pessary is lubricated and inserted into the vagi-na. A Gehrung pessary would be adjusted 45 degrees so that it sits like a bridge holding up the anterior wall and flattening any rectocele. All pessaries must be small enough to allow one finger-breadth between the pessary and the vaginal wall. The patient should use the Valsalva maneuver in the standing position to check that the pessary does not immediately fall out. She should void before leaving the office and return within 1 week to check for erosions and discharge.

Antibacterial vaginal creams or estrogen creams are useful to prevent vaginal mucosal ulcerations and discharge. The patient should return to the office to check the device at least every 3 months unless she can remove and clean it regularly herself, leaving it out at night. Some physicians work with visiting nurses to minimize the need for office visits. Pessaries provide an excellent solution for many patients who wish to avoid surgery. In one study, 73% of patients with symptomatic prolapse were successfully fitted and 92% of these patients were still satisfied after 2 months. Pessaries may be less successful for women with incontinence, with half of patients discontinuing after 6 months.

**TABLE 149–152-1.** Commonly Used Pessaries

| Pessary Type | Primary Uses | Special Considerations |
|---|---|---|
| Ring incontinence or donut | 1° and 2° uterine prolapse<br>Cystocele<br>(Ring incontinence type used to partially obstruct the urethra in incontinence) | |
| Lever | Uterine support and repositioning<br>Has been used for cervical incompetence | Requires narrow pubic arch |
| Gehrung | Cystocele or rectocele | Difficult to insert |
| Gellhorn | 3° uterine or vaginal prolapse or procidentia | Requires capacious vagina |
| Cube | 3° uterine or vaginal prolapse or procidentia with rectocele or cystocele | Difficult to remove |
| Ball | Nonspecific | Size must be greater than defect |

**TABLE 149–152-2.** Indications for Use of Common Pessaries

| Indication | Pessary |
|---|---|
| Malposition | Lever type (Smith-Hodge) |
| Prolapse/pelvic relaxation | |
|    Uterine | Gellhorn, ring, donut, cube |
|    Vaginal | Gellhorn, donut, cube, ball |
|    Cystocele or rectocele | Gehrung |
| Incompetent cervix | Lever, ring |
| Incontinence | Donut, lever, ring incontinence |
| Preoperative | Based on defect |
| Drug delivery | Ring (17β-estradiol, medroxyprogesterone) |

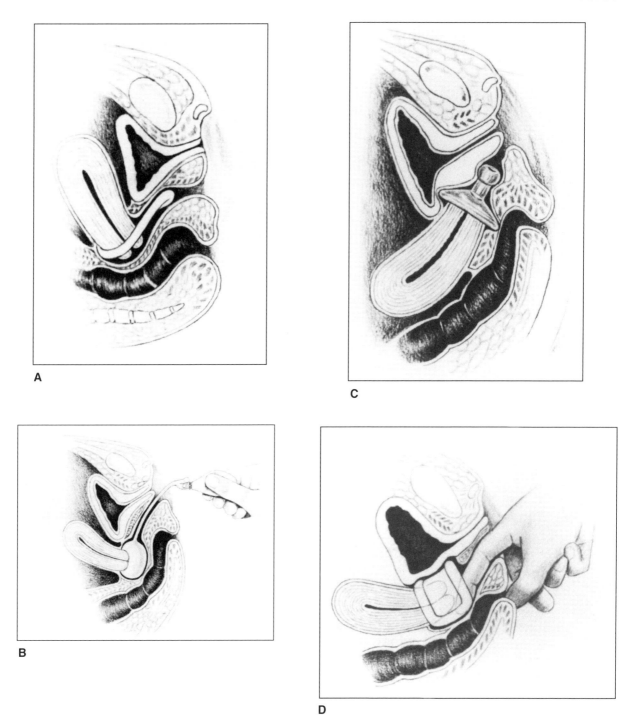

**FIG. 149–152-1.** Diagrams illustrating insertion of different types of pessaries in the vagina. **A.** The ring and lever pessary should fit behind the cervix and rest in the retropubic notch. **B.** Once in position, the ball pessary is inflated to gently occlude the upper vagina, thereby lifting the vaginal apex and uterus. **C.** In a case of uterine prolapse, the Gellhorn pessary should rest with the plate above the levator plane as shown; the stem of the pessary should be contained entirely within the vagina. **D.** The limbs of the Gehrung pessary should sit on the levator plane lateral to the cervix at the apex of the vagina. **E.** Pessaries specifically designed to help control urinary incontinence, such as the ring incontinence pessary shown here, should provide more support to the urethra and periurethral tissues. **F.** The cube pessary must be compressed before it is inserted into the vagina. **G.** When correctly positioned, the cube pessary should occupy the upper vagina and rest against the cervix (when present). (Pessary drawings courtesy of Milex Products, Inc., Chicago, Illinois 60634-1403.)

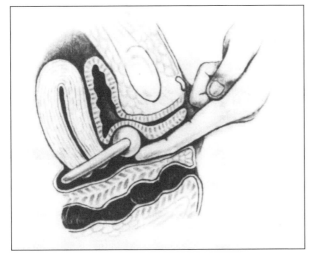

**E**

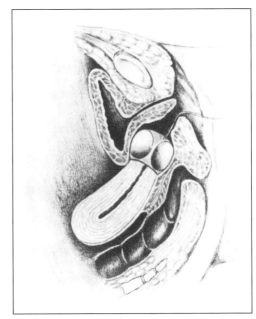

**G**

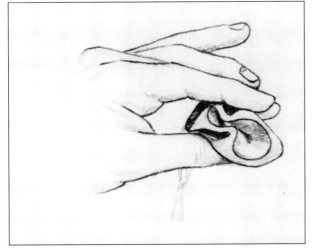

**F**

Clemons JL, Aguilar VC, Tillinghast TA, Jackson ND, Myers DL. Patient satisfaction and changes in prolapse and urinary symptoms in women who were fitted successfully with a pessary for pelvic organ prolapse. Am J Obstet Gynecol 2004;190:1025–9.

Donnelly MJ, Powell-Morgan S, Olsen AL, Nygaard IE. Vaginal pessaries for the management of stress and mixed urinary incontinence. Int Urogynecol J Pelvic Floor Dysfunct 2004;15:302–7.

Miller DS. Contemporary use of the pessary. In: Sciarra JJ, editor. Gynecology and obstetrics. Vol. 1. Philadelphia (PA): JB Lippincott; 1999. p. 1–13.

Smith RP, Ling FW. Pessary fitting. In: Procedures in women's health. Baltimore (MD): Williams & Wilkins; 1997. p. 127–36.

Sulak PJ, Kuehl TJ, Shull BL. Vaginal pessaries and their use in pelvic relaxation. J Reprod Med 1993;38:919–23.

# 153–155
## Hormone therapy options

Match the patient scenario (153–155) with the best hormonal therapy option (A–D).

(A) oral conjugated equine estrogen
(B) low-dose oral contraceptive
(C) transdermal estradiol-17β
(D) esterified estrogen

B    **153.** A 48-year-old woman, gravida 2, para 2, reports heavy menses occurring every 21–24 days with no intermenstrual bleeding. Before the onset of her menses, she also experiences headaches, occasional hot flushes and night sweats, and mood swings. She feels depressed because she has been healthy all her life and her heavy menses are disruptive to her active lifestyle. Medical history is negative for any illnesses or risk factors. Examination, including pelvic examination, is normal.

C    **154.** A 49-year-old woman with type 2 diabetes mellitus is taking oral hypoglycemic agents and a lipid-lowering drug for elevated triglycerides and an elevated high-sensitivity c-reactive protein (hs-CRP). She presents with severe hot flushes and distressing night sweats. She has tried multiple over-the-counter herbal preparations and has been prescribed a selective serotonin reuptake inhibitor (SSRI) for depression. She requests estrogen therapy.

C    **155.** A 52-year-old woman, gravida 1, para 1, complains of severe hot flushes and night sweats. She is unresponsive to an antidepressant, a progesterone cream, and herbal therapies. She has a history of deep vein thrombosis (DVT) postpartum 30 years ago that was treated with anticoagulants for several months. She has had no recurrent episodes. She requests estrogen because night sweats disrupt her sleep and hot flushes interfere with her job as a television reporter.

The perimenopause is associated with a multitude of symptoms resulting from declining ovarian function. Although the average age of menopause is 51–52 years, the perimenopausal period can begin many years earlier. Detailed evaluation of hormonal levels of women in their forties documents the hormonal changes known to occur in many women during perimenopause. Although menopause is associated with an increased follicle-stimulating hormone (FSH) level, estrogen deficiency, and amenorrhea, before this occurs, many patients produce increased estrogen and experience heavier menses that occur every 21–24 days rather than the usual expected 28–30 days. This shortened cycle results from increased estrogen secretion throughout the cycle with an accompanying reduced progesterone secretion in the luteal phase leading to an elevated estrogen-to-progesterone ratio. This results in a shortened follicular phase of the cycle and often is associated with heavier menses (Patient 153). These patients are often effectively managed with low-dose oral contraceptives. Because all oral contraceptives are progestin-dominant, these formulations decrease the estrogen–progesterone ratio, often alleviating the problems of heavy menses while simultaneously lowering the

risk of endometrial cancer. Healthy, normotensive women who do not smoke can use oral contraceptives safely up to menopause.

As patients become more estrogen deficient, they often experience severe vasomotor symptoms not relieved by herbal therapies or nonestrogen pharmacologic management. Before prescribing hormone therapy, contraindications must be assessed and risks vs benefits discussed with the patient. Patient 154 has diabetes and severe vasomotor symptoms that are unresponsive to alternative therapies. Because of her history of increased triglycerides, a transdermal preparation is the best option if estrogen is to be used to manage her symptoms. Although oral and transdermal agents increase high-density lipoprotein (HDL) cholesterol and decrease low-density lipoprotein (LDL) cholesterol, oral estrogen formulations are associated with an increase in triglycerides. An increase in triglycerides is not seen with transdermal estrogen preparations. The estrogen patch with the lowest dose should be used for Patient 154.

Patient 155 presents with a clinical dilemma. Her personal history of a DVT while pregnant decades ago is a listed contraindication to estrogen use. If estrogen is to be prescribed, the patient must be counseled thoroughly regarding the risks vs benefits with written documentation in the medical record. If estrogen is prescribed, an ultra low-dose (0.025 mg estradiol) transdermal patch is the best option based on current information. In a case–control study evaluating the incidence of venous thromboembolic events, oral estrogen was associated with an increased risk (odds ratio [OR] = 3.5; 95% confidence interval [CI], 1.8–6.8). The transdermal patch did not increase the risk (OR = 0.9; 95% CI, 00.5–1.6).

American College of Obstetricians and Gynecologists. Prevention of deep vein thrombosis and pulmonary embolism. ACOG Practice Bulletin 21. Washington, DC: ACOG; 2000.

Godsland IF. Effects of postmenopausal hormone replacement therapy on lipid, lipoprotein, and apolipoprotein (a) concentrations: analysis of studies from 1974–2000. Fertil Steril 2001;75:898–915.

McKinlay SM, Brambilla DJ, Posner JG. The normal menopause transition. Maturitas 1992;14:103–15.

Santoro N, Brown JR, Adel T, Skurnick JH. Characterization of reproductive hormonal dynamics in the perimenopause. J Clin Endocrinol Metab1996;81:1495–501.

Scarabin PY, Oger E, Plu-Bureau G. Differential association of oral and transdermal oestrogen-replacement therapy with venous thromboembolism risk. EStrogen and THromboEmbolism Risk Study Group. Lancet 2003;362:428–32.

Use of hormonal contraception in women with coexisting medical conditions. ACOG Practice Bulletin No. 73. American College of Obstetricians and Gynecologists. Obstet Gynecol 2006;107:1453–72.

# 156–159
## Health maintenance choices

For each of the following patients (156–159), select the most appropriate test or vaccination (A–D).

(A) Tuberculin skin testing
(B) Pneumococcal vaccination
(C) Influenza vaccination
(D) Chest X-ray

A  **156.** A 42-year-old asymptomatic woman who recently moved to the United States from Haiti

A  **157.** A 24-year-old asymptomatic woman who works in a homeless shelter

D  **158.** A 37-year-old woman who presents with a productive cough, fever, and rales on pulmonary auscultation

B  **159.** A 15-year-old adolescent who recently had a splenectomy following a motor vehicle accident

Annually, 8 million to 9 million new cases of tuberculosis (TB) occur worldwide. Most of these cases involve residents of countries in the developing world. Latent TB infection refers to the presence of *Mycobacterium tuberculosis* organisms without symptoms or radiographic evidence of disease. Identification and treatment of individuals with latent disease prevents active tuberculosis.

Proteins characteristic of *M tuberculosis* include those in tuberculin, used for skin testing. Tuberculin skin testing is most useful for detecting latent infection. To perform the tuberculin skin test, 5 tuberculin units (TU) of purified protein derivative (PPD) tuberculin solution are injected intradermally on the volar surface of the lower arm using a 27-gauge needle, to produce a weal 6–10 mm in diameter. In 48–72 hours, induration and erythema should be assessed. In individuals with no TB risk factors, 15-mm induration is considered positive. In recent immigrants, injection drug users, residents or employees of congregate settings, mycobacteriology laboratory personnel, and individuals with clinical conditions that place them at high risk, 10-mm induration is considered positive. Induration of 5 mm is considered positive in HIV-infected individuals, those with close contact to an infectious TB case, individuals with chest X-rays consistent with prior untreated TB, organ transplant recipients, and other immunosuppressed patients.

Because the prevalence of tuberculosis is high in Haiti, skin testing is appropriate for women who have emigrated from that country within the past 5 years, as in Patient 156. Likewise, tuberculosis is prevalent among homeless individuals, so a woman working in a homeless shelter merits skin testing (Patient 157). Given their risk factors, a skin test with induration of 10 mm or more would be considered positive for latent infection in these individuals.

A chest X-ray is not indicated for the three women free of symptoms of pulmonary disease. An X-ray would be appropriate for the woman with symptoms and signs suggestive of pneumonia, as with Patient 158.

*Streptococcus pneumoniae* (pneumococcus) is a bacterial pathogen that affects children and adults worldwide. It is most likely to cause illness and death among those with certain underlying conditions as well as the elderly. Use of pneumococcal polysaccharide (inactivated) vaccine prevents invasive bacteremic pneumococcal infections. Pneumococcal vaccine is administered intramuscularly or subcutaneously as one 0.5-mL dose. Asplenia predisposes individuals to pneumococcal infection. As a consequence, whether the asplenia is functional, as in a person with hemoglobinopathy, or surgical, as in Patient 159 who had undergone splenectomy, vaccination is appropriate. Influenza vaccination, particularly for high-risk indi-

viduals such as pregnant women, is appropriate during the influenza season. However, it is not indicated for any of the described patients.

Keusch GT, Bart KJ, Miller M. Immunization principles and vaccine use. In: Kasper DL, Fauci AS, Longo DL, Braunwald E, Hauser SL, Jameson JL, editors. Harrison's principles of internal medicine. 16th ed. New York; McGraw-Hill, 2005. p. 713–25.

Centers for Disease Control and Prevention. Targeted tuberculin testing and treatment of latent tuberculosis infection, 2005. Atlanta (GA): CDC; 2005. Available at: http://www.cdc.gov/NCHSTP/tb/pubs/slidesets/LTBI/default.htm. Retrieved August 4, 2006.

Prevention of pneumococcal disease: recommendations of the Advisory Committee on Immunization Practices (ACIP). MMWR Recomm Rep 1997;46(RR-8):1–24.

Primary and preventive care: periodic assessments. ACOG Committee Opinion No. 292. American College of Obstetricians and Gynecologists. Obstet Gynecol 2003;102:1117–24. Washington, DC: ACOG; 2002.

Raviglione MC, O'Brien RJ. Tuberculosis. In: Kasper DL, Fauci AS, Longo DL, Braunwald E, Hauser SL, Jameson JL, editors. Harrison's principles of internal medicine. 16th ed. New York (NY): McGraw-Hill; 2005. p. 953–66.

# 160–163

## Risks for deep vein thrombosis

Clinical assessment for suspected deep vein thrombosis (DVT) can be inaccurate, but it can be used to stratify patients using a pretest probability of DVT. To complete the workup for each patient (160–163) described, select the most likely pretest probability of DVT (A–C).

    (A) Low probability of DVT (approximately 5%)
    (B) Intermediate probability of DVT (approximately 20–25%)
    (C) High probability of DVT (approximately 70–80%)

C    160.   A 56-year-old woman, 2 weeks after vaginal hysterectomy and vault suspension, has tenderness along the right deep venous system and unilateral pitting, pretibial edema.

A    161.   A moderately obese 39-year-old woman with a temperature of 38.6°C (101.5°F) has trace bilateral ankle edema and a 10 × 14-cm erythematous, indurated swelling on the lateral right calf.

A    162.   A 19-year-old woman has an 8-cm vulvar hematoma and mild pain and bruising on the left thigh following a straddle injury.

C    163.   A 47-year-old woman with stage III A squamous cell cancer of the cervix has had radiation treatment and presents with a swollen right leg.

The diagnosis of DVT is complicated by the fact that no individual symptom or sign is unique to the disorder or is invariably found in the presence of thrombosis. In addition, the criterion standards for assessing thromboses (venography or angiography) are expensive and invasive. Therefore, noninvasive diagnostic strategies that are not as sensitive nor as specific have largely replaced the invasive tests. The probability that a patient has a disease following a diagnostic test is determined by both the accuracy of the test and the estimated probability that the patient had the disease before having the test, based on clinical and historical data. This means that the predictive power of diagnostic tests is critically dependent on the pretest probability of disease. Stratification of patients with possible venous thromboembolism into low-, intermediate-, and high-pretest probability subgroups has been shown to optimize the positive and negative predictive values, improving the clinical usefulness of noninvasive diagnostic tests. A well-recorded history and physical examination are crucial parts of the diagnostic pathway.

Several methods of stratifying patients into risk subgroups have been developed, including empirical assessments by experienced clinicians and simpler clinical scoring models. A formalized strategy based on appropriate verification of its reliability at individual institutions allows for optimal use of resources and more accurate diagnosis. The exact choice of assessment tool is less important than the necessity of performing a careful

pretest probability. One commonly used score for suspected DVT is shown in Box 160-163-1. When pooling patient data by one of these methods, 39% of patients can be classified as low risk for DVT, 45% can be classified as intermediate risk, and 16% as high risk. This translates to prevalence of DVT in the subgroups of 5%, 23%, and 74%, respectively.

Patient 160, the 56-year-old posthysterectomy patient, is at high risk for DVT because of recent surgery, localized tenderness, and unilateral pitting edema. An important additional factor is that there is no clear, alternative diagnosis that would account for her symptoms.

Patient 161, the 39-year-old woman, is at low-risk for DVT (approximately 5%) because she has bilateral leg edema and cellulitis. She does not have tenderness over the distribution of the deep venous system or other clear risk factors.

Patient 162, the 19-year-old woman, has a clear cause, which is trauma. Although there is direct trauma with tenderness on the thigh and vulva, she otherwise has no additional signs or symptoms that would place her in the high-risk category.

Patient 163, the 47-year-old patient with cancer, has classic risk factors of active cancer and unilateral leg–calf swelling. Additional workup and confirmation of DVT in this high-risk patient is warranted.

Venous compression ultrasonography is the most widely used noninvasive test for suspected DVT. In patients with symptomatic DVT, approximately 80% have throm-

BOX 160–163-1

**Revised Clinical Model for Predicting Pretest Probability for Deep Vein Thrombosis\***

Score one point for affirmative responses to the following points:

1. Active cancer (treatment ongoing or within previous 6 months or palliative)
2. Paralysis, paresis or recent plaster immobilization of the lower extremities
3. Recently bedridden for greater than 3 days or major surgery within 4 weeks
4. Localized tenderness along the distribution of the deep venous system
5. Thigh and calf swollen (should be measured)
6. Calf swelling 3 cm greater than asymptomatic side (measured 10 cm below tibial tuberosity)
7. Pitting edema; symptomatic leg only
8. Dilated superficial veins (nonvaricose) in symptomatic leg only

\*Score minus 2 points for an alternative diagnosis as likely as or more likely than deep vein thrombosis. Clinical probability calculated as follows: high, greater than or equal to 3 points; moderate, 1–2 points; low, less than or equal to 0 points.

Wells PS, Hirsh J, Anderson DR, Lensing AW, Foster G, Kearon C, et al. A simple clinical model for the diagnosis of deep-vein thrombosis combined with impedance plethysmography: potential for an improvement in the diagnostic process. J Intern Med 1998;243:20.

bus that involves the popliteal or more proximal veins. In the remainder of patients, a thrombus is limited to the distal calf veins and can progress to involve the proximal veins within 1 week of presentation.

If the clinical probability of DVT is low and a noninvasive test result is negative, the posttest probability is sufficiently low to exclude the diagnosis of DVT. Therefore, a patient with a low or moderate pretest probability of DVT who has a negative venous ultrasonogram result can be followed safely without additional testing unless the clinical scenario changes. In contrast, if the findings of pretest probability and the noninvasive test are discordant, further testing such as venography or angiography should be considered. D-dimer, another tool in the diagnosis of venous thromboembolism, has not been evaluated as a test for thromboembolism in pregnancy.

D-dimer is a degradation product of a cross-linked fibrin blood clot that is typically elevated in a patient with an acute venous thromboembolism. There are both qualitative and quantitative D-dimer tests and several generations of the tests. Overall, the D-dimer is a sensitive test. However, it is not a specific test. Its real value is that it provides a negative test result to exclude the diagnosis of venous thromboembolism in the proper setting. If the D-dimer is to be used, one must know which test is being used and how to interpret the results. For example, D-dimer can be increased by other conditions such as recent major surgery, hemorrhage, trauma, malignancy, or sepsis. The D-dimer is not a substitute for a good medical history and physical examination nor a substitute for a good determination of the clinical pretest probability of venous thromboembolism. Randomized trials have evaluated the use of qualitative D-dimer assays when the pretest probability of disease is low. When this pretest probability is low, a negative qualitative D-dimer test can exclude the diagnosis of venous thromboembolism.

Kearon C, Ginsberg JS, Douketis J, Crowther MA, Turpie AG, Bates SM, et al. A randomized trial of diagnostic strategies after normal proximal vein ultrasonography for suspected deep venous thrombosis: D-dimer testing compared with repeated ultrasonography. Ann Intern Med 2005;142:490–6.

Kelly J, Hunt BJ. The utility of pretest probability assessment in patients with clinically suspected venous thromboembolism. J Thromb Haemost 2003;1:1888–96.

Miron MJ, Perrier A, Bounameaux H. Clinical assessment of suspected deep vein thrombosis: comparison between a score and empirical assessment. J Intern Med 2000;247:249–54.

Perrier A, Desmarais S, Miron MJ, de Moerloose P, Lepage R, Slosman D, et al. Non-invasive diagnosis of venous thromboembolism in outpatients. Lancet 1999;353:190–5.

Wells PS, Owen C, Doucette S, Fergusson D, Tran H. Does this patient have deep vein thrombosis? JAMA 2006;295:199–207.

Wicki J, Perneger TV, Junod AF, Bounameaux H, Perrier A. Assessing clinical probability of pulmonary embolism in the emergency ward: a simple score. Arch Intern Med 2001;161:92–7.

# 164–167
## Types of headache

For each patient with headache (164–167), select the most likely diagnosis (A–E).

(A) Common migraine
(B) Classic migraine
(C) Cluster headache
(D) Tension headache
(E) Intracranial hemorrhage

B  **164.** A 26-year-old woman with a history of unilateral, throbbing headaches associated with photophobia, nausea, and occasional emesis. She usually experiences minor visual changes just before the onset of a headache.

D  **165.** A 40-year-old woman with frequent headaches that occur late in the afternoon and are characterized by a band-like pain with pressure and tightness.

E  **166.** A 50-year-old woman with an excruciating occipital headache she describes as "the worst pain I've ever had," with nausea, blurred vision, vomiting, and anisocoria.

C  **167.** A 32-year-old woman who describes intense, unilateral, periorbital headaches associated with runny nose and a "droopy eyelid." The attacks usually occur several times a day for 1–2 hours at a time.

Headache is a common complaint encountered by physicians in office practice. It is estimated that 90% of the population will experience headache at some time each year, and headache alone accounts for up to 17 billion health care dollars annually. When confronted by a patient who complains of headache, it is always important to take a careful and complete history that includes onset, duration, quality, location, and intensity of pain. The patient should be encouraged to describe the pain and any aggravating factors in her own words, and the physician should note any associated findings (eg, nausea, vomiting, and visual disturbances). A history of her headaches should be elicited, and the patient questioned as to how this episode of headache may be different from prior episodes. A clear understanding of different types of headache is essential to ensure that potentially life-threatening causes of headache are not overlooked.

Approximately 23 million individuals in the United States suffer from recurrent migraine headaches. Migraineurs are three times more likely to be women than men, and the frequent association of migraines with the menstrual cycle makes migraine a familiar complaint to most gynecologists. The International Headache Society classifies migraine into two main categories:

1. Migraine without aura (formerly known as common migraine)

2. Migraine with aura (formerly known as classic migraine)

The older terms are familiar to patients and physicians and remain in the vernacular.

Migraine without aura is a vascular type of headache that typically presents as unilateral throbbing pain of moderate to severe intensity. Associated symptoms may include nausea, vomiting, photophobia, and phonophobia. Physical activity aggravates the condition.

Patient 164 has migraine with aura, a less common form of migraine, characterized by an array of prodromal symptoms that can occur up to an hour before the onset of headache. These symptoms may include visual scotomata, paresthesias, paresis, and dysphasia. The ensuing headache tends to be unilateral, throbbing, and similar to common migraine. Migraine headaches of both types may last 4–72 hours and can be debilitating in intensity.

Patient 165 has a tension headache, the most common type of headache, which occurs in 69% of the population. The pain is usually mild to moderate, bilateral, and constant. Nausea, vomiting, and photophobia are typically absent. Tension headaches are gradual in onset and may last from several hours to several days. Patients often describe the pain as a "band-like" pressure around the head that may extend to the neck and shoulders. Tension headaches frequently occur later in the day and may be related to situational stress. Another common type of headache is rebound headache from overuse of oral analgesics.

Patient 166 has a headache that is strongly suggestive of intracranial hemorrhage, a potentially life-threatening condition. Ruptured cerebral aneurysm is the most common cause of bleeding in the subarachnoid space and accounts for up to two thirds of all episodes of spontaneous intracranial hemorrhage. Patients relate a very sudden and abrupt onset of intense headache "like a thunder clap" and often describe the pain as "the worst headache of my life." The pain is frequently occipital and associated with ptosis, diplopia, and anisocoria. Vomiting is common. Headache from intracranial hemorrhage has high morbidity and mortality and should be considered a medical emergency.

Patient 167 suffers from cluster headaches. This type of headache is much less common in women and is characterized by sudden severe, unilateral throbbing pain in the orbital region. These short, intense headaches last 1–3 hours and are frequently associated with acute rhinorrhea, tearing, and nasal congestion. Unlike migraines, movement does not aggravate cluster headaches and patients will tend to pace back and forth. Attacks can happen several times throughout the day and will usually occur in "clusters" that can last for several weeks.

Evans RW, Olesen J. Migraine classification, diagnostic criteria, and testing. Neurology 2003;60(suppl 2):S24–S30.

Gaini SM, Fiori L, Cesana C, Vergani F. The headache in the emergency department. Neurol Sci 2004;25(suppl 3):S196–S201.

Weitzel KW, Thomas ML, Small RE, Goode JV. Migraine: a comprehensive review of new treatment options. Pharmacotherapy 1999; 19:957–73.

# Appendix A

## Normal Values for Laboratory Tests*

| Analyte | Conventional Units |
|---|---|
| Alanine aminotransferase, serum | 8–35 units/L |
| Alkaline phosphatase, serum | 15–120 units/L |
| Menopause | |
| Amniotic fluid index | 3–30 mL |
| Amylase | |
| 60 years or younger | 20–300 units/L |
| Older than 60 years | 21–160 units/L |
| Aspartate aminotransferase, serum | 15–30 units/L |
| Bicarbonate | |
| Arterial blood | 21–27 mEq/L |
| Venous plasma | 23–29 mEq/L |
| Bilirubin | |
| Total | 0.3–1 mg/dL |
| Conjugated (direct) | 0.1–0.4 mg/dL |
| Newborn, total | 1–10 mg/dL |
| Blood gases (arterial) and pulmonary function | |
| Base deficit | Less than 3 mEq/L |
| Base excess, arterial blood, calculated | –2 to +3 mEq/L |
| Forced expiratory volume | 3.5–5 L |
| | More than 80% of predicted value |
| Forced vital capacity | 3.5–5 L |
| Oxygen saturation ($So_2$) | 95% or higher |
| $Pao_2$ | 80 mm Hg or more |
| $Pco_2$ | 35–45 mm Hg |
| $Po_2$ | 80–95 mm Hg |
| Peak expiratory flow rate | Approximately 450 L/min |
| pH | 7.35–7.45 |
| $Pvo_2$ | 30–40 mm Hg |
| Blood urea nitrogen | |
| Adult | 7–18 mg/dL |
| Older than 60 years | 8–20 mg/dL |
| CA 125 | Less than 34 units/mL |
| Calcium | |
| Ionized | 4.6–5.3 mg/dL |
| Serum | 8.6–10 mg/dL |
| Chloride | 98–106 mEq/L |
| Cholesterol | |
| Total | |
| Desirable | 140–199 mg/dL |
| Borderline high | 200–239 mg/dL |
| High | 240 mg/dL or more |
| High-density lipoprotein (HDL) | 40–85 mg/dL |
| Low-density lipoprotein | |
| Desirable | Less than 130 mg/dL |
| Borderline high | 140–159 mg/dL |
| High | More than 160 mg/dL |
| Total cholesterol-to-HDL ratio | |
| Desirable | Less than 3 |
| Borderline high | 3–5 |
| High | More than 5 |

*Values listed are specific for adults or women, if relevant, unless otherwise differentiated.

*(continued)*

## Normal Values for Laboratory Tests *(continued)*

| Analyte | Conventional Units |
|---|---|
| Cholesterol *(continued)* | |
| Triglycerides | |
| 20 years and older | Less than 150 mg/dL |
| Less than 20 years | 35–135 mg/dL |
| Cortisol, plasma | |
| 8 AM | 5–23 mcg/dL |
| 4 PM | 3–15 mcg/dL |
| 10 PM | Less than 50% of 8 AM value |
| Creatinine, serum | 0.6–1.2 mg/dL |
| Dehydroepiandrosterone sulfate | 60–340 mcg/dL |
| Erythrocyte | |
| Count | 3,800,000–5,100,000/mm$^3$ |
| Distribution width | 10 plus or minus 1.5% |
| Sedimentation rate | |
| Wintrobe method | 0–15 mm/h |
| Westergren method | 0–20 mm/h |
| Estradiol-17β | |
| Follicular phase | 30–100 pg/mL |
| Ovulatory phase | 200–400 pg/mL |
| Luteal phase | 50–140 pg/mL |
| Child | 0.8–56 pg/mL |
| Ferritin, serum | 18–160 mcg/L |
| Fibrinogen | 150–400 mg/dL |
| Follicle-stimulating hormone (FSH) | |
| Premenopause | 2.8–17.2 mIU/mL |
| Midcycle peak | 15–35 mIU/mL |
| Postmenopause | 24–170 mIU/mL |
| Child | 0.1–7 mIU/mL |
| Glucose | |
| Fasting | 70–105 mg/dL |
| 2-hour postprandial | Less than 120 mg/dL |
| Random blood | 65–110 mg/dL |
| Hematocrit | 36–48% |
| Hemoglobin | 12–16 g/dL |
| Fetal | Less than 1% of total |
| Hemoglobin A$_{1C}$ (nondiabetic) | 5.5–8.5% |
| Human chorionic gonadotropin | 0–5 mIU/mL |
| Pregnant | More than 5 mIU/mL |
| 17α-Hydroxyprogesterone | |
| Adult | 50–300 ng/dL |
| Child | 32–63 ng/dL |
| 25-Hydroxyvitamin D | 10–55 ng/mL |
| Iron, serum | 65–165 mcg/dL |
| Binding capacity total | 240–450 mcg/dL |
| Lactate dehydrogenase, serum | 313–618 units/L |
| Leukocytes | |
| Total | 5,000–10,000/mm$^3$ |
| Differential counts | |
| Basophils | 0–1% |
| Eosinophils | 1–3% |
| Lymphocytes | 25–33% |
| Monocytes | 3–7% |
| Myelocytes | 0% |
| Band neutrophils | 3–5% |
| Segmented neutrophils | 54–62% |

*(continued)*

## Normal Values for Laboratory Tests (*continued*)

| Analyte | Conventional Units |
| --- | --- |
| Lipase | |
|   60 years or younger | 10–140 units/L |
|   Older than 60 years | 18–180 units/L |
| Luteinizing hormone | |
|   Follicular phase | 3.6–29.4 mIU/mL |
|   Midcycle peak | 58–204 mIU/mL |
|   Postmenopause | 35–129 mIU/mL |
|   Child | 0.5–10.3 mIU/mL |
| Magnesium | |
|   Adult | 1.6–2.6 mg/dL |
|   Child | 1.7–2.1 mg/dL |
|   Newborn | 1.5–2.2 mg/dL |
| Mean corpuscular | |
|   Hemoglobin | 27–33 pg |
|   Hemoglobin concentration | 33–37 g/dL |
|   Volume | 80–100 cubic micrometers |
| Partial thromboplastin time | 30–45 s |
|   Activated | 21–35 s |
| Phosphate, inorganic phosphorus | 2.5–4.5 mg/dL |
| Platelet count | 140,000–400,000/mm$^3$ |
| Potassium | 3.5–5.3 mEq/L |
| Progesterone | |
|   Follicular phase | Less than 3 ng/mL |
|   Luteal phase | 2.5–28 ng/mL |
|   On oral contraceptives | 0.1–0.3 ng/mL |
|   Secretory phase | 5–30 ng/mL |
|   Older than 60 years | 0–0.2 ng/mL |
|   1st trimester | 9–47 ng/mL |
|   2nd trimester | 16.8–146 ng/mL |
|   3rd trimester | 55–255 ng/mL |
| Prolactin | 0–17 ng/mL |
|   Pregnant | 34–386 ng/mL by 3rd trimester |
| Prothrombin time | 10–13 s |
| Reticulocyte count | Absolute: 25,000–85,000 mm$^3$ |
| | 0.5–2.5% of erythrocytes |
| Semen analysis, spermatozoa | |
|   Antisperm antibody | % of sperm binding by immunobead technique; More than 20% = decreased fertility |
|   Count | 20 million/mL or more |
|   Motility | 60% or more |
|   Morphology | 60% or more normal forms |
| Sodium | 135–145 mEq/L |
| Testosterone, female | |
|   Total | 6–86 ng/dL |
|     Pregnant | 3–4 × normal |
|     Postmenopause | ½ of normal |
|   Free | |
|     20–29 years old | 0.9–3.2 pg/mL |
|     30–39 years old | 0.8–3 pg/mL |
|     40–49 years old | 0.6–2.5 pg/mL |
|     50–59 years old | 0.3–2.7 pg/mL |
|     Older than 60 years | 0.2–2.2 pg/mL |
| Thyroid-stimulating hormone | 0.3–3.0 µU/mL |

(*continued*)

## Normal Values for Laboratory Tests *(continued)*

| Analyte | Conventional Units |
| --- | --- |
| Thyroxine | |
|   Serum free | 0.9–2.3 ng/dL |
|   Total | 1.5–4.5 mg/dL |
| Triiodothyronine uptake | 25–35% |
| Urea nitrogen, blood | |
|   Adult | 7–18 mg/dL |
|   60 years or older | 8–20 mg/dL |
| Uric acid, serum | 2.6–6 mg/dL |
| Urinalysis | |
|   Epithelial cells | 0–3/HPF |
|   Erythrocytes | 0–3/HPF |
|   Leukocytes | 0–4/HPF |
|   Protein (albumin) | |
|     Qualitative | none detected |
|     Quantitative | 10–100 mg/24 hours |
|   Specific gravity | |
|     Normal hydration and volume | 1.005–1.03 |
|     Concentrated | 1.025–1.03 |
|     Diluted | 1.001–1.01 |

# Appendix B

## Diagnostic Criteria for Metabolic Syndrome

| Measure (Any Three of Five Criteria Constitute Diagnosis of Metabolic Syndrome) | Categorical Cut Points |
|---|---|
| Elevated waist circumference*† | 102 cm or more (40 in. or more) in men<br>88 cm or more (35 in. or more) in women |
| Elevated triglycerides | 150 mg/dL or more (1.7 mmol/L or more)<br>*or*<br>Drug treatment for elevated triglycerides |
| Reduced high-density lipoprotein Cholesterol (HDL-C) | Less than 40 mg/dL (less than 1.03 mmol/L) in men<br>Less than 50 mg/dL (less than1.3 mmol/L) in women<br>*or*<br>Drug treatment for reduced HDL-C‡ |
| Elevated blood pressure (BP) | 130 mm Hg or higher systolic BP<br>*or*<br>85 mm Hg or higher diastolic blood pressure<br>*or*<br>Drug treatment for hypertension |
| Elevated fasting glucose | 100 mg/dL or more<br>*or*<br>Drug treatment for elevated glucose |

*To measure waist circumference, locate top of right iliac crest. Place a measuring tape in a horizontal plane around the abdomen at level of iliac crest. Before reading tape measure, ensure that tape is snug but does not compress the skin and is parallel to floor. Measurement is made at end of normal expiration.

†Some U.S, adults of non-Asian origin (eg, white, black, Hispanic) with marginally increased waist circumference (eg, 94–101 cm [37–39 in.] in men and 80–87 cm [31–34 in.] in women) may have a strong genetic contribution to insulin resistance and should benefit from changes in lifestyle habits, similar to men with categorical increases in waist circumference. Lower waist circumference cut point (eg, 90 cm [35 in.] in men and 80 cm [31 in.] in women) appears to be appropriate for Asian Americans.

‡Fibrates and nicotinic acid are the most commonly used drugs for elevated triglycerides and reduced HDL-C. Patients who take one of these drugs are presumed to have high triglycerides and low HDL.

Grundy SM, Cleeman JI, Daniels SR, Donato KA, Eckel RH, Franklin BA, et al. Diagnosis and management of the metabolic syndrome: an American Heart Association/National Heart, Lung, and Blood Institute scientific statement. Circulation 2005;112:2739. Reproduced with permission. AHA Scientific Statement: Diagnosis and Management of Metabolic Syndrome © 2005, American Heart Association.

# Appendix C

Stepwise Approach for Managing Asthma During Pregnancy and Lactation: Treatment

| Classify Severity | Clinical Features Before Treatment or Adequate Control | | Medications Required to Maintain Long-Term Control |
|---|---|---|---|
| | Symptoms/Day Symptoms/Night | PEFR or FEV$_1$ PEFR Variability | |
| Step 4 Severe Persistent | Continual Frequent | 60% or less More than 30% | Preferred treatment: High-dose inhaled corticosteroid* *and* Long-acting β$_2$-agonist *and* If needed, corticosteroid tablets or syrup long-term, 82 mg/kg per day, generally not to exceed 60 mg per day. (Make repeat attempts to reduce systemic corticosteroid and maintain control with high-dose corticosteroid.*) Alternative treatment: High-dose inhaled corticosteroid* Sustained-release theophylline to serum concentration of 5–12 mcg/mL |
| Step 3 Moderate Persistent | Daily More than 1 night per week | More than 60% but less than 80% More than 30% | Preferred treatment: Low-dose inhaled corticosteroid* *and* Long-acting β$_2$-agonist *or* Medium-dose inhaled corticosteroid* If needed (particularly in patients with recurring severe exacerbations): Medium-dose inhaled corticosteroid* *and* Long-acting β$_2$-agonist Alternative treatment: Low-dose inhaled corticosteroid* and either theophylline or leukotriene receptor agonist[†] |
| Step 2 Mild Persistent | More than 2 days per week but less than daily | 80% or more 20–30% | Preferred treatment: Low-dose inhaled corticosteroid* Alternative treatment (listed alphabetically): cromolyn, leukotriene receptor agonist[†] *or* sustained-release theophylline concentration of 5–12 mcg/mL |
| Step 1 Mild Intermittent | 2 days per week or less Less than 2 nights per month | 80% or more Less than 20% | No daily medication needed Severe exacerbations may occur, separated by long periods of normal lung function and no symptoms. A course of systemic corticosteroid is recommended. |

*(continued)*

## Stepwise Approach for Managing Asthma During Pregnancy and Lactation: Treatment *(continued)*

| Classify Severity | Clinical Features Before Treatment or Adequate Control | | Medications Required to Maintain Long-Term Control |
|---|---|---|---|
| | Symptoms/Day Symptoms/Night | PEFR or FEV$_1$ PEFR Variability | |
| Quick Relief<br>All Patients | | | Short-acting bronchodilator: 2–4 puffs short-acting inhaled β$_2$-agonist[‡] as needed for symptoms. |
| | | | Intensity of treatment will depend on severity of exacerbation; up to three treatments at 20-minute intervals or a single nebulizer treatment as needed. Course of systemic corticosteroid may be needed. |
| | | | Use of short-acting inhaled β$_2$-agonist[‡] more than two times per week in intermittent asthma (daily, or increasing use in persistent asthma) may indicate the need to initiate (increase) long-term control therapy. |

PEFR, peak expiratory flow rate, measured as percent of personal best; FEV$_1$, forced expiratory volume in 1 second, measured as percent predicted.

↓Step down. Review treatment every 1–6 months; a gradual stepwise reduction in treatment may be possible.

↑Step up. If control is not maintained, consider step up. First, review patient medication technique, adherence, and environmental control.

Goals of therapy:

• Minimal or no chronic symptoms day or night

• Minimal or no exacerbations

• No limitations on activities; no schoolwork missed (in the case of children or adolescents)

• Maintain (near) normal pulmonary function

• Minimal use of short-acting inhaled β$_2$-agonist[‡]

• Minimal or no adverse effects from medications

*There are more data on using budesonide during pregnancy than on using other inhaled corticosteroids.

†There are minimal data on using leukotriene receptor agonists in humans during pregnancy, although reassuring animal data have been submitted to the U.S. Food and Drug Administration.

‡There are more data on using albuterol during pregnancy than on using other short-acting inhaled β$_2$-agonists.

Notes: The stepwise approach is meant to assist, not replace, the clinical decision-making required to meet individual patient needs. Classify severity: assign patient to the most severe step in which any feature occurs. Gain control as quickly as possible (consider a short course of systemic corticosteroid), then step down to the least medication necessary to maintain control. Minimize use of short-acting inhaled β$_2$-agonist (eg, use of approximately one canister a month even if not using it every day indicates inadequate control of asthma and the need to initiate or intensify long-term control therapy). Provide education on self-management and controlling environmental factors that make asthma worse (eg, allergens, irritants). Refer to an asthma specialist if there are difficulties controlling asthma or if Step 4 care is required. Referral may be considered if Step 3 care is required.

# Appendix D

Management of Asthma Exacerbations During Pregnancy and Lactation: Home Treatment

**Assess severity**

Measure PEF: Value less than 50% of personal best or predicted suggests severe exacerbation.

Note signs and symptoms: Degrees of cough, breathlessness, wheeze, and chest tightness correlate imperfectly with severity of exacerbation.

Accessory muscle use and suprasternal retractions suggest severe exacerbation.

Note presence of fetal activity.*

↓

**Initial treatment**

Administer short-acting inhaled $\beta_2$-agonist: up to three treatments of two to four puffs by metered-dose inhaler at 20-minute intervals or single nebulizer treatment.

**Good response**

Mild exacerbation:

PEF more than 80% of predicted or personal best

No wheezing or shortness of breath

Response to short-acting inhaled $\beta_2$-agonist sustained for 4 hours

Appropriate fetal activity*

Treatment:

Continue short-acting inhaled $\beta_2$-agonist every 3–4 hours for 24–48 hours.

For patients on inhaled corticosteroid, double dose for 7–10 days.

↓

Contact clinician for follow-up instructions.

**Incomplete response**

Moderate exacerbation:

PEF 50–80% of predicted or personal best

Persistent wheezing and shortness of breath

Decreased fetal activity*

Treatment:

Add oral corticosteroid.

Continue short-acting inhaled $\beta_2$-agonist.

↓

Contact clinician urgently (this day) for instructions.

**Poor response**

Severe exacerbation:

PEF less than 50% of predicted or personal best

Marked wheezing and shortness of breath

Decreased fetal activity*

Treatment:

Add oral corticosteroid.

Repeat short-acting inhaled $\beta_2$-agonist immediately.

If distress is severe and nonresponsive, call your clinician immediately and proceed to emergency department; consider calling ambulance or 911.

↓

Proceed to emergency department.

---

*Fetal activity is monitored by observing whether fetal kick counts decrease over time.

MDI, metered-dose inhaler; PEF, peak expiratory flow.

Reprinted from Journal of Allergy & Clinical Immunology, Vol. 115(1): 34–46, "NAEPP Expert Panel Report: Managing Asthma During Pregnancy: Recommendations for Pharmacologic Treatment–2004 Update. National Heart, Lung, and Blood Institute; National Asthma Education and Prevention Program Asthma and Pregnancy Working Group." © 2005 American Academy of Allergy, Asthma, and Immunology.

# Appendix E

## Classes of Nonsteroidal Antiinflammatory Drugs

| Class | Drug |
| --- | --- |
| Propionic acids | Fenoprofen |
| | Flurbiprofen |
| | Ibuprofen |
| | Ketoprofen |
| | Naproxen |
| | Naproxen sodium |
| | Oxaprozin |
| Acetic acids | Diclofenac sodium |
| | Etodolac |
| | Indomethacin |
| | Ketorolac |
| | Nabumetone |
| | Sulindac |
| | Tolmetin |
| Fenamates (anthranilic acids) | Meclofenamate |
| | Mefenamic acid |
| Oxicams | Piroxicam |

# Index

**NOTE: Numbers refer to questions, not pages.**

**NOTE: Numbers refer to questions, not pages.**

**NOTE: Numbers refer to questions, not pages.**

**NOTE: Numbers refer to questions, not pages.**

**NOTE: Numbers refer to questions, not pages.**

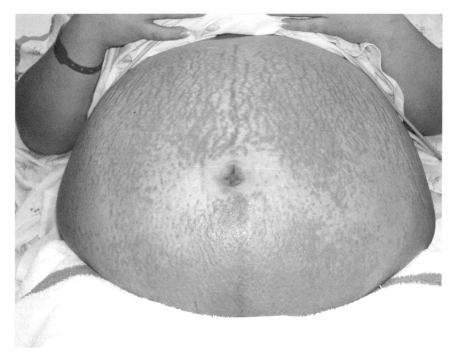

**FIG. 6-1.** Generalized erythematous skin eruption.

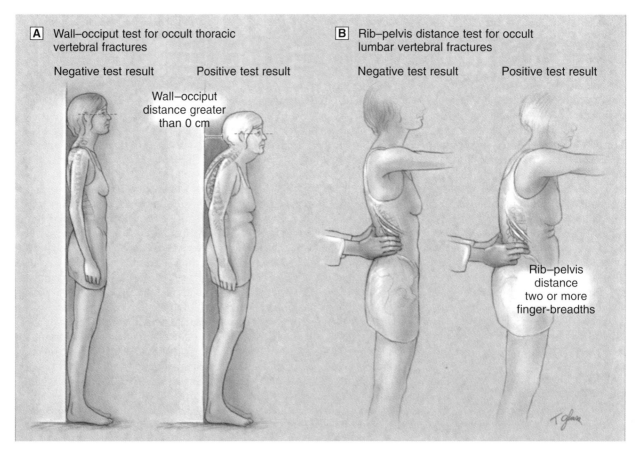

**FIG. 7-1.** Physical examination tests for detection of occult vertebral fractures. **A.** Wall–occiput test is used to detect occult thoracic vertebral fractures. A positive test result in this review is defined as being unable to touch the wall with the occiput when standing with the back and heels against the wall and the head positioned such that an imaginary line from the lateral corner of the eye to the superior junction of the auricle is parallel to the floor. **B.** Rib–pelvis distance test is used to detect occult lumbar vertebral fractures. A positive test result is defined as a distance of two finger-breadths or less between the inferior margin of the ribs and the superior surface of the pelvis in the midaxillary line. (Green AD, Colon-Emeric CS, Bastian L, Drake MT, Lyles KW. Does this woman have osteoporosis? JAMA 2004;292:2892. Copyright © 2004. American Medical Association. All rights reserved.)

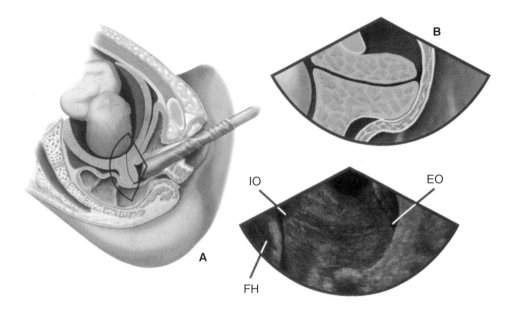

**FIG. 13-1. A**. Diagrams and sonogram of the female pelvis demonstrating placement of the transvaginal transducer in the vagina (IO, internal os; EO, external os; FH, fetal head). (Illustration by James A. Cooper, MD, San Diego, CA.) **B.** Uterine cervix as seen by transvaginal ultrasonography. (Reprinted from Scheerer LJ, Bartolucci L. Ultrasound evaluation of the cervix. In: Callen P. Ultrasonography in obstetrics and gynecology. 4th ed. Philadelphia (PA): WB Saunders; 2000. p. 579. Copyright © 2000, with permission from Elsevier.)

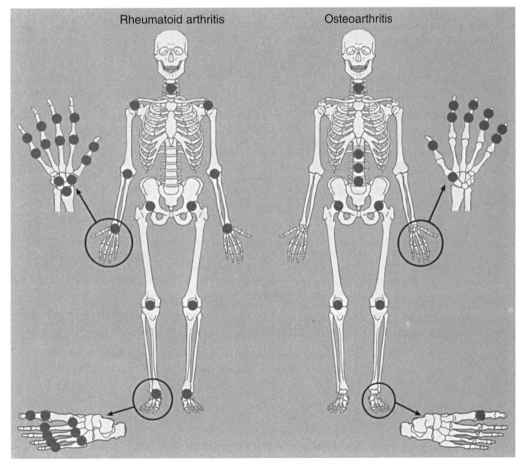

**FIG. 15-1.** The joint distribution of the two most common forms of arthritis—rheumatoid arthritis and osteoarthritis—are compared and contrasted. Joints involved in these arthritides are noted by black circles over the involved joint areas. (Reprinted from O'Dell JR. Rheumatoid arthritis. In: Goldman L, Ausiello D, editors. Cecil textbook of medicine. 22nd ed. Philadelphia (PA): WB Saunders; 2004. p. 1647. Copyright © 2004, with permission from Elsevier.)

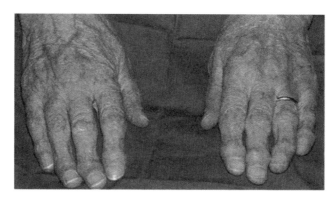

**FIG. 15-2.** Typical hand deformities in osteoarthritis. (Reprinted from Schnitzer TJ, Lane NE. Osteoarthritis. In: Goldman L, Ausiello D, editors. Cecil textbook of medicine. 22nd ed. Philadelphia (PA): WB Saunders; 2004. p. 1701. Copyright © 2004, with permission from Elsevier.)

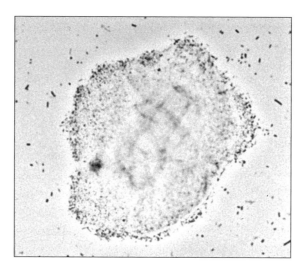

**FIG. 22-1.** Pattern of bacterial vaginosis on wet mount.

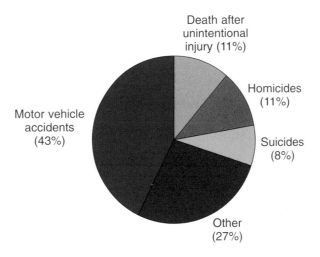

**FIG. 41-1.** Mortality, by percent, among females aged 10–24 years. Centers for Disease Control and Prevention, National Centers for Injury Prevention and Control. MVA, motor-vehicle accident. Web-based Injury Statistics Query and Reporting System (WISQARS). Available at: http://www.cdc.gov/ncipc/wisqars/. Retrieved June 4, 2005.

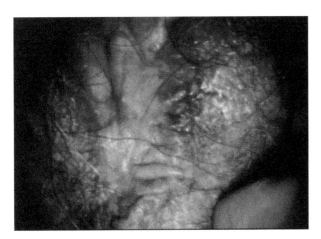

**FIG. 44-1.** Pigmentation of vulva.

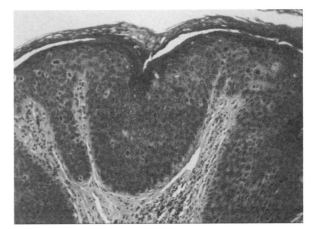

**FIG. 44-2.** Punch biopsy of vulvar lesion.

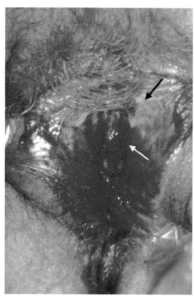

**FIG. 54-1.** Erosions and erythema of the vestibule.

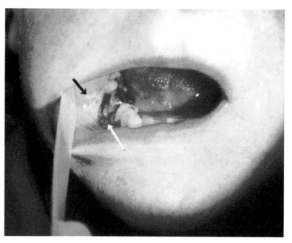

**FIG. 54-2.** Oral lichen planus lesions.